Auditory Electrophysiology

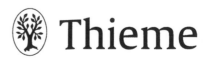

Auditory Electrophysiology
A Clinical Guide

Samuel R. Atcherson, PhD
Assistant Professor
Department of Audiology and Speech Pathology
University of Arkansas at Little Rock
University of Arkansas for Medical Sciences
Little Rock, Arkansas

Tina M. Stoody, PhD
Assistant Professor
Audiology and Speech Language Sciences
University of Northern Colorado
Greeley, Colorado

Thieme
New York · Stuttgart

Thieme Medical Publishers, Inc.
333 Seventh Ave.
New York, NY 10001

Acquisitions Editor: Emily Ekle
Managing Editor: Elizabeth D'Ambrosio
Editorial Assistant: Chris Malone
Editorial Director, Clinical Reference: Michael Wachinger
Production Editor: Sonia Kulshreshtha, DiTech Process Solutions
International Production Director: Andreas Schabert
Senior Vice President, International Marketing and Sales: Cornelia Schulze
Vice President, Finance and Accounts: Sarah Vanderbilt
President: Brian D. Scanlan
Compositor: DiTech Process Solutions

Library of Congress Cataloging-in-Publication Data

Auditory electrophysiology: a clinical guide / [edited by] Samuel R. Atcherson, Tina M. Stoody.
    p.; cm.
  Includes bibliographical references and index.
  ISBN 978-1-60406-363-9 (alk. paper) — ISBN 978-1-60406-364-6 (EISBN)
  I. Atcherson, Samuel R. II. Stoody, Tina M.
  [DNLM: 1. Evoked Potentials, Auditory—physiology. WV 270]

  612.8'51—dc23
              2012009840

Important note: Medical knowledge is ever-changing. As new research and clinical experience broaden our knowledge, changes in treatment and drug therapy may be required. The authors and editors of the material herein have consulted sources believed to be reliable in their efforts to provide information that is complete and in accord with the standards accepted at the time of publication. However, in view of the possibility of human error by the authors, editors, or publisher of the work herein or changes in medical knowledge, neither the authors, editors, nor publisher, nor any other party who has been involved in the preparation of this work, warrants that the information contained herein is in every respect accurate or complete, and they are not responsible for any errors or omissions or for the results obtained from use of such information. Readers are encouraged to confirm the information contained herein with other sources. For example, readers are advised to check the product information sheet included in the package of each drug or device they plan to administer or use to be certain that the information contained in this publication is accurate and that changes have not been made in the recommended dose or in the contraindications for administration. This recommendation is of particular importance in connection with new or infrequently used drugs. Some of the product names, patents, and registered designs referred to in this book are in fact registered trademarks or proprietary names even though specific reference to this fact is not always made in the text. Therefore, the appearance of a name without designation as proprietary is not to be construed as a representation by the publisher that it is in the public domain.

Printed in Germany by Beltz Grafische Betriebe
ISBN 978-1-60406-363-9
EISBN 978-1-60406-364-6

Dedication

To our spouses,
and to our children

Contents

Foreword

I was truly honored and delighted when Sam Atcherson and Tina Stoody asked me to write the foreword for this book. Who would have guessed more than a decade ago, when they were both doctoral students at the University of Memphis, they would master the literature, technology, and the application and interpretation of so many matters related to auditory electrophysiology? Not me. As an assistant professor of otolaryngology then, I noticed these two students often hung out together at conferences, shared notes and thoughts, conferred, reflected, and asked brilliant and insightful questions to which I likely responded, "I'll get back to you." They were two of the nicest and brightest students whom I had ever taught, but auditory electrophysiology as their areas of expertise? Really?

Today they are each assistant professors at their respective institutions training the future generation of our profession. Luckily for the students (and professionals) reading this book, Sam and Tina chose perhaps the most important area of audiology as their particular area of expertise. It is not only their depth of understanding and their respect for knowledge learned and yet-to-be-learned that make this text the most practical and pragmatic guide to auditory electrophysiology, but their ability to review, reveal, and *vitalize* the information is why this book will quickly become the go-to book with regard to pragmatics issues and answers in auditory electrophysiology.

Of note, the many contributing authors are not mainstream household names—at least not yet. In conversation with Sam and Tina, I learned that they selected authors based on their experience and expertise, more so than their pre-established notoriety. The result is a fresh and invigorating text with a multiplicity of new and exciting explanations, revelations, and viewpoints.

This book takes an unusual and very welcomed approach to auditory electrophysiology. It combines the "quick, elevator story" with scholarly, academic, and clinical information and seamlessly weaves them into a text that goes from deep, to deeper, to deepest across a multitude of fascinating audiology-based electrophysiology topics.

Of tremendous importance, this text truly "stands on the shoulders of giants" as it addresses vast contemporary topics such as auditory neuropathy spectrum disorder (ANSD), chirp stimuli, vestibular evoked myogenic potentials (VEMPs), auditory steady-state responses (ASSR), and much more within the context of classic auditory electrophysiology, while adding fresh insight and updating the reader along the way, and concluding with a comprehensive presentation.

Douglas L. Beck, AuD
Board Certified Audiologist
Director of Professional Relations
Oticon Inc.
Somerset, New Jersey
and
Web Content Editor
American Academy of Audiology
Reston, Virginia

Preface

We proudly stand on the shoulders of a number of giants with this textbook, *Auditory Electrophysiology: A Clinical Guide*. Our academic lineage in auditory electrophysiology can be traced back to Hallowell Davis, father of auditory evoked potentials. Our first tracing begins with our academic and research advisor at the University of Memphis, Herbert Jay Gould, who was trained by Albert Derbyshire at the University of Illinois at Urbana–Champaign. Derbyshire, as a student in 1929, brought to the attention of Davis a paper by Hans Berger on the recording of the alpha wave using an invention that he called the electroencephalogram. After several years of work, in 1934, Davis, Derbyshire, Pauline Davis, and H.N. Simpson recorded the first human alpha rhythm in the United States. Using this technology, Pauline Davis is credited for the discovery of the auditory evoked potential in 1939 of cortical origin. Hallowell Davis and various colleagues worked relentlessly through the 1960s to see if the cortical potential could be used as an objective audiometric tool for infants and children, and to a large extent, it fell short because successful recordings depended on long recording times, minimal physical movement, and an awake/alert patient. With the discovery, description, and wave nomenclature of the auditory brainstem response (ABR) by two different teams in the 1960s and 1970s (H. Sohmer and M. Feinmesser, and D. Jewett, M. Romano, and J. Williston), the auditory evoked potential landscape changed drastically (at least for a time). Gould frequently jokes with his students about how, in 1975 (the year he completed his doctorate degree), he read every single published paper on ABR—all 12 of them.

Our academic lineage can be traced back a second way through Maurice Mendel, who is currently Dean of the School of Communication Sciences and Disorders at the University of Memphis and served on our respective dissertation committees. Mendel was trained by Robert Goldstein at the University of Wisconsin–Madison, and Goldstein worked collaboratively with Davis. Mendel enjoys sharing stories with students about his involvement with the historic and classic middle latency response (MLR) study published in 1977 that settled the debate on whether the MLR had myogenic origin from muscles around the ear or had neurogenic origin that was a true response of the auditory system. The subject of this study (one of the co-authors) allowed himself to be injected with succinylcholine (a muscle relaxer), and while unable to move a single muscle in his body, the MLR was recorded. This lineage has an interesting mix of clinician-scholar physicians and audiologists.

How much has our literature exploded since then? How much more knowledge are we responsible for in this day and age of evidence-based practice? How much more is still yet to be learned? The good news is that the use of auditory evoked potentials in the clinic is generally well-established and through continued research (basic, translational, and applied), we fully expect that it will remain with us for a long time to come. Not only are we using evoked potentials to study the auditory system, but we are also using it to evaluate the vestibular system as well. We hope that this textbook serves its purpose well as an educational and practical guide for students and clinicians who have the interest and opportunity to add these various techniques to their clinical practice. As you read through this text, you will learn from numerous individuals who have contributed over the years to our current understanding of auditory evoked potentials (some with a similar lineage or not at all). We are indebted to the work of so many.

Acknowledgments

You don't choose your family. They are God's gift to you, as you are to them.
~Desmond Tutu

Knowledge is gained through instruction, observation, and application. We have to give credit to some of the teachers early in our careers who exposed us to the underpinnings of auditory electrophysiology in the classroom, clinic, or lab: Herbert Jay Gould, Maurice Mendel, Monique Pousson, T.K. Parthasarathy, Kevin Ohlemiller, Albert De Chicchis, Robert Nozza, Holly Kaplan, Alice Sanderson, and Judy Schafer. These individuals laid the foundation for our future research and practice of audiology.

The seeds of this textbook were first planted by former Thieme Acquisitions Editor, Beth Campbell, during an office meeting with Sam and later with Tina at an American Academy of Audiology meeting. She gave us the inspiration and motivation to write this book. Former Thieme Managing Editor, Dominik Pucek, helped with early questions and organization; however, it was our current Thieme team, Emily Ekle, Elizabeth (Liz) D'Ambrosio, and Chris Malone, who carried us through to fruition. We are grateful for the support and guidance that they provided. We thank Timothy Lim and Jennifer Rigsby for their contributions to this book in the form of artwork and clinical protocols. We are also indebted to Julie Fitzer who read through several of the chapters, offering a critical review with fresh eyes and to several AuD students who read through early drafts of this work and helped to improve it (Elyssa Doom, Raven Brasseux, Carlos Minaya, Josh Spann, and Stephanie Machen).

Finally, we have to acknowledge our families. Sam thanks his wife Rebecca and children Calleigh and Bayleigh, for lost time with them during holidays, vacations, early mornings, or late evenings, in the past two years for the distraction of trying to get this book done. But this book would also not have been possible with the generosity of his mother-in-law, Ruth Zellmer, for finding time for him to write by taking the girls. Tina would like to thank her husband Cullen and daughter Becca, for indulging in "Daddy and Becca time" while she devoted time to this book. Tina also thanks her father-in-law, John Stoody, for keeping her honest and consistently checking up on the book's progress. We love each and every one of you! *Soli Deo Gloria.*

Contributors

Radhika Aravamudhan, PhD
Associate Professor
George S. Osborne College of Audiology
Salus University
Elkins Park, Pennsylvania

Rebecca S. Atcherson, AuD
Department of Audiology and Speech
Pathology
Arkansas Children's Hospital
Little Rock, Arkansas

Samuel R. Atcherson, PhD
Assistant Professor
Department of Audiology and Speech
Pathology
University of Arkansas at Little Rock
University of Arkansas for Medical
Sciences
Little Rock, Arkansas

Shaum P. Bhagat, PhD
Associate Professor
School of Audiology and Speech
Pathology
University of Memphis
Memphis, Tennessee

Paul M. Brueggeman, AuD
Audiologist
Children's Care Hospital and School
Sioux Falls, South Dakota

John L. Dornhoffer, MD
Professor and Director
Division of Otology and Neurotology
Department of Otolaryngology
University of Arkansas for Medical Sciences
Little Rock, Arkansas

Ashley W. Harkrider, PhD
Associate Professor
Department of Audiology and Speech
Pathology
College of Allied Health Sciences
University of Tennessee Health Science
Center
Knoxville, Tennessee

Cathy C. Henderson, AuD
University of Arkansas at Little Rock
Speech and Hearing Clinic
Little Rock, Arkansas

Gayle Hicks, PhD, D.ABNM, ABA
President
Audioscope Audiology Group, APC
Neurodynamics, Inc.
San Diego, California

Annette Hurley-Larmeu, PhD
Assistant Professor
Louisiana State University Health Sciences
Center
Department of Communication Disorders
New Orleans, Louisiana

Yell Inverso, AuD, PhD
Audiology Program Coordinator
Nemours/Alfred I. duPont Hospital for
Children
Wilmington, Delaware

Elizabeth D. Leigh-Paffenroth, PhD
Audiologist
James H. Quillen Veterans Affairs Medical
Center
Mountain Home, Tennessee

Marni Johnson Martin, AuD
Assistant Professor
Department of Communication
Disorders
University of South Dakota
Vermillion, South Dakota

Patti F. Martin, PhD
Director
Audiology and Speech Pathology
Arkansas Children's Hospital
Little Rock, Arkansas

Alyssa Needleman, PhD
Manager
Department of Audiology
Rady Children's Hospital of San Diego
San Diego, California

Nannette Nicholson, PhD
Associate Professor
Department of Audiology and Speech
Pathology
University of Arkansas at Little Rock
University of Arkansas for Medical Sciences
Little Rock, Arkansas

Abby R. Nolder, MD
Resident
Department of Otolaryngology
University of Arkansas for Medical
Sciences
Little Rock, Arkansas

Christina L. Runge, PhD
Associate Professor
Chief, Communication Sciences
Director, Koss Cochlear Implant Program
Department of Otolaryngology and
Communication Sciences
Medical College of Wisconsin
Milwaukee, Wisconsin

Todd B. Sauter, MA
Director
Department of Audiology
University of Massachusetts Memorial
Medical Center
Worcester, Massachusetts

Sheryl S. Shoemaker, AuD, PhD
Professor
Head of Department of Speech
Louisiana Tech University
Ruston, Louisiana

Tina M. Stoody, PhD
Assistant Professor
Audiology and Speech Language Sciences
University of Northern Colorado
Greeley, Colorado

Julie Strickland, MS
Department of Audiology
Rady Children's Hospital of San Diego
San Diego, California

Matthew E. Wester, AuD
Instructor and Clinical Audiologist
Mayo College of Health Sciences
Mayo Clinic Arizona
Scottsdale, Arizona

Letitia White, PhD
Associate Professor
Department of Communication Sciences and
Disorders
Missouri State University
Springfield, Missouri

Chapter 1

Introduction to Auditory Evoked Potentials

Samuel R. Atcherson and Tina M. Stoody

[R]ecording of electrical activity provides an objective method of inferring how the brain goes about its business. (Goff, Allison, and Vaughn, 1978)

The study of auditory evoked potentials (AEPs) has a long and rich history, and both scientific and clinical exploration of the auditory system will continue in the years to come. With some basic knowledge and clinical training, the recording of AEPs can be relatively straightforward, and the goal of this text is to provide fast clinical information about a variety of AEPs commonly used in clinics, as well as those that have strong potential for future clinical use. Therefore, the purpose of this chapter is to provide an orientation to this textbook, an overview and classification of AEPs, some history, and a discussion of clinical competencies. These topics should help set the stage for the entire textbook. Because of obvious limitations of space and the underlying goal of this text, not all topics are reviewed. Clinicians desiring more detail or assistance with protocol design and development must consult other excellent texts and are highly encouraged to do so. Much information is presented in this textbook, with the information divided into easily digestible sections.

◆ What's in This Text?

For clinicians new to AEPs, **Section I** provides a fast summary of information related to instrumentation, stimulus and recording parameters, and neuroanatomy and neurophysiology related to AEPs. It is assumed that the reader will have some prior background knowledge in anatomy and physiology, hearing science, psychoacoustics, and basic diagnostics.

Section II is a compendium of literature reviews of major classes (or types) of AEPs. Readers are encouraged to explore these chapters to better understand the description of various AEPs, their neurologic or myogenic origin, and some of their recording and analysis considerations. Clinicians requiring a crash course may skip this section for now and concentrate on **Section III**.

Section III gets the reader right in the clinical trenches with specific information about current clinical protocols, equipment setup, patient-related factors, common clinical interpretations, and case studies, which should help both new and returning clinicians. The AEPs that have made it into Section III represent those that appear to be in regular clinical use at the time of this writing. AEPs such as the frequency-following response (FFR) and the

P1/N1/P2 complex and mismatch negativity (MMN) of the cortical event–related potentials (CERPs) have strong possibilities for clinical application in the near future, however, they are largely still in the realm of research for the study of the central auditory nervous system with respect to spectrotemporal processing, maturation, and aging. Interested readers will find relevant information for potential clinical application within dedicated chapters in Section II. For example, we expect to see the return of P1/N1/P2 responses in the estimation of hearing sensitivity (Lightfoot and Kennedy, 2006). Also, we expect to see routine and clinically feasible studies of P1 as a maturational biomarker in children with hearing loss, particularly those whose auditory implants are producing stimulus artifacts during recordings (e.g., Gilley, Sharma, Dorman, Finley, Panch, and Martin, 2006; Sharma, Martin, Roland, Bauer, Sweeney, Gilley, et al, 2005).

Section IV contains information that would not quite align well with the themes of the other sections or chapters but were considered clinically useful and practical "how to" applications and concepts relevant to AEPs.

◆ Overview of Auditory Evoked Potentials

From a simplistic point of view, AEPs are electrophysiologic responses arising from one or more sources within the peripheral and/or central auditory system structures in response to the presentation of acoustic stimuli. These responses, recorded from specific sites on the scalp, on the ears, or within the ears, appear as waveforms with both positive and negative voltage deflections at successive time points after the presentation of stimuli. These deflections are often referred to as waves, peaks, or components. The height or depth of a peak provides amplitude information, whereas the time of appearance of a peak provides latency information. One or both of these general measures may be of interest to the clinician. Other AEPs, however, are analyzed in the frequency domain, particularly if the AEP has the ability to follow or phase-lock to a repetitive pattern in a stimulus.

In a normal functioning brain, there is spontaneous neurophysiologic activity that is present whether or not there is direct external stimulation; this is apparent on an electroencephalogram (EEG). The EEG measures brain activity; it can depict one of several states of alertness, such as a drowsy brain oscillating around 10 Hz, a sleeping brain oscillating around 3 Hz, or an alert brain oscillating at or above 20 Hz. When recording from electrodes placed on the scalp, the EEG activity is recorded along with the AEPs. Compared with typical AEPs, EEGs are on the order of several times larger in amplitude. As a result, one cannot actually "see" the AEPs unless the EEG is submitted to a signal averaging process made possible through the use of digital signal processing (DSP). Through the signal averaging process, the otherwise quasi-random EEG signal begins to cancel itself out, whereas the AEP "sums" together. Although signal averaging is clearly an important piece for the recording of AEPs, several other technical considerations must be followed as well, such as filtering and amplification.

Another signal that can be recorded is large amplitude myogenic (muscle) activity that can occur with or without direct external stimulation. In general, myogenic activity is often unwanted because it can contaminate AEP recordings. Blinking of the eyes, jaw clenching, swallowing, and tension in the neck are some of the most common forms of unwanted myogenic activity, but they can often be reduced or eliminated with proper electrode placement and/or instruction to the patient. Other unwanted myogenic activity may in fact be an auditory-sensitive response to loud acoustic stimulation, such as that seen in the postauricular muscle (PAM) behind the ear or the temporalis muscle just above the ear. More recently, however, there has been clinical interest in the vestibular evoked myogenic potential (VEMP), which is the high-intensity acoustic stimulation of the saccule of the inner ear giving rise to a measure of inhibition of the contracted sternocleidomastoid (SCM) muscle of the tense neck. The VEMP test assesses the function of the saccule and vestibulocollic and vestibulospinal reflexes, which has been shown to be abnormal in a variety of vestibular and some cochlear disorders. In this case, the myogenic response is of interest, and not the auditory response. We include the VEMP in this text because it is evoked by auditory stimuli, and its assessment is well within the scope of practice of audiologists.

We live in the world of electricity, and there will always be subtle electromagnetic signals that can also be picked up in AEP or VEMP recordings. One common example is the 60-Hz line noise (50 Hz in some countries) of electrical outlets in the wall or from light sources in the room. Through signal averaging, good patient control, and firm protocols, quality recordings can commence with the primary goal of reducing or eliminating background noise and capturing the desired, small-amplitude AEP. In effect there would be an increase in the signal-to-noise ratio.

◆ Classification of Auditory Evoked Potentials

AEPS can be classified in several different ways. Usually, classifications are handled by latency, by anatomical site of generation, and by relationship to the stimulus (**Table 1.1**). The most popular means of AEP classification is by latency, which includes short latency potentials (<15 msec), middle latency potentials (15–80 msec), and late, long, or slow latency potentials (>80 msec). Another classification of AEPs is whether they are considered exogenous, endogenous, or both. Exogenous potentials are obligatory, sensory evoked potentials largely elicited and subsequently affected by the physical parameters of the stimulus (Donchin, Ritter, and McCallum, 1978), such as stimulus intensity, rise time, frequency, and duration. These potentials generally comprise all of the AEPs up to the long-latency, late auditory evoked potentials (LAEPs). The auditory brainstem response (ABR) is a classic example of an exogenous potential.

Endogenous potentials, in contrast, depend less on stimulus features and more on the contextual factors related to the stimulus (Donchin et al, 1978). These potentials have very long latencies. Endogenous potentials arise to demands placed on psychological processes (i.e., attention and memory) to a particular event, such as listening for a rare (or deviant) stimulus in a sequence of repetitive stimuli (Duncan-Johnson and Donchin, 1977; Swick, Kutas, and Neville, 1994). Because of the contextual, nonobligatory nature of these potentials, endogenous potentials are more often referred to as event-related potentials (ERPs) rather than evoked potentials. The P300 is a classic example of an ERP. Higher-order cognition can influence ERPs. For example, the P300 amplitude could be made larger by simply attending to the stimulus, whereas ignoring the stimulus could make it smaller. Also, the degree of difficulty of the listening task could alter the shape of the P300 for one person but not for another. It is for this reason that Jacobson (1994) refers to the P300 as a perceptual potential. In general, the longer the latency of the AEP, the more likely it will have endogenous influences.

One important distinction is that some AEPs are transient or onset potentials, and others are steady-state or sustained potentials. Transient potentials are those that occur at the onset of the stimulus, and there is generally no one-to-one correlation between the waveform of the stimulus and the waveform of the AEP. Classic examples of transient AEPs are the compound action potential (CAP) of the electrocochleogram (ECochG), the ABR, the middle latency response (MLR) arising from subcortical and cortical structures, cortical potentials (e.g., P1/N1/P2 complexes), and the P300 cognitive potential. Steady-state potentials typically arise from repetitive or continuous stimulation, and the AEP waveform either follows the stimulus waveform, or the AEP waveform takes on a voltage shift and maintains it throughout the duration of the stimulus. Examples of steady-state potentials include the summating potential (SP) of the ECochG, the FFR arising primarily in the brainstem, and the auditory steady-state response (ASSR) arising potentially from multiple but segregated areas of the central auditory nervous system. The cochlear microphonic (CM) can be thought of as a steady-state potential if recorded very near the cochlea, or it can be revealed in some cases of auditory neuropathy spectrum disorder, in which case the CM appears to "ring" even in response to a click stimulus. Below, a limited selection of AEPs is described briefly for the reader to develop an appreciation for some of the major differences among classes.

Table 1.1 Classification of Auditory Evoked Potentials

Common Name	Latency Range (msec)	Analysis Method	Physiologic Description	Anatomical Generator	Stimulus Response	Exogenous or Endogenous
ECochG (CM, SP, CAP)	0–2	Time	Cochlear, neurogenic	Hair cells, auditory nerve	Steady state, transient	Exogenous
ABR (I, III, V)	1–10	Time	Neurogenic	Auditory nerve, brainstem	Transient	Exogenous
FFR	N/A	Time, frequency	Neurogenic	Brainstem	Steady state	Exogenous
MLR (Na, Pa)	15–35	Time	Neurogenic	Subcortical, cortical	Transient	Exogenous
LAEP (or LLR) (P1, N1, P2)	50–250	Time	Neurogenic	Cortical	Transient	Exogenous,* endogenous
MMN	150–300	Time, subtraction	Neurogenic	Cortical	Transient	Exogenous, endogenous*
P300	250–400	Time	Neurogenic	Cortical	Transient	Exogenous, endogenous*
N400	350–500	Time	Neurogenic	Cortical	Transient	Endogenous
ASSR (<20, ~40, >60 Hz)	10–30	Frequency, phase	Neurogenic	Brainstem, subcortical, cortical	Steady state	Exogenous,* endogenous
VEMP (P1, N1)	12–27	Time	Myogenic	Vestibulocolic reflex	Transient	Exogenous

Abbreviations: ABR = auditory brainstem response; ASSR = auditory steady-state potential; CAP = compound action potential; CM = cochlear microphonic; FFR = frequency-following response; LAEP = late auditory evoked potential; LLR = late latency response; MLR = middle latency response; MMN = mismatch negativity; SP = summating potential; VEMP = vestibular evoked myogenic potential

* Predominant classification of the two descriptions

◆ A Brief History of Auditory Evoked Potentials

The starting point of AEPs in the field of audiology begins with Hallowell Davis, MD (1896–1992), who is often called the father of auditory evoked responses. Many have credited him with introducing the EEG to America. For more than 50 years, Dr. Davis published extensively on cortical potentials and the physiology of the cochlea. Davis's first wife, Pauline Davis, however, also deserves some recognition. It was she who described (and solely published) transient changes in an ongoing EEG in response to external stimuli (Davis, 1939). This observable change later became known as a vertex potential and the auditory late response (ALR) of cortical origin. Several years earlier, however, Wever and Bray (1930) stumbled on what later became known as the CM when they placed an electrode on the auditory nerve near the medulla of a cat and another wire from the cat to an amplified telephone receiver. Rather than recording AEPs, they indirectly recorded steady state potentials from the cat's ear by presenting acoustic stimuli to the cat's ear. As they spoke into the cat's ear and presented tonal stimuli with tuning forks, the cat's inner ear reproduced the signals with remarkable fidelity through the telephone receiver. A neurophysiologist by the name of Dawson (1951, 1954) is largely credited with developing the signal-averaging computer that made it possible to extract the AEP from the ongoing EEG. From Dawson's work, other investigators worked diligently to develop their own signal-averaging computers, such that Jerome Cox, Maynard Engebretson, and Hallowell Davis at the Central Institute of the Deaf came up with the histogram average ogive calculator (HAV-OC), and Wesley Clark at the Massachusetts Institute of Technology developed the average response computer (ARC). Davis and his colleagues conducted numerous cortical potential studies in the 1960s and 1970s, including trying to determine the feasibility of using cortical potentials to estimate audiogram thresholds in young cooperative children. This diagnostic method became popularized as evoked response audiometry. Using Clark's ARC system, Dan Geisler completed his dissertation and earned his claim to fame by publishing the first study on the MLR using signal averaging (Geisler, Frishkopf, and Rosenblith, 1958). The ECochG with its three subcomponents (CM, SP, and action potentials [APs]) has been described in animals and humans. The earliest report of the CM recording was probably described by Fromm, Nylen, and Zotterman (1935) when they sought to understand the Wever and Bray effect. The SP was described by Davis, Fernández, and McAuliffe (1950) in animals; a clearly visible SP in the human ear canal by Coats (1974); and the AP in animals by Tasaki (1954) and in humans by Ruben and colleagues (1959, 1960; Ruben and Walker, 1963).

Today, we are seeing wide use of various AEPs that had been discovered and described many years ago. Jewett and his colleagues (1970, 1971), were among the first to describe the ABR that is used today to estimate hearing thresholds in infants and young children, as well as to identify neurologic lesions in the auditory nerve and brainstem. Variations of the ABR have included Stacked ABR (used to screen for acoustic tumors < 1 cm), Cochlear Hydrops Masking Procedure (CHAMP; used to access Meniere disease), and a synthetic /da/ stimulus), and the Biological Marker of Auditory Processing (BioMARK; which is showing promise for detecting underlying timing deficits in patients suspected of having auditory processing disorders [APD]). Manny Don and his colleagues (1997, 2005a, 2005b) are credited for the work related to Stacked ABR and CHAMP, whereas BioMARK is credited to Nina Kraus and her colleagues (Johnson, Nicol, and Kraus, 2005; Russo, Nicol, Musacchia, and Kraus, 2004; Song, Banai, Russo, and Kraus, 2006). The 40-Hz response, an accidental technical variation of the MLR using click stimuli, was described by Galambos, Makeig, and Talmachoff (1981) as probably the first ASSR. However, the 40-Hz response is not used clinically, but newer amplitude-, frequency-, or mixed-modulated stimuli are being used today to elicit the ASSR. Numerous investigators from several countries are to be credited for our current understanding and application of ASSRs, but the earliest reports point to Geisler (1960) and Campbell, Atkinson, Francis, and Green (1977). Unlike most other AEPs, ASSR waveforms are not read, but rather are submitted to frequency or phase analysis techniques to determine whether or not there is a response. While Pauline Davis (1939) first described the cortical potential, Ostroff, Martin, and Boothroyd (1998) described a variant called the acoustic change complex (ACC) that has been found to be sensitive to midstream changes in auditory stimuli, and Sharma and colleagues (2005) described the use of the immature P1 response as a sensitive biomarker for cortical auditory development in children. Each of these may help guide treatment and management related to hearing aids and cochlear implants. Some investigators and clinicians have described the use of the P300 and MMN, which are unique responses that arise to an acoustic difference between two stimuli where there is some uncertainty about when one of the two stimuli will be presented. The P300 was initially described by Davis (1964) and Sutton, Braren, Zubin, and John (1965), while the MMN was discovered by Näätänen, Gaillard, and Mäntysalo (1978).

As can be appreciated, AEPs have been around for a long time. Some AEPs are already in wide clinical use, whereas others still require further study and refinement to be used clinically with reasonable validity and reliability. Some AEPs have been abandoned (permanently or temporarily), whereas others appear to be reemerging with the development of sophisticated software programs and/or improvements in hardware providing opportunity for novel uses. Simply put, history is still being written.

◆ Competencies in Auditory Evoked Potential Measurement

An ad hoc committee on AEPs put together by the American Speech-Language-Hearing Association (2003) produced and published a set of guidelines for what they felt were knowledge and skill competencies necessary for successful clinical AEP use. Divided into four major areas, this document lists competencies for identification of patients for whom AEP evaluations are appropriate, identification and administration of appropriate test procedures and strategies, analysis and interpretation of AEP findings, and reporting of findings and recommendations. The reader is encouraged to browse quickly through this document, as these themes will surface throughout this entire textbook, with certain topics presented in specific sections or chapters.

References

American Speech-Language-Hearing Association (2003). *Guidelines for competencies in auditory evoked potential measurement and clinical applications.* Retrieved from http://www.asha.org/docs/pdf/KS2003-00020.pdf.

Campbell, F. W., Atkinson, J., Francis, M. R., & Green, D. M. (1977). Estimation of auditory thresholds using evoked potentials: A clinical screening test. *Progress in Clinical Neurophysiology, 2,* 68–78.

Coats, A. C. (1974). On electrocochleographic electrode design. *Journal of the Acoustical Society of America, 56,* 708–711.

Davis, H. (1964, July). Enhancement of evoked cortical potential in humans related to a task requiring a decision. *Science, 145,* 182–183. PubMed

Davis, H., Fernández, C., & McAuliffe, D. R. (1950, October). The excitatory process in the cochlea. *Proceedings of the National Academy of Sciences USA, 36*(10), 580–587. PubMed

Davis, P. A. (1939). Effects of acoustic stimuli on the waking human brain. *Journal of Neurophysiology, 2,* 494–499.

Dawson, G. D. (1951). A summation technique for detecting small signals in a large irregular background. *Journal of Physiology, 115*(1), 2–3. PubMed

Dawson, G. D. (1954, February). A summation technique for the detection of small evoked potentials. *Electroencephalography and Clinical Neurophysiology, 6*(1), 65–84. PubMed

Don, M., Kwong, B., & Tanaka, C. (2005). A diagnostic test for Meniere's disease and cochlear hydrops: Impaired high-pass noise masking ABRs. *Otology and Neurotology, 26,* 711–722. PubMed

Don, M., Kwong, B., Tanaka, C., Brackmann, D. E., & Nelson, R. A. (2005, September–October). The stacked ABR: A sensitive and specific screening tool for detecting small acoustic tumors. *Audiology and Neuro-Otology, 10*(5), 274–290. PubMed

Don, M., Masuda, A., Nelson, R. A., & Brackmann, D. E. (1997). Successful detection of small acoustic tumors using the stacked derived band ABR amplitude. *American Journal of Otology, 18*, 608–621.

Donchin, E., Ritter, W., & McCallum, W. C. (1978). Cognitive psychophysiology: The endogenous components of the ERP. In E. Callaway, P. Tueting, & S. Koslow (Eds.), *Event-related brain potentials in man.* pp. 349–411. New York: Academic Press.

Duncan-Johnson, C. C., & Donchin, E. (1977, September). On quantifying surprise: The variation of event-related potentials with subjective probability. *Psychophysiology, 14*(5), 456–467. PubMed

Fromm, B., Nylen, C. O., & Zotterman, Y. (1935). Studies in the mechanism of the Wever and Bray effect. *Acta Oto-Laryngologica, 22*, 477–486.

Galambos, R., Makeig, S., & Talmachoff, P. J. (1981, April). A 40-Hz auditory potential recorded from the human scalp. *Proceedings of the National Academy of Sciences USA, 78*(4), 2643–2647. PubMed

Geisler, C. D. (1960). *Average responses to clicks in man recorded by scalp electrodes* (Technical Report No. 380). Cambridge, MA: MIT Research Laboratory of Electronics.

Geisler, C. D., Frishkopf, L. S., & Rosenblith, W. A. (1958, November). Extracranial responses to acoustic clicks in man. *Science, 128*(3333), 1210–1211. PubMed

Gilley, P. M., Sharma, A., Dorman, M., Finley, C. C., Panch, A. S., & Martin, K. (2006, August). Minimization of cochlear implant stimulus artifact in cortical auditory evoked potentials. *Clinical Neurophysiology, 117*(8), 1772–1782. PubMed

Goff, W. R., Allison, T., & Vaughn, H. G. (1978). The functional neuroanatomy of event related potentials. In E. Callaway, P. Tueting, & S. H. Koslow (Eds.), *Event related potentials in man.* pp. 1–79. New York: Academic Press.

Jacobson, J. T. (1994). *Principles and applications in auditory evoked potentials.* Needham Heights, MA: Allyn & Bacon.

Jewett, D. L., Romano, M. N., & Williston, J. S. (1970, March). Human auditory evoked potentials: Possible brain stem components detected on the scalp. *Science, 167*(924), 1517–1518. PubMed

Jewett, D. L., & Williston, J. S. (1971). Auditory-evoked far fields averaged from the scalp of humans. *Brain, 94*(4), 681–696. PubMed

Johnson, K. L., Nicol, T., & Kraus, N. (2005). The brainstem response to speech: A biological marker of auditory processing. *Ear and Hearing, 26*(5), 424–434. PubMed

Lightfoot, G., & Kennedy, V. (2006, October). Cortical electric response audiometry hearing threshold estimation: Accuracy, speed, and the effects of stimulus presentation features. *Ear and Hearing, 27*(5), 443–456. PubMed

Näätänen, R., Gaillard, A. W., & Mäntysalo, S. (1978, July). Early selective-attention effect on evoked potential reinterpreted. *Acta Psychologica, 42*(4), 313–329. PubMed

Ostroff, J. M., Martin, B. A., & Boothroyd, A. (1998, August). Cortical evoked response to acoustic change within a syllable. *Ear and Hearing, 19*(4), 290–297. PubMed

Ruben, R. J., Bordley, J. E., Nager, G. T., Sekula, J., Knickerbocker, G. G., & Fisch, U. (1960, June). Human cochlea responses to sound stimuli. *Annals of Otology, Rhinology, and Laryngology, 69*, 459–479. PubMed

Ruben, R. J., Knickerbocker, G. G., Sekula, J., Nager, G. T., & Bordley, J. E. (1959, June). Cochlear microphonics in man: A preliminary report. *Laryngoscope, 69*(6), 665–671. PubMed

Ruben, R. J., & Walker, A. E. (1963, November). The VIIIth nerve action potential in Ménière's disease. *Laryngoscope, 73*, 1456–1464. PubMed

Russo, N., Nicol, T., Musacchia, G., & Kraus, N. (2004, September). Brainstem responses to speech syllables. *Clinical Neurophysiology, 115*(9), 2021–2030. PubMed

Sharma, A., Martin, K., Roland, P., Bauer, P., Sweeney, M. H., Gilley, P., et al. (2005, September). P1 latency as a biomarker for central auditory development in children with hearing impairment. *Journal of the American Academy of Audiology, 16*(8), 564–573. PubMed

Song, J. H., Banai, K., Russo, N. M., & Kraus, N. (2006). On the relationship between speech- and nonspeech-evoked auditory brainstem responses. *Audiology and Neuro-Otology, 11*(4), 233–241. PubMed

Sutton, S., Braren, M., Zubin, J., & John, E. R. (1965, November). Evoked-potential correlates of stimulus uncertainty. *Science, 150*(700), 1187–1188. PubMed

Swick, D., Kutas, M., & Neville, H. (1994). Localizing the neural generators of event-related brain potentials. In A. Kertesz (Ed.), *Localization and neuroimaging in neuropsychology* (pp. 73–121). San Diego, CA: Academic Press.

Tasaki, I. (1954, March). Nerve impulses in individual auditory nerve fibers of guinea pig. *Journal of Neurophysiology, 17*(2), 97–122. PubMed

Wever, E. G., & Bray, C. W. (1930). The nature of the acoustic response: The relations between sound frequency and frequency of impulses in the auditory nerve. *Journal of Experimental Psychology, 13*, 373–387.

Chapter 2

Basic Instrumentation, Acquisition, and Recording Considerations

Tina M. Stoody and Samuel R. Atcherson

The instrumentation involved in recording auditory evoked potentials (AEPs) may have evolved tremendously over the last 50 to 60 years, but the core concepts regarding the recording of AEPs generally have not. Today's instrumentation typically includes a desktop or laptop computer, an amplifier box, an electrode box, electrodes, and one or more transducers (e.g., insert earphones, supra-aural headphones, bone oscillators, and speakers). The transducers are used to present a variety of stimuli to one or both ears, whereas the electrodes act like antennas, picking up voltage changes from underneath the skin surface. The amplifier is necessary to bring the small-amplitude electroencephalogram (EEG), and subsequently the AEP, into the voltage range of the computer. The computer is initially involved in analog-to-digital conversion of the incoming EEG but then it will also filter unwanted signal frequencies and perform signal averaging so that the AEP can be extracted. However, there can be no AEP unless the computer also presents stimuli with specific physical characteristics at necessary intensity levels, stimulation rates, and so on. This chapter provides more information about the basic science behind stimulus generation and presentation, AEP instrumentation, and various subject-based factors to consider for the acquisition of AEPs. With an increased familiarity of how AEP equipment functions and basic knowledge regarding recording parameters, one can confidently set up protocols and record all the AEPs discussed within this text.

♦ Signal versus Noise

When there is no direct sensory stimulation (e.g., acoustic stimuli to the ears), the neuronal activity of the cortex is quite dominant compared with noncortical neurons and can easily be recorded with electrodes placed on the scalp. This cortical activity is called the electroencephalogram (EEG). As with any signal that can be represented by simple or complex waves, the ongoing EEG is a biologic wave that is somewhat noiselike in appearance and can exhibit voltages as high as 50 to 100 µV. In a relaxed person, the EEG can be as low as 10 to 20 µV. A spectral analysis of the EEG in a person who is awake would show frequencies ~20 Hz and higher. However, when a person becomes drowsy and then falls asleep, the EEG drops to ~10 and 3 Hz, respectively. Conversely, when a sensory system (e.g., the auditory system) is stimulated, there is a propagation of neuronal activity through the peripheral and central nervous systems (PNS and CNS). Sensory stimulation produces what is called an evoked potential (EP) or evoked response (ER). In contrast to the EEG, EP signals are much smaller in amplitude (i.e., usually no more than a few microvolts). Indeed, any EP would be virtually lost against the larger EEG without sophisticated techniques to extract the EP (desired signal) from the EEG (noise, or unwanted signal). The signal of interest is recorded using a digital computer for later processing, analysis, and interpretation. Basic tenets of digital signal processing (DSP) are described in the next section.

◆ Digital Signal Processing

To understand how digital computers aid in the recording of AEPs, it is helpful to understand the dichotomy between continuous (analog) and discrete (digital) signals. Continuous signals are those that can be represented by a value at all points in time, no matter how small or how many decimal points there are (Johnson, 1997). Both EEGs and AEPs coming from the head surface and all stimuli presented acoustically, by nature, are continuous signals. Discrete signals have a limited number of decimal places (Johnson, 1997); as a result, some information about an otherwise continuous signal may be lost once converted to a discrete signal. Discrete signals can undergo DSP. Stimuli presented from a computer through earphones and all visual displays of the AEP and/or EEG on a computer monitor screen will be in the form of a discrete signal; thus, conversion from analog-to-digital (A-D) and from digital-to-analog (D-A) can be appreciated during routine AEP testing.

A-D conversion is a two-step process involving sampling and quantization (Finan, 2010; Johnson, 1997; Lagerlund, 1996). Sampling involves breaking a continuous signal down into a limited number of manageable units, called samples, each having equal time duration. As an example, the auditory brainstem response (ABR) is commonly recorded using a time window of 10 msec and a fixed number of sampling points (usually 256). This means that the ABR will be divided into 256 pieces, with each piece (sample) having a duration of 0.0390625 msec. Quantization involves breaking down a continuous signal into manageable amplitude units, called steps. From the point of view of electronic or biologic signals, amplitude values

are really voltage values. Computers process information in binary digits (or bits) with strings of 0s and 1s, and a 16-bit computer has the ability to quantize amplitude values into 65,536 discrete amplitude steps.

Perhaps the most important aspect of DSP for AEP testing is sampling rate (also called sampling frequency). Sampling rate is important because it determines the maximum signal frequency that can be digitized (Lagerlund, 1996). The Nyquist theorem states that the sampling rate should be at least two times the highest frequency in the signal of interest (Finan, 2010; Hyde, 1994; Lagerlund, 1996; Ruchkin, 1988). The highest frequency of interest in the signal is called the Nyquist frequency. If this requirement is not satisfied, a situation called aliasing occurs in the A-D process, and the digital waveform will misrepresent the analog signal (Johnson, 1997; Lagerlund, 1996). A distortion is created by the folding of frequency components higher than the frequency of interest onto lower frequency components (Lagerlund, 1996). For example, a 75-Hz sine wave sampled at a rate of 100 samples per second will erroneously be digitized as a 25 Hz sine wave. However, to achieve a reasonably faithful representation of a continuous signal, sampling rates higher than a factor of 2 may be necessary (Hall, 1992; Hyde, 1994; Lagerlund, 1996). This discussion surfaces again later in this chapter with respect to filtering and signal averaging.

◆ Time and Frequency Domain

Auditory stimuli and AEPs both occur in time as waveforms, and both can be analyzed in the time and frequency domains. It may be helpful to understand that both auditory stimuli and AEPs are often referred to as signals to differentiate them from noise. A time domain analysis evaluates the amplitude of a signal over time, and the signal appears as a waveform with alternating positive and negative values. In contrast, a frequency domain analysis (e.g., a spectrum) removes the element of time to reveal the spectral energies of the signal as the waveform is translated to its respective amplitude values across frequencies. An AEP is nothing more than a complex waveform (i.e., a

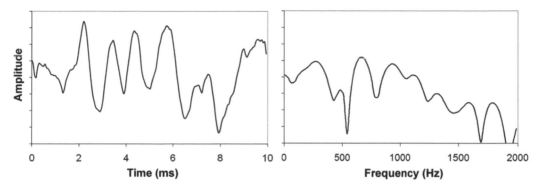

Fig. 2.1 The auditory brainstem response (ABR) in the time (*left*) and frequency (*right*) domains. The time domain shows the ABR as having a series of several waves within a 10-msec time window. The frequency domain shows the spectral energies within the ABR with the element of time removed. Notice that spectral energy is greatest between ~200 and 1000 Hz, with major spectral peaks around 250, 600, and 900 Hz.

combination of many frequencies or sine wave components). Thinking about an AEP in terms of its spectral energy is a concept that is not always intuitive for clinicians who are used to visualizing an AEP represented in the time domain. However, it is important to understand this concept, which will become particularly evident in later sections discussing filter settings. **Figure 2.1** illustrates an example of an AEP in its respective time and frequency domains.

♦ Instrumentation

Stimulus Generator

Most AEP systems are capable of generating a variety of stimuli, and the clinician may have some control and flexibility in defining certain physical parameters of a stimulus. Clinically, the most commonly used stimuli include 100-μsec clicks and short-duration tone bursts. With auditory steady-state responses (ASSRs), signals are typically amplitude or frequency modulated tones, or they may use a combination of both, referred to as mixed modulation. Other AEPs may be evoked by simple speech stimuli (e.g., /da/). Typically, the equipment allows the clinician to import stimulus files (e.g., .wav files) that are not default selections within the software, as is often the case if a speech stimulus is desired. The type of stimulus used and its characteristics have important effects on AEPs;

these stimulus effects vary depending on the signal of interest and therefore are discussed throughout the text for each individual AEP.

Transducers

Although the choice of transducer is up to the clinician, tubal-style insert earphones (e.g., ER-3A; Etymotic Research Inc., Elk Grove Park, IL) are more commonly used for AEPs compared with supra-aural headphones (e.g., TDH-49; Telephonics Corporation, Huntington, NY). However, both are commonly reported in the literature and used by clinics around the world. As with audiometry, the same advantages for the use of insert earphones with AEPs generally apply (e.g., sanitary and comfortable), but the most important advantage is the physical and temporal separation of the transducer box from the ear and electrodes. The tube produces a small time delay of ~0.8 msec and permits a separation of any stimulus-related artifact from contaminating the AEP as it is being recorded. In most cases, the stimulus artifact will not affect the recordings when insert earphones are used; however, a ringing stimulus artifact from a TDH-49 supra-aural headphone may obscure or even enhance wave I artificially. For ABR, in particular, care must be taken to physically separate the insert earphone transducer box from the electrode wires as much as possible. In some cases, it is possible for the stimulus artifact to be so large as to cause the artifact rejection to overreact, thereby affecting the averaging process. **Figure 2.2** shows an example

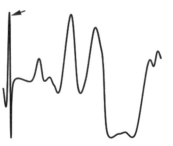

Transducer Box
too Close to
Electrode Wires

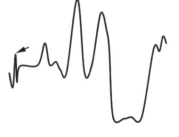

Transducer Box
Distant from
Electrode Wires

Fig. 2.2 The physical relationship of the insert earphone transducer box and the electrodes on the magnitude of the stimulus artifact (*arrows*) seen in an auditory brainstem response (ABR) recording.

of stimulus artifact when the insert earphone transducer is close to the electrode wires and when it is placed at a distance.

Trigger

The trigger is key to the recording of all AEPs and works in tandem with signal averaging. In general, the trigger is a digital pulse or word that lets the averaging computer know precisely when each stimulus is being presented. Once the recording time window is defined, the trigger and stimulus onset are essentially synonymous with time zero in the analysis time window. While all commercially available EP systems have their own self-contained triggers as each stimulus is presented, some EP systems may accept a trigger from another computer system (or stimulus generator) that is not associated with the recording system. In this way, novel stimuli and/or stimulus paradigms often seen in research may be used to evoke the AEP without having to acquire research-grade equipment.

♦ Acquisition Parameters

The primary technical problem of recording brain electrical activity from the scalp is that the ongoing EEG contains both the AEP of interest (i.e., signal) and various sources of noise, both physiologic and nonphysiologic. Sources of physiologic noise include spontaneous brain activity, electromyogenic potentials, corneoretinal potentials, and electrodermal potentials. Some nonphysiologic noise sources are electromagnetically induced potentials (e.g., 60-Hz line noise), internal electrical instrument noise, and electrode polarization. With few exceptions, AEPs are smaller in amplitude than the background EEG, and thus they have a poor signal-to-noise ratio (SNR). To extract the smaller AEP signal and attenuate noise (i.e., improve SNR), several techniques are necessary to condition the AEP signal for later analysis: amplification, filtering, and averaging. The use of metal electrodes placed on the scalp permits the collection of brain electrical voltages into the recording equipment. Specific details regarding acquisition parameters of individual AEPs are located throughout this text; general information regarding SNR techniques and application of electrodes is addressed in this section.

Differential Amplification

Amplification of AEPs serves two purposes: to reduce background noise through differential recording and to bring the signal of interest into the range of the A-D converter (Durrant and Ferraro, 1999; Misulis, 1989; Misulis and Fakhoury, 2001). For a basic differential recording, a minimum of three electrodes is required: noninverting, inverting, and ground electrodes (Hyde, 1994). Electrode terminology can be confusing, as multiple terms are used interchangeably to describe the different electrode sites (see **Table 2.1** for a summary). During amplification, any signal (and noise) that is common at the scalp to the positive and negative inputs will be reduced, while signals

Table 2.1 Interchangeably Used Terminology for Electrode Sites

Noninverting	Inverting	Ground
Active	Reference	Common/ground
Positive (+)	Negative (−)	Common/ground
Input 1	Input 2	Common/ground

that differ between these inputs are amplified (Duffy, Iyer, and Surwillo, 1989; Durrant and Ferraro, 1999; Hall, 1992; Misulis and Fakhoury, 2001). The process of canceling signals common to both inputs is referred to as common-mode rejection (CMR) (**Fig. 2.3**).

How the CMR process works within the operation of the differential amplifier is frequently confused. Specifically, why is the negative input of the differential amplifier called the inverting input? Additionally, how are the signals combined within the differential amplifier? The first question can be answered by understanding the physical design of the

differential amplifier. Within the differential amplifier are two single-ended amplifiers that are mirror images of one another, each sharing a common ground (Duffy et al, 1989). One of the amplifiers forces the incoming signal at the input to become inverted. Thus, any electrode connected to this input will be referred to as the inverting electrode. The second question can be answered in the way the CMR process works within the differential amplifier. Although the goal is to obtain the difference between the two inputs, the differential amplifier does not perform any subtraction; it can only add signals. With

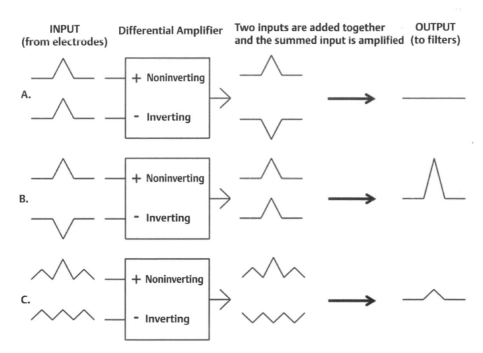

Fig. 2.3 Function of the differential amplifier and common mode rejection. Tracings on the left-hand side of the figure are inputs from the electrodes. Positive (+) input is noninverting, and negative (−) input is inverting. Tracings on the right-hand side of the figure are outputs of the differential amplifier to the filters. (**A**) Signals common to both inputs (+ and −) cancel at the output. (**B**) Signals uncommon to both inputs amplify at the output. (**C**) Signals common to both inputs (low-amplitude peaks) were canceled at output, whereas the slightly larger peak at the noninverting input is preserved and amplified.

the "mirror image" setup of the single-ended amplifiers, the differential amplifier will add the inverted input to the noninverted input, thereby "amplifying the difference" between the voltages present simultaneously at the two inputs (Duffy et al, 1989). Thus, the voltage output of the amplifier will be zero whenever the voltages at the two inputs upon entering the differential amplifier are identical (hence common mode).

Although differential amplification greatly improves SNR, it is not sufficient alone for the enhancement of AEPs and attenuation of noise. There are at least two primary reasons for this dilemma. First, noise has only a moderate correlation between the two amplifier inputs, which implies that noise will not cancel out entirely (Hyde, 1994). Second, the recording of AEPs reflects a potential (i.e., voltage) difference between two sites, not over a single site. For this reason, CMR works best when

the inputs record activity at electrodes placed at sites of opposite bioelectric polarity (Hyde, 1994) or in the appropriate plane relative to the signal's neuroanatomical dipole (see Chapter 4 regarding dipoles). **Figure 2.4** illustrates the effect of proper electrode placement with respect to the differential amplifier and neuroanatomic dipoles of the ABR.

In addition to differential amplification, there is additional amplification, referred to as gain, that can be applied to the recorded response. The AEP software will include gain as a parameter that can be modified within the acquisition parameters. Remember that AEPs are quite small (e.g., no more than a few microvolts); therefore, gain settings are set to magnify the response to values to 50,000, 75,000, or 100,000 times. Amplification settings depend not only on the AEP of interest, but also on other protocol parameters (e.g., electrode placement). For example, gain does not need

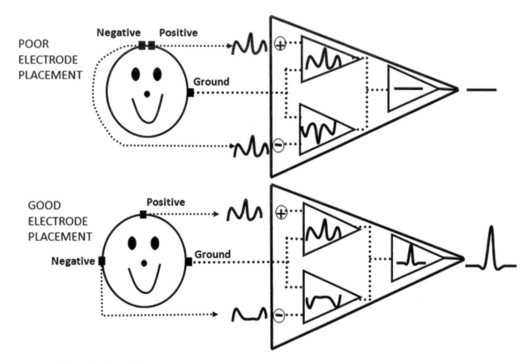

Fig. 2.4 Effect of electrode placement on common mode rejection/differential amplification for the auditory brainstem response (ABR). In the top half of the figure, electrodes are placed close together on the scalp, resulting in similar activity being received by both. By inverting the input from the negative electrode and adding it to the input from the positive electrode, essentially everything is canceled out, and the output of the amplifier is zero. In the lower half of the figure, the positive electrode is at vertex, whereas the negative electrode is on the ipsilateral ear. This electrode placement will ensure different that activity relative to the evoked response is recorded, as the electrodes are on opposite ends of the signal pathway; however, the noise should be similar. When the inputs are added together, the noise (common activity between the electrodes) is canceled, whereas the signal is amplified.

to be nearly as high for tympanic membrane electrode placement (e.g., gain = 50,000) as it does for ear canal electrode placement (e.g., gain – 75,000) with electrocochleography (ECochG) (see Chapter 12).

Filtering

Filtering is the next technique that is used for improving SNR. As with complex sound waves, all biological signals can be broken down into component frequencies, with each frequency having its own amplitude (Misulis, 1989). Because the signal of interest may occur together with unwanted noise (Elberling and Don, 1984; Hyde, 1994; Ruchkin, 1988), filtering provides a means of suppressing noise that is not in the frequency band associated with the AEP. Filters, by definition, attempt to pass signals of interest while rejecting noise. Noise can be defined as any part of a signal detected by the electrodes that is not of interest (Hall, 1992; Misulis and Fakhoury, 2001). What is preserved and what is suppressed during AEP recording depends on the filter settings. The spectral (frequency) composition of the AEP of interest, which will help to determine appropriate filter settings. To determine the spectral composition of an AEP, and thus its greatest spectral energy, can be determined by performing a fast Fourier transform (FFT) to break down the AEP into component frequencies. **Figure 2.5** illustrates an FFT on a cortical event–related potential

(CERP) waveform with energy between 1 and 50 Hz.

Analog versus Digital Filters

Both analog and digital filters are frequently used in AEP recordings, each with major differences. Analog filters are physical devices that take any real numerical value (plus and minus infinity) of an electrical signal that varies continuously in voltage and time (Hyde, 1994). Analog filters are used in differential amplifiers because the brain's electrical signal is continuous. Digital filters, by contrast, are numerical algorithms performed by a computer. Digital filtering is particularly useful after A-D conversion has taken place and discrete numerical values are stored in memory. A-D conversion has more relevance in the statistical averaging process, which is discussed in the section on signal averaging.

Filter Designs

Filters are characterized by the range of frequencies that they allow to pass and those they reject or stop. There are four basic filter designs specified by cutoff frequencies: high-pass, low-pass, bandpass, and notch (band-reject) filters. High-pass filters attenuate low-frequency signals, such as direct current (DC) signals, whereas low-pass filters attenuate high-frequency signals, such as myogenic artifact and radio transmissions (Duffy et al, 1989). Using both high-pass and low-pass filters together in the appropriate way can create either a bandpass or notch filter.

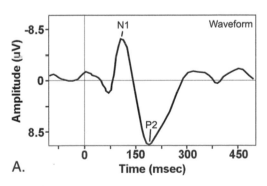

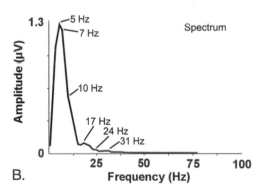

Fig. 2.5 Illustration of fast Fourier transform (FFT) on a cortical event–related potential (CERP) waveform. (**A**) Averaged waveform represented in the time domain (msec). (**B**) Applying FFT on the waveform, the spectral energy is represented in the frequency domain (Hz) with energy up to ~50 Hz. The greatest spectral energy occurs ~5 Hz. Thus, the bandpass filter during acquisition should have cutoffs as low as 0.01 Hz and as high as 100 Hz (i.e., twice the Nyquist frequency).

Signal Averaging

After differential amplification and filtering, the third way of improving SNR is signal averaging AEP signals time-locked to presented stimuli. The basis for the SNR improvement by signal averaging is due to noise (i.e., EEG) not being time-locked to the external stimulus (Durrant and Ferraro, 1999; Hyde, 1994; Ruchkin, 1988). The EEG is assumed to be random and statistically stationary (e.g., values normally-distributed around the mean) at all time intervals through the averaging process. Thus, noise will cancel itself out, whereas time-locked signals sum together. **Figure 2.6** shows a simplified example of how signal averaging works to minimize noise.

When the incoming signal is sampled from the surface of the head, only a set amount of the signal is sampled for a fixed duration of time. Generally, the entire EEG is not recorded. Instead, the EEG is chunked into time-limited epochs during which the AEP is expected to appear following stimulus presentation. The duration of the epoch should be at least as long as the period of the lowest frequency of interest for the AEP waveform of interest to be seen clearly. The beginning of each epoch should coincide with the presentation of the stimulus in a predetermined manner so that the unaveraged responses (i.e., signal embedded in EEG) elicited by the stimulus are time-locked to one another in the averaging process (Duffy et al, 1989). Recall that the EEG contains the AEP of interest, but it is buried within the noise, and the entire epoch has been digitized. During signal averaging, the digitized epochs are mathematically averaged into the singular response waveform seen on the computer monitor screen.

The rate of improvement of SNR is proportional to the square root of the number of epochs, or the square root of the number of stimulus presentations (or $\sqrt{N}$) (Hyde, 1994; Ruchkin, 1988). The amount of SNR depends on the type of signal being averaged and the amount of concurrent noise (Ruchkin, 1988). For example, the ABR may require several thousand stimulus presentations because of signal amplitudes <0.5 μV, which are on the order of 50 to 100 times smaller than the amplitude of noise (~50 μV). Long-latency potentials (e.g., N1/P2), on the other hand, require only hundreds of sweeps or fewer as their amplitudes are larger (~5 μV). **Figure 2.7** illustrates an example of SNR improvement for the ABR with 50, 500, and 1500 stimulus presentations.

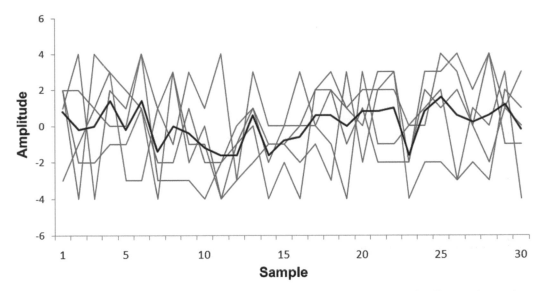

Fig. 2.6 A simplified example of how noise is minimized with signal averaging. Five separate noise waveforms made up of 30 samples each are shown as gray lines. Notice that they appear quite different from each other, with random values in whole integers varying between −4 and 4. The black line is the mathematical average of the five gray lines. Although still somewhat random and zagged, the black line is smoother in appearance, with values in a narrower range between −2 and 2. This reduction in overall amplitude accomplished by averaging is in effect how the random noise signals are gradually canceled out.

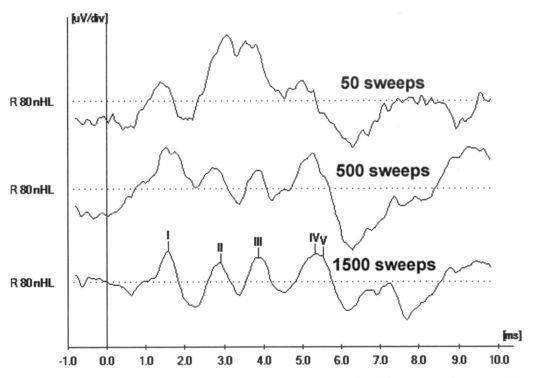

Fig. 2.7 Examples of signal-to-noise ratio (SNR) improvement in the auditory brainstem response with 50 (*top*), 500 (*middle*), and 1500 (*bottom*) sweeps. Although the middle and bottom recordings are similar, these were obtained from a very relaxed patient.

♦ Electrodes

Electrodes form the primary connection between the patient and the AEP recording equipment. Mere application of an electrode to the skin or scalp is not suitable for recording bioelectrical activity because the outermost skin layer (i.e., the stratum corneum) acts as an electrical insulator (Durrant and Ferraro, 1999; Geddes, 1972). To improve the electrical conductivity, the skin is abraded to remove dead skin cells, and an electrolyte gel or paste (usually a sodium chloride solution) is applied. However, this interface between the electrode and the skin will continue to have some degree of electrical opposition known as electrode impedance (Durrant and Ferraro, 1999; Geddes, 1972; Misulis, 1989).

Electrode Impedance

The electrode impedance is determined by several factors, including the surface area of the electrode, the tissue to which it is attached, any debris in between (e.g., oil, dirt, and sweat), the electrolyte solution, and the type of metal used for the electrode. The type of metal used is of particular importance in terms of voltages and impedances that are developed when used in conjunction with electrolytes (Duffy et al, 1989). Good conducting metals are silver, gold, platinum, lead, tin, and stainless steel; because they have low impedances and low electrode potentials (Duffy et al, 1989; Durrant and Ferraro, 1999). Some electrodes can be designed that allow free exchange of ions across an electrical double layer. An example is the silver–silver chloride (Ag-AgCl) electrode formed by silver plated with salt, which lowers impedances further.

Pearl

As a general rule, Ag-AgCl electrodes will work with most AEPs, from ABR to CERP, and will remain stable regardless of recording time (McPherson, Ballachanda, and Kaf, 2007).

For optimal recording, electrical impedances should not exceed 5 kΩ (Duffy et al, 1989; Durrant and Ferraro, 1999). Because a minimum of three electrodes is required for differential recording (Hyde, 1994), it is imperative that the electrode impedances be balanced between all electrodes employed. The reason that the impedances must be balanced is because bias can be implicated in the frequency sensitivity and the optimization of the common-mode rejection of noise (Duffy et al, 1989; Durrant and Ferraro, 1999). As a rule, it has been suggested that interelectrode impedances not exceed 2 kΩ (Durrant and Ferraro, 1999).

Electrode Types

In general, electrodes are long metal wires with insulative coating. At one end of the electrode is a connecting plug to the recording equipment, and the other end connects to the patient. The end that is connected to the patient comes in several different shapes, sizes, and styles and will vary depending on the clinical application or the type of AEP desired. Except for needle electrodes that may be used for intraoperative monitoring purposes, most scalp electrodes are either disk- or cup-shaped, or they are pre-gelled disposable types. **Figure 2.8** features several electrode types commonly used by audiologists.

Electrode Placement

To facilitate laboratory comparison of AEP data, Jasper (1958) developed the international 10–20 system of electrode placement (or 10–20 system). The 10–20 system has been the standard for electrode placement for many years, and it provides guidelines for the placement of 21 electrodes. The electrodes are placed manually following measurement from standard positions on the scalp—that is, nasion, inion, and preauricular points. The strength of this system is that by making such proportional measurements, variations in head size and shape are accommodated. Each electrode is given a designation based on brain area as well as a subscript letter or number to indicate midline or homologous areas of the left and right hemispheres. Brain areas are designated frontal (F), parietal (P), occipital (O), temporal (T), and central (C).

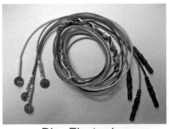
Disc Electrodes

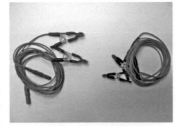
Alligator Clip Electrodes

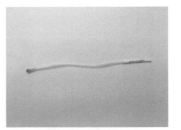
TM Electrode

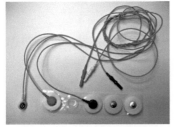

Snap-On Gel Electrodes

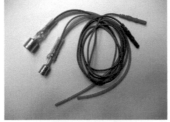
Goil-Foiled TIPtrodes

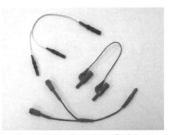
Electrode Jumper Cables

Fig. 2.8 Some examples of electrodes and connectors used by audiologists. Note that adult and pediatric ear clip electrodes are both shown, as are adult and pediatric gold foil TIPtrode inserts. The bottom right box has examples of electrode jumper cables.

Even numbers are associated with the right hemisphere and odd numbers, with the left. Midline electrode locations are labeled with a "z" (zero). Also included in the 10–20 system are electrodes Fpz (frontal pole), A1 and A2 (earlobes), Cb1 and Cb2 (cerebellar), and Pg1 and Pg2 (pharyngeal). Other designations later used in audiology include M1 and M2 (mastoids), Ai (ipsilateral earlobe), Ac (contralateral earlobe), and C7 (nape of the neck) (McPherson et al, 2007). **Figure 2.9** shows the organization of commonly used electrode sites in audiology.

A review of the vast scalp-recorded evoked potential literature will convey a wide variety of reference electrode sites employed. A reference is required in recording AEPs because voltages can be measured only as a difference between two scalp points. With respect to scalp AEP recordings, Wolpaw and Wood (1982) suggest that the optimal site is a place on the head or body where the potential field is most stable. Whenever possible, the reference electrode should not be close to the generator site of interest and should not favor one generator over another, particularly in hemispheric studies (Cacace and

McFarland, 2001; Wolpaw and Penry, 1975). Wolpaw and Wood (1982) have shown that nasion, earlobes, and mastoids work well as reference sites. McPherson and Starr (1993) also advocate the use of a noncephalic site on the nape of the neck (C7). **Table 2.2** shows the most common electrode montages employed for different AEPs.

Number of Electrodes versus Number of Channels

Beginning clinicians often confuse the number of recording channels with the number of electrodes that are needed. Generally, a minimum of three electrodes are required to complete the circuit for one channel (Hyde, 1994). Two electrodes go into each of the inputs of the differential amplifier, and the remaining electrode goes to ground. Many AEPs can be recorded with a single channel setup using either Cz or Fz (noninverting), Ai (inverting), and Ac (ground). The most common example of a two-channel setup is the simultaneous ipsilateral and contralateral ABR recording where each ear serves as the inverting input for separate differential amplifiers, Cz is

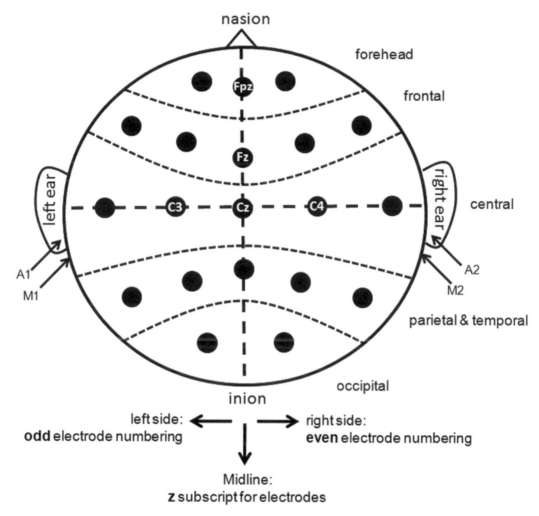

nasion

forehead

frontal

left ear

right ear

central

A1

M1

A2

M2

parietal & temporal

inion

occipital

left side: ⟵   ⟶ right side:
odd electrode numbering   **even** electrode numbering

Midline:
z subscript for electrodes

Fig. 2.9 Illustration of 10–20 system of electrode placement. Electrodes are placed on the scalp in designated areas based on measurements between nasion, inion, and preauricular points. See the text for a description of the electrode nomenclature based on the 10–20 electrode placement system.

Table 2.2 Commonly Used Electrode Montage for Major AEPs

AEP	Noninverting	Inverting	Common/Ground
Electrocochleography	Ac	Ipsilateral TM or ear canal	Fz
ABR	Cz or Fz (avoid Cz for infant testing)	Mi or Ai	Mc or Ac
MLR	Cz or Fz for single channel, C3 and C4 to investigate electrode effects	Ai (avoid mastoid due to PAM artifact)	Ac
CERP	Cz (Pz for P300)	Mi or Ai (some use linked mastoids)	Fz

Abbreviations: ABR, auditory brainstem response; AEP, auditory evoked potential; CERP, cortical event–related potential; MLR, middle latency response; PAM, postauricular muscle; TM, tympanic membrane.

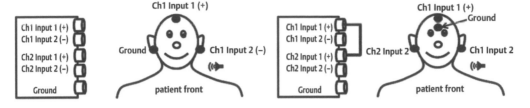

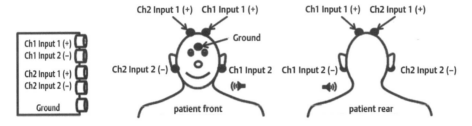

Fig. 2.10 Illustration of different electrode montages. (**A**) Single-channel auditory brainstem response (ABR) using three electrodes. (**B**) Two-channel ABR using four electrodes (Input 1 of both channels is jumpered). (**C**) Two-channel middle latency response (MLR) using five electrodes. See the text for more information.

physically linked by a jumper cable plugged into both noninverting inputs, and ground is Fpz. Thus, four electrodes and a jumper are required, but only two channels are involved. Here a single noninverting electrode site is used (Cz); however, clinicians are using the independent references that may be used in interpretation.

A different two-channel setup is often used with middle latency responses (MLRs) is recorded simultaneously from both temporal lobe regions. In it, C3 (left temporal lobe) and C4 (right temporal lobe) serve as noninverting inputs to separate differential amplifiers, the ears (A1/A2 or M1/M2) serve as reference electrodes and ground is on Fpz. In this example, five electrodes were required for only two channels. In preplanning, it often helps to draw your desired electrode montage on paper and stick with commonly used protocols, particularly with placement of the noninverting and inverting electrodes. Here independent recordings on each side of the head is possible to evaluate hemispheric symmetry (or lack thereof). All three montages are illustrated in **Fig. 2.10.**

◆ Recording Considerations for Auditory Evoked Potentials

Electrode Array and Number of Channels

The way in which the different electrodes are arranged on the individual being tested is dependent on the anatomy and physiology behind the AEP of interest. This arrangement is commonly referred to as the electrode array. Remember, for differential amplification to be maximally beneficial, it is important to plan out your electrode array (montage) based on the neuroanatomical organization of the underlying dipoles. The number of channels necessary for recording depends on the AEP of interest and the reason for testing. Most AEPs can provide sufficient information with a single recording channel. A single recording channel is the simplest electrode setup, with one noninverting (active) electrode, one inverting electrode (reference), and one ground electrode. There are, however, certain test protocols that require extra channels (i.e., additional active electrode sites) to obtain all the necessary information for appropriate test interpretation. For example, multiple channels are often used to record an MLR for neurodiagnostic purposes to check for the presence of electrode effects (see Chapter 9). Additional channels are also recommended to monitor eyeblink artifact during CERP recordings (see Chapter 10).

Time Window

The time window is defined by the amount of time both before and after the presentation of the stimulus that will be analyzed in the recording. Therefore, the time window will be chosen based on the expected latencies of the AEP of interest. It is important to choose a time window that is sufficiently long enough to capture the entire AEP while not including much response information beyond the components of interest. For example, waves I to V of the ABR are typically recorded within the first 6 msec after the stimulus. A time window of 10 msec is often chosen for neurodiagnostic ABR testing. However, there are stimulus and subject factors that can increase the latency of the response (e.g., low-frequency stimuli, decreased stimulus intensity, infants with immature central auditory nervous systems). In these cases, the time window will be increased, but only enough to account for the small change in latency (e.g., time windows of 15–25 msec). It is important to choose an appropriate time window. Too short a time window may cut off relevant waves. Too

long a time window will decrease the sampling rate and thereby decrease your time resolution (i.e., increase sample duration).

Sampling Rate

Sampling rate has an intimate relationship with the time window, especially when a fixed number of sampling points are chosen: 256, 512, and sometimes 1024. Most commercially available AEP systems give at least two of these choices. Sampling rate can then be determined by dividing the time window (in seconds) into the number of points. For example, the ABR is often recorded using a time window of 10 msec (or 0.01 s). If we chose 256 sample points, 256/.01 = 25,600 samples per second (or Hz). If the Nyquist frequency in the ABR is around 1000 Hz, it must be sampled at least 2000 Hz, which means that a sampling rate of 25,600 Hz is more than plenty to sample the ABR with high temporal resolution. In fact, at this sampling rate, each sample duration is ~0.039 msec. Realize, however, as the time window increases, the sampling rate will decrease, and it will be important to ensure that the Nyquist theorem is never violated by knowing beforehand the spectrum of the AEP of interest (recall from Fig. 2.1). Some authors suggest that the sampling rate be no less than four times the Nyquist frequency. **Figure 2.11** illustrates how 64 and 256 sampling points differ in terms of their resolution.

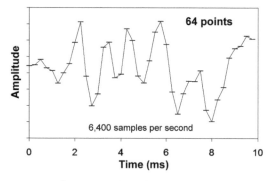

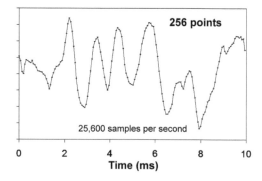

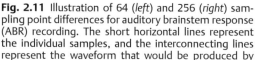

Fig. 2.11 Illustration of 64 (*left*) and 256 (*right*) sampling point differences for auditory brainstem response (ABR) recording. The short horizontal lines represent the individual samples, and the interconnecting lines represent the waveform that would be produced by the number of sampling points available. Notice the increase in sampling rate resulting from the increase in the number of sampling points. Sampling points of 256, 512, or 1024 are standard.

Number of Sweeps (Stimulus Repetitions)

The number of sweeps needed for an average AEP is inversely proportional to the SNR and the amplitude of the AEP of interest. As the SNR improves and the amplitude of the AEP increases, the number of sweeps required for testing decreases. In general, the longer the latency of the response, the greater the amplitude (i.e., CERP > MLR > ABR); therefore, the higher up in the central auditory nervous system being tested, the fewer the number of sweeps that will be necessary to adequately view the AEP response. Generally, sweeps of 200, 1000, and 2000 are needed for CERP, MLR, and ABR, respectively, though some protocols may call for many more and sometimes less. If the SNR is good, the clinician may stop averaging and quickly move on to the next step in the protocol. However, if the SNR is poor, more sweeps are necessary. A technique used often with ABR threshold estimation is Fsp, which adds a statistical confidence component to the recordings by helping clinicians decide whether more or fewer sweeps are needed. The technique is described further in Chapters 3 and 6.

Stimulation Rate

The stimulation rate is dependent on the time window as well as the duration of the stimulus, because the goal during AEP testing is to avoid presenting more than one stimuli in the same time window. When there is more than one stimulus in the same time window, the recording will contain overlapping responses and distort the waveform. Stimulation rates are often much slower for later AEPs (e.g., CERPs) than for earlier AEPs (e.g., ECochG and ABR). For example, during ABR testing, the time window is usually 10 msec, and the stimuli are very brief (e.g., 100 μsec click). Although the clinician could present clicks up to 100 per second for an ABR time window of 10 msec without overlapping responses, the ABR waveform will be severely degraded. During CERP testing, you might have a much longer time window (e.g., 500 msec or 0.5 s), and the stimulus you are presenting may be much longer (e.g., 400 msec). In this case, you can present up to a rate of 1.25 stimuli per second. If you present at a faster rate, both the first and second stimuli will occur within the time window, which is not desirable. To increase the stimulation rate, you would have to decrease either the duration of the stimulus or the time window accordingly. If the selected stimulation rate is incompatible with the time window selected, the AEP software will often alert the clinician to this error after the stimulus type and duration have been defined. However, it is best to know the relationship of your stimulation rate, time window, and stimulus duration before selecting your protocol.

Pearl

Associated with stimulation rate are two other terms often seen in the literature: *interstimulus interval* (ISI) and *stimulus onset asynchrony* (SOA). The ISI is the time duration between the end of the preceding stimulus and the start of the following stimulus. The SOA is the time duration between the start of the preceding stimulus and the start of the following stimulus. When stimuli are long, the SOA will be longer than the ISI.

Filter Settings

Filter settings are employed to eliminate spectral energy (i.e., noise) not contained within the AEP of interest in an effort to maximize the SNR of the recording. Typically, a bandpass filter is used where there is a specified high-frequency and low-frequency cutoff for the recording. Remember that AEPs are nothing more than complex waveforms that can be plotted in both the time and frequency domains. The filter settings employed are simply based on the frequencies that constitute the AEP (i.e., spectral energy). Therefore, filter settings are different for every AEP because the spectral energy or frequency composition of each waveform is different. For example, CERPs are much lower in frequency than the ABR such that bandpass filter settings for a given CERP may be 0.1 to 30 Hz, but those filter settings are changed to 100 to 3000 Hz for the ABR.

Amplification

Gain is the AEP acquisition feature used to amplify and in turn visualize the recorded response. Refer back to the differential amplification section earlier in this chapter for information regarding gain settings.

Artifact Rejection

Even with all of the aforementioned measures in place to reduce SNR and suppress noise/signals outside the frequency band of the AEP of interest, artifact can still make visualization of the AEP response challenging. Therefore, there is an additional acquisition parameter called "artifact reject," which can be set to eliminate any epochs in which the electrical activity exceeds a predetermined criterion. This is especially helpful for eliminating epochs during which time there might have been excessive movement and/or muscle activity. In some cases, the clinician may want to turn off artifact rejection or set it to more aggressive levels. For example, the vestibular evoked myogenic potential (VEMP) is a myogenic response with high levels of activity. If the artifact reject is not turned off, most if not all of the responses would be eliminated, rendering the clinician unable to collect enough samples for an averaged response.

◆ General Subject Factors

Several subject-related factors that need to be considered when choosing the most appropriate stimulus acquisition parameters for a given AEP. These subject factors are generally addressed in this section. More information regarding protocol adjustments based on various subject effects for specific AEPs can be found in Section II of this text.

Age

The central auditory nervous system is not fully mature until adolescence. Clinicians need to take maturation effects into consideration, particularly when testing infants and children. For example, the ABR is not adult-like until 18 to 24 months of age. Typically, the most common effects of lack of maturation are longer latencies that would call for a longer time window to be chosen. In addition, auditory systems that are either immature or perhaps degenerating are often more negatively affected by faster stimulation rates. In later adulthood, there is typically an age effect on latency for most AEPs such that latency increases slightly with age. Therefore, clinics would be wise to develop age-related normative values.

Gender

Most of the literature with respect to gender effects has centered on the ABR. Specifically, women have shorter latencies and larger amplitude responses than men (Hall, 2007). Although some researchers have postulated that these are due to differences in head size and scalp/skull thickness, the differences due to these factors is negligible. Others suggest gender differences are related to differences in cochlear anatomy, specifically that the basilar membrane is longer in men than women. This difference yields longer travel times for acoustic stimuli within the male cochlea, as well as reduced synchronicity of nerve fiber responses resulting from distribution of frequency bands over a longer length (Picton, 2010).

Muscle Activity

For all AEPs discussed in this text (with the exception of the VEMP), the desired activity is neuronal, not myogenic. Therefore, it is critical to avoid measuring any excess muscle activity, which can obscure the AEP response waveform. Unfortunately, there are many muscles that innervate the head and neck, which can cause problems during AEP recordings. Probably the best known is the postauricular muscle (PAM) artifact, which is most problematic during MLR recordings. To reduce muscle artifact contamination, the clinician can alter the electrode montage, choosing an earlobe rather than the mastoid for the site of the active electrode. Another technique to reduce the chances of muscle artifact contaminating the response waveform is to adjust the artifact reject parameter or implement a stricter cutoff criterion if too much artifact seems to be present during recording.

Attention

For many AEPs, attention is not a factor during recording. For example, a patient will be encouraged to relax with eyes closed or sleep during ABR recordings. However, attention plays a larger role in some of the CERPs, particularly the P300 response. Although the clinician does not need to change any stimulus acquisition parameters to account for attention effects per se, the level of attention may have an effect on the morphology of the response. See Chapter 10 for more information regarding the effects of attention on the P300 and other CERP responses.

Temperature

In most instances, temperature will not be a concern during AEP testing. It is only in special circumstances (i.e., during intraoperative monitoring or anesthetization) that body temperature changes should be considered. Certain populations, such as comatose patients and premature infants, are also prone to hypothermia (Arnold, 2007). Because lower body temperature can prolong latencies, it may be advisable to use longer time windows when testing these patient populations.

References

Arnold, S. A. (2007). The auditory brainstem response. In R. J. Roesser, M. Valente, & H. Hosford-Dunn (Eds.) *Audiology diagnosis* (2nd ed., pp. 426–442). New York: Thieme.

Cacace, A. T., & McFarland, D. J. (2001). Middle latency auditory evoked potentials: Basic issues and potential applications. In J. Katz (Ed.), *Handbook of clinical audiology* (5th ed., pp. 349–377). Baltimore: William & Wilkins.

Duffy, F. H., Iyer, V. G., & Surwillo, W. W. (1989). *Clinical electroencephalography and topographic brain mapping.* New York: Springer-Verlag.

Durrant, J. D., & Ferraro, J. A. (1999). Short-latency auditory evoked potentials. In F. E. Musiek & W. F. Rintelmann (Eds.), *Contemporary perspectives in hearing assessment* (5th ed., pp. 197–242). Boston: Allyn & Bacon.

Elberling, C., & Don, M. (1984). Quality estimation of averaged auditory brainstem responses. *Scandinavian Audiology, 13*(3), 187–197. PubMed

Finan, D. S. (2010). Get hip to the data acquisition scene: Principles of digital signal recording. *Perspectives on Speech Science and Orofacial Disorders, 20*(1), 6–13.

Geddes, L. A. (1972). *Electrodes and the measurement of bioelectric events.* New York: John Wiley & Sons.

Hall, J. W. (1992). *Handbook of auditory evoked responses.* Boston: Allyn & Bacon.

Hall, J. W. (2007). *New handbook of auditory evoked responses.* Boston: Allyn & Bacon.

Hyde, M. L. (1994). Signal processing and analysis. In J. T. Jacobson (Ed.), *Principles and applications in auditory evoked potentials* (pp. 47–83). Boston: Allyn & Bacon.

Jasper, H. H. (1958). The ten twenty electrode system of the international federation. *Electroencephalography and Clinical Neurophysiology, 10,* 371–375.

Johnson, K. (1997). *Acoustic and auditory phonetics.* Malden, MA: Blackwell Publishing.

Lagerlund, T. D. (1996). Digital signal processing. In T. D. Lagerlund (Ed.), *Clinical neurophysiology* (pp. 40–49). Philadelphia: F. A. Davis.

McPherson, D. L., Ballachanda, B. B., & Kaf, W. (2007). Middle and long latency auditory evoked potentials. In R. J. Roesser, M. Valente, & H. Hosford-Dunn (Eds.), *Audiology diagnosis* (2nd ed., pp. 443–47). New York: Thieme.

McPherson, D. L., & Starr, A. (1993). Auditory evoked potentials in the clinic. In A. M. Halliday (Ed.), *Evoked potentials in clinical testing* (pp. 359–381). New York: Churchill Livingston.

Misulis, K. E. (1989). Basic electronics for clinical neurophysiology. *Journal of Clinical Neurophysiology, 6*(1), 41–74. PubMed

Misulis, K. E., & Fakhoury, T. (2001). *Spehlmann's evoked potential primer.* Boston: Butterworth-Heinemann.

Picton, T. W. (2010). *Human auditory evoked potentials.* San Diego: Plural Publishing.

Ruchkin, D. S. (1988). Measurement of event-related potentials: Signal extraction. In T. W. Picton (Ed.), *Handbook of electroencephalography and clinical neurophysiology* (Vol. 3, pp. 7–43). Amsterdam: Elsevier.

Wolpaw, J. R., & Penry, J. K. (1975). A temporal component of the auditory evoked response. *Electroencephalography and Clinical Neurophysiology, 39*(6), 609–620. PubMed

Wolpaw, J. R., & Wood, C. C. (1982). Scalp distribution of human auditory evoked potentials: 1. Evaluation of reference electrode sites. *Electroencephalography and Clinical Neurophysiology, 54*(1), 15–24. PubMed

Chapter 3

Principles of Analysis and Interpretation

Samuel R. Atcherson and Tina M. Stoody

In Chapter 2, the emphasis was on auditory evoked potential (AEP) instrumentation and acquisition parameters. In this chapter, we focus on the principles of analysis and interpretation techniques that may be applied across the scope of AEPs. Generally, most analysis and interpretation techniques take place following the completed, averaged recording. This is the case when the clinician is expected to mark (or label) portions of the waveforms to obtain certain time of occurrence (latency) and amplitude measures. Most recorded AEPs will undergo this process. Some analysis and interpretation techniques are performed "on the fly" as the averaging process is taking place, which may allow the clinician to make judgments about whether to terminate the recording early or continue averaging. This approach is used most commonly in auditory brainstem response (ABR) threshold estimation applications, which do not depend on precise latency or amplitude values. Finally, the auditory steady-state response (ASSR) is analyzed spectrally through a time-to-frequency conversion process, even though averaged waveforms are recorded behind the scenes. In this chapter, we are concerned with questions, such as the following:

- Is a response present, or is it just artifact or noise?

- Is the response reliable and repeatable?

- If the response is present, how does it compare with others obtained from individuals with normal hearing and auditory processes?

- How confident am I that the recorded response will help me with differential diagnosis or threshold estimation?

- Are there internal or external factors that explain the outcome of the recording?

Although the averaged AEP can be thought of as an objective record of the underlying neurophysiology, in many cases it will still depend on final subjective judgment from the clinician. It is for this reason that we must treat all AEPs from a statistical perspective. Recognize first that the recorded waveform has undergone one of the most basic statistical procedures: averaging. Specifically, each recorded waveform is composed of a finite number of samples and the averaging process during recording attempts to cause random background noise (i.e., electroencephalogram, or EEG) to cancel out while allowing the desired AEP (i.e., the response or signal) to continue to develop in the average. For example, the ABR is commonly recorded with 256 points in a 10-msec time window. Dividing 10 msec by 256, each individual point (or sample) is ~0.039 msec in duration. Each and every 0.039-msec sample in the waveform holds a single amplitude value, which contains both the response and noise, and is going through averaging with each and every stimulus presentation. Next, appreciate that any part of a recorded waveform may be selected and compared with normative data collected from a larger group of individuals. Normative data typically yield the central tendency of the group (mean), as well as the variability of the group (standard deviation, SD). If, for example, a patient has a measurement that exceeds 2 SD above or below the mean, there is a greater likelihood that there is an abnormality. Finally, there are objective response detection techniques that depend on the use of statistics to provide a confidence measure of whether or not a response is actually there. Therefore, this chapter also addresses the following question:

- Are there techniques available that will improve response detection or measurement and minimize the subjective aspect of analysis and interpretation?

◆ Transient versus Steady-State Responses

Most AEPs that we find in the literature are of the transient type; that is, they are evoked to the onset of mostly short-duration stimuli with reasonably fast acoustic changes, and the response waveform generally looks nothing like the stimulus waveform. These AEPs include the electrocochleogram (ECochG), ABR, middle latency response (MLR), cortical event–related potential (CERP), and vestibular evoked myogenic potential (VEMP). Example stimuli for evoking transient AEPs include clicks, tone bursts, noise bursts, and synthetic and natural speech stimuli. Transient AEPs each have a characteristic waveform with somewhat predictable positive and negative voltage patterns. How this voltage pattern appears will depend to a large extent on the analysis time window, the filter settings, and the recording electrode locations. As the waveform varies over time about the zero voltage baseline, any positive or negative voltage swing can come to a maximal point. This maximal point is generally referred to

as a "peak" or a "wave." Sometimes, these peaks or waves are called "components." When voltages are displayed with positive up and negative down, the negative peaks are sometimes called "troughs." Throughout this chapter and text, these terms may be interchangeable. Transient AEPs make up the bulk of this textbook, with literature reviews and clinical applications of more commonly known AEPs in Sections II and III. As such, the majority of this chapter focuses largely on analysis and interpretation techniques for transient AEPs.

AEPs such as the ASSR and the frequency-following response (FFR) have the ability to mimic (or follow) periodic spectral or envelope patterns. Because of the repetitive nature of these AEPs, marking peaks has limited value, and other techniques are implemented for analysis and interpretation. One of the most commonly used measures with steady-state AEPs involves a time-to-frequency conversion process called a fast Fourier transformation (FFT) to reveal the dominant spectral energies in the recorded response. ASSRs are evoked to stimulus types that have a repetitive nature, such as amplitude-modulated tones, tone pairs, repeated clicks and tone bursts, and stimuli that combine amplitude and frequency modulations (Purcell and Dajani, 2008). FFRs can be evoked by sinusoids, tone pairs, vowels, and consonant-vowel (CV) stimuli with simple and complex formant and harmonic relationships that vary in time and frequency (Krishnan, 2007). FFR is still under investigation with some promising clinical applications (see Chapter 8), whereas ASSR is available on many clinical evoked potential systems with research that is ongoing to better understand its strengths and limitations (see Chapters 8 and 15). Because the ASSR is in mainstream clinical use, it assumes the focus of this chapter on the analysis of steady-state AEPs in the frequency domain. It should be noted that in recent years, some attention has been drawn to a brainstem response that contains an initial transient portion (ABR) followed by a steady-state (FFR) portion when evoked by a synthetic CV stimulus (/da/) (Russo, Nicol, Musacchia, and Kraus, 2004). This speech-evoked brainstem response can be analyzed in both the time and frequency domains.

◆ Analyses in the Time Domain

This section of the chapter considers two commonly used time-domain analysis and interpretation approaches. The first involves analysis and interpretation techniques that follow the collection of the averaged response. That is, the averaged response waveform is saved to the hard drive and ready for measurement marking and other post hoc or offline processing, if needed. The second involves techniques that are used during the averaging process that is ongoing and the recording is not yet complete. These two techniques are described in greater depth as follows.

Analysis Techniques Following Signal Averaging

Measurement techniques following the completion of an averaged recording are a form of offline processing. That is, the original data are usually stored on the computer hard drive, and the clinician can apply several different manual techniques to the waveform. The clinician has an opportunity to scale, smooth, and/or apply additional filtering to the recorded waveform, if needed. Some AEPs require additional mathematical calculations to be applied to the waveforms (i.e., subtraction, addition, and averaging of multiple waveforms) before the final waveform is subjected to measurements. Generally, these offline recordings will be marked at select peaks to derive latency and/or amplitude measurements. **Table 3.1** lists some of the more common time-domain measurements obtained for the various classes of AEPs covered in this text.

> **Pearl**
>
> For transient AEPs, many commercial systems allow one to mark (or label) the individual peaks during the averaging process rather than having to wait until the recording is completed. This can help to shorten the overall analysis time by making these measurements "on the fly," such as with ECochG and ABR. However, be sure to do a quick final measurement check for accuracy.

Latency and Amplitude

Once a peak (or trough) is identified, two measurements can be obtained and interpreted: latency and amplitude (**Table 3.2**).

Table 3.1 Commonly Used Clinical Analysis Techniques in Auditory Evoked Potentials

	Analysis Techniques Employed
ECochG	• Marking of primary waves SP and AP; baseline is also marked to determine baseline-peak amplitude measures
ABR	• Marking of primary waves I, III, and V, although other waves may be marked, such as II and IV • Marking wave V only and tracking its presence to decreasing intensity levels • Looking for signs of ringing cochlear microphonic in an absent or grossly malformed ABR waveform, as in the case of auditory neuropathy spectrum disorder (ANSD)
ASSR	• Amplitude or phase analysis by fast Fourier transform (FFT; time-to-frequency conversion)
MLR	• Marking of primary waves Na and Pa, although other waves may also be marked, such as Po, Nb, Pb, and Nc
CERP	• Marking of primary waves P1, N1, and P2 in cortical potential • Marking of N1 and P2 and tracking its presence to decreasing intensity levels • Marking of P1 only and tracking its latency/presence as a child ages • Marking of P300 in cognitive auditory paradigm
VEMP	• Marking of P13 (P1) and N23 (N1)

Abbreviations: ABR, auditory brainstem response; ANSD, auditory neuropathy spectrum disorder; AP, action potential; ASSR, auditory steady-state response; CERP, cortical event-related potential; ECochG, electrocochleogram; MLR, middle latency response; SP, summating potential; VEMP, vestibular evoked myogenic potential.

The measurement of absolute latency is generally thought of as the time at which a peak appears relative to when the stimulus began (or stimulus onset), and it is usually reported in milliseconds (msec). For example, wave V of the ABR usually appears around 5.6 msec following the onset of a moderately high-intensity click, and the N1 component of the CERP usually appears around 100 msec following the onset of virtually any abrupt stimulus. In addition to absolute latencies, there are interpeak (or interwave) and interaural latencies. The term *interpeak latency* (IPL) refers to the time duration between successive peaks, usually of the same voltage polarity (i.e., not peak to trough). Interpeak latencies are often analyzed for neurodiagnostic ABR testing; as an example, the conduction time between waves I and V is normally ~4 msec.

Interaural latencies are also often analyzed in neurodiagnostic ABR testing where the absolute latencies of wave V for each ear are compared. It should be noted that different classes of AEPs will designate which positive or negative peaks are deemed important for neurodiagnostic purposes. Additionally, when the recording window size is increased from 10 to 500 msec (e.g., ABR to CERP, respectively), the duration of each sample will often increase. Recall that the entire AEP has undergone analog-to-digital (A-D) conversion, and both latency and amplitude are represented by a limited number of samples, with each sample having a fixed duration. For example, if 256 points are used to record the ABR in a 10-msec window, then each sample is ~0.039 msec in duration. That is, the 10-msec ABR waveform will be divided into 256 samples. These

Table 3.2 Latency and Amplitude Utility for Time-Domain Auditory Evoked Potentials

	Latency	Amplitude
ECochG	Useful for wave identification but may be diagnostically irrelevant unless delayed.	SP and AP measurements relative to baseline are critically important here.
ABR	Absolute and relative latencies for waves I, III, V, I–III, III–V, and I–V are deemed most important; interaural latency difference (ILD or IT5) for wave V between ears.	Absolute amplitudes are too variable to be used clinically; however, wave V/I ratio and wave V can be used for threshold estimation and stacked ABR.
FFR (BioMARK)	Latencies are important in examining potential timing deficits when compared with a normative template.	The overall amplitude and slope of the wave V to wave A (following trough) complex is used as a neurodiagnostic criteria in the BioMARK.
MLR	Latencies are generally not important; however, recorded waves should fall within certain latency ranges. Check to be sure that postauricular muscle (PAM) artifact is not confused for MLR.	Amplitudes are important generally only in the context of absence or presence and typically when comparing hemispheric sites.
CERP (P1/N1/P2)	Latencies are generally not important; however, recorded waves should fall within certain latency ranges. The latency of P1 in young children may be used as a biomarker of auditory system development.	Amplitudes are important generally in the context of absence or presence and when comparing hemispheric sites; they will be useful for threshold estimation.
CERP (P300)	Latencies are generally variable in normals but may be significantly delayed in certain sensory, language, learning, and cognitive impairments.	Amplitude is generally not important, although it may signal deficits.
VEMP	Latencies are generally irrelevant, although they are expected to fall within a certain range.	Amplitude is important, P1–N1 (P13–N23) amplitude ratio between ears is used as a diagnostic criterion.

Abbreviations: ABR, auditory brainstem response; AP, action potential; CERP, cortical event–related potential; ECochG, electrocochleogram; FFR, frequency-following response; MLR, middle latency response; SP, summating potential; VEMP, vestibular evoked myogenic potential.

settings would correspond to a sampling rate of 25,600 samples per second. Although this is more than sufficient for the ABR, one could increase the number of sampling points to 512 in a 10 msec analysis window, which would correspond to 51,200 samples per second, or 0.019-msec duration samples. Increasing the number of sampling points, by definition, will increase the sampling rate and vice versa. The point of the discussion on the number of sample points, sample duration, and sampling rate is that it will affect the precision of the latency (and amplitude) measurements, and clinicians are not likely to find fewer than 256 points on a commercially available system. However, they may have the option of raising the number of points to 512 or 1024.

For some classes of AEPs, amplitude measurements are important. The amplitude of a peak can be determined in one of two ways. The first method is to measure the peak amplitude relative to the zero baseline. For some classes of AEPs, the clinician can artificially create a zero baseline by setting up what is called a prestimulus window (Lopes da Silva, 1976). That is, the recording window will include an interval of time before the stimulus is presented and is part of the designated time window. For example, if a prestimulus time period of −10 msec is desired for an MLR analysis time window of 80 msec, then the actual time window will be −10 to 70 msec (not −10 to 80 msec). When the AEP is averaged, it is assumed (and desirable) that the prestimulus activity averages to a flat line around the zero baseline. When a prestimulus time period is added, latency will be not be affected because the onset of the stimulus (as well as the trigger) is still at 0 msec.

The second method for measuring amplitude involves a peak-to-trough (also referred to as peak-to-peak) amplitude measure, where the overall voltage of the peak of interest and voltage of the following peak (usually in the opposite direction of polarity) is calculated. For the ABR, measuring the peak-to-trough for waves I and V will aid in the calculation of the wave V/I ratio measurement. As another example, measuring the trough-to-peak amplitude of Na and Pa will aid in assessing the degree of symmetry (or asymmetry) between the MLR recorded over the right temporal lobe area and over the left temporal lobe area.

Marking or Labeling Waves

Marking or labeling waves is a learned skill. At times, peaks to be marked are obvious. At other times, peaks to be marked are vague or obscured. Recall that all AEPs are recorded through an averaging process, and each waveform is composed of a fixed number of sampling points. That is, each individual sample's latency and amplitude value will be influenced by the overall signal-to-noise ratio (SNR) achieved during the averaging process. Noisy waveforms may produce several spurious bumps in the vicinity of the desired peak and make the marking of peaks difficult for AEPs that may depend on precise latency measurements.

Prior to marking a waveform, it helps to have a visual or mental template of what the waveform morphology should look like with a given stimulus type and other recording parameters. This visual or mental template should also give you a general idea of where various peak latencies would be expected. Once you can anticipate where the peaks are that require marking, then you can proceed. On most commercial systems, you will use the computer mouse to click on the peak and a button or pull-down menu to locate the label of the peak you are marking.

Pearl

Because of signal-to-noise issues that affect every recording, no two recordings will ever appear exactly alike. Thus, the repetition of every recording is a practice that is strongly encouraged to increase confidence that a response is present or absent. In addition, having two or more recordings can help with marking the waveforms.

Because the interpretation of neurodiagnostic ABR tends to rely on precise latency measurements, it is recommended that normative data be collected and that there be a consistent method for marking peaks. Peak picking would be easy if there were a single sample that defines the maximum amplitude of that peak. Complications arise in picking peaks when more than one sample has the same maximal amplitude in the expected vicinity of the peak of interest. Here is a dilemma: if there is an odd number of samples with the same amplitude value (e.g., three or five), one might choose the middle sample. But if there is an even number of samples with the same amplitude value (e.g., two or four), there is no middle sample leaving the clinician in a quandry. Therefore, it is our recommendation that anytime there are two or more samples in the vicinity of an ABR peak, you select the right-most sample before the amplitude begins to decrease. **Figure 3.1** illustrates this recommendation using a blowup of the vicinity of the wave V peak. Ideally, this strategy should be applied to all marked waves. When wave V is on the following shoulder of a larger wave IV, select the point on the shoulder before the biggest drop in amplitude.

Another difficulty related to the ABR is the appearance of a wave IV/V complex. Sometimes the two waves are very distinguishable and have clearly defined latency differences. Sometimes the wave IV/V complex is fused and takes on the latency that would be expected of either wave IV or V alone. Sometimes wave IV is on the leading shoulder of wave V; other

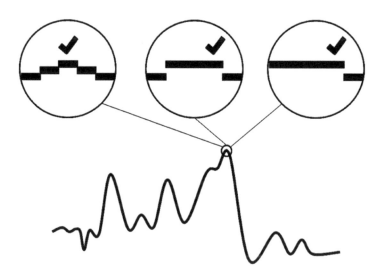

Fig. 3.1 Example strategy for picking auditory brainstem response peaks. Each circle represents a blow-up (*or* magnification) of three hypothetical sampling patterns having the same maximal amplitude that might be observed for wave V. The first (*left*) has a single maximal peak, the second (*middle*) has three samples, and the third (*right*) has four samples. To avoid ambivalence with picking peaks, it is recommended that the right-most sample be used, as seen in the middle and right circles.

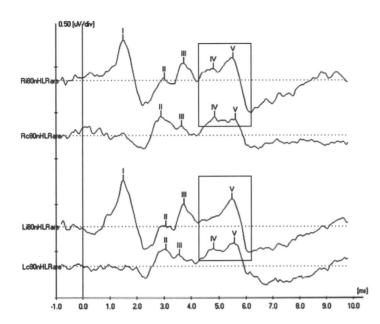

Fig. 3.2 Contralateral auditory brainstem response (ABR) may help resolve wave IV/V complex issues (Mizrahi, Maulsby, and Frost, 1983). The two top waves are the ipsilateral and contralateral waves to right ear stimulation; the bottom two are the same to left ear stimulation.

times wave V is on the following shoulder of wave IV. One potentially helpful solution is to record simultaneously both the ipsilateral and contralateral ABRs (**Fig. 3.2**). In some patients with obscure ipsilateral wave IV/V complexes, the contralateral ABR may be useful, as the separation of the two waves may be accentuated. With the exception of wave I, which is absent in the contralateral ABR, waves III, IV, and V are generally comparable between the ipsilateral and contralateral recordings.

Post Hoc Filtering and Smoothing

Filtering is predetermined or set prior to all recordings to restrict certain frequency ranges that would be considered unrelated to the AEP of interest. In some cases, such as with ECochG and ABR recordings, no further post hoc processing is necessary (or even desired) after the recording is complete. In other cases, more commonly with MLR and later AEPs, clinicians may opt to "clean up" the waveforms using additional filtering or smoothing. Filtering generally involves applying a more restricted filter bandwidth to remove additional low or high frequencies. Although some filtering is helpful, any aggressive filtering (i.e., too restricted bandwidth) can lead to waveform distortions (**Fig. 3.3**). These distortions usually come in the form of amplitude reduction and latency shifts.

Smoothing involves the clumping of several adjacent samples and forces them into a common value and does so throughout the entire recorded waveform (**Fig. 3.4**). Earlier AEPs, such as ECochG and ABR, generally do not require additional filtering or smoothing for at least two reasons: (1) the spectral information contained within the ECochG and ABR (>100 Hz) is much higher than the spectral information contained within the ongoing EEG (<100 Hz), and (2) the initial filter settings restrict most of the EEG activity. Later AEPs, which generally have lower spectral information, may overlap with the EEG spectrum.

Pearl

Additional post hoc filtering should involve frequency cutoffs that are set to be at least the same as or narrower than the initial filter settings at the time of the recording. For example, the CERP is typically recorded with a bandpass filter setting of 0.1 to 100 Hz. To clean up the waveforms, the clinician could lower the low-pass frequency cutoff to 30 Hz while leaving the high-pass frequency cutoff intact. Changing the low-pass filter will have a smoothing effect.

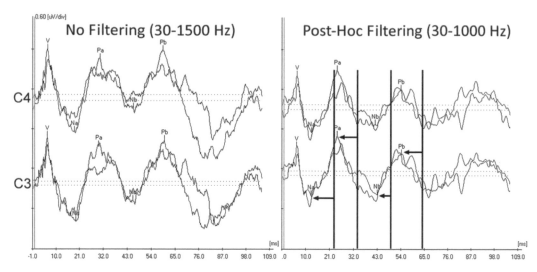

Fig. 3.3 Middle latency response recordings without (*left*) and with (*right*) post hoc filtering. With post hoc filtering (lowering low-pass cutoff from 1500 to 1000 Hz), the resultant waveform is distorted with the short-ening of latencies and a reduction of overall amplitude. The vertical line with arrows shows the amount of latency shift caused by filtering, which is not equal for all peaks.

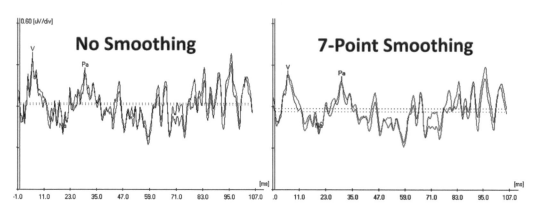

Fig. 3.4 Middle latency response recordings without (*left*) and with (*right*) seven-point smoothing.

Scaling

Scaling is a technique in which the amplitude axis of an averaged waveform is changed to make the waves a little larger or smaller. Scaling is a display parameter; it is not the same as changing the gain, which is part of the actual recording protocol. Instead, scaling is used like a microscope or telescope to change the magnification of the averaged waveform. Sometimes the recordings are too large on the screen, and you will want to make them smaller to fit better to the screen. Other times, you may want to stack several waveforms together in the same window, and the only way they will all fit is by making the overall amplitudes smaller. In some cases, the recordings may look too small to appreciate the overall waveform morphology, so you will want to make the responses larger. As you change the scale, there will be an inverse relationship between projected waveform amplitude and the amplitude divisions of the x-axis. For example, the x-axis of the ABR analysis window may initially be 0.5 μV per division. Increasing the scaling value to 0.75 μV per division will make the waveform smaller, whereas decreasing the scalping value to 0.25 μV per division will make the waveform larger. The reason this is occurring is because the number of amplitude divisions may be fixed on the screen. **Figure 3.5** illustrates an example of how scaling affects the same waveform and appears to assist with detection of wave V on the shoulder.

Latency-Intensity Functions

Following ABR threshold estimation recordings, for example, wave V, can be plotted on a latency-intensity function (LIF) graph (**Fig. 3.6**) to observe shifts in peak latency with decreases in stimulus intensity. This technique was

first proposed by Galambos and Hecox (1978) as a way of differentiating types of hearing loss. Prior to the use of a LIF graph, the normative data that had previously been collected with certain stimulus and recording parameters would be superimposed on the graph. On the abscissa (x-axis) is the stimulus intensity, and on the ordinate (y-axis) is the absolute latency. Given that latencies become longer with decreasing intensity, a certain pattern

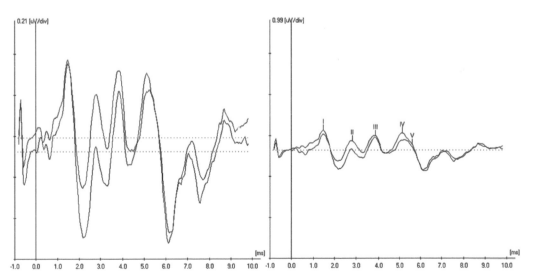

Fig. 3.5 Normal repeated auditory brainstem response to response recordings on two different scales. In this particular case, the larger waveform (*left*; 0.21 μV/division)

makes wave V detection somewhat difficult, whereas the smaller waveform (*right*; 0.99 μV/division) shows a clear wave V shoulder that is distinct from wave IV.

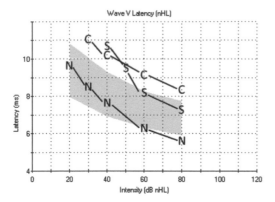

Fig. 3.6 Hypothetical latency-intensity function (LIF) curves for wave V for normal (N), sensorineural hearing loss (S), and conductive hearing loss (C). The shaded gray area represents the region of normal for adult listeners. The normal LIF begins at a latency slightly below the gray area at 80 dB nHL (normal hearing level) but would be considered within normal limits at that level and all other intensity levels. The LIF for sensorineural hearing loss shows normal latency at high levels (80 dB nHL) but quickly deviates from the gray area with progressive decrease of intensity level. For the conductive hearing loss, the LIF mirrors both the normal LIF and the gray area.

or configuration of ABR waves plotted on the LIF will be expected to fall within the normative range. Sensorineural hearing loss is indicated when the LIF shows latencies within the normative range at higher intensity levels but progressively falls outside the normative range at lower intensity levels. Conductive hearing losses can also be indicated by a LIF that mirrors the configuration of the normative range, but all latencies are prolonged regardless of the stimulus intensity.

Pitfall

Clinicians must be aware that the normative ranges on a LIF graph may change based on different age groups, gender, and right versus left ear stimulation. Unless all of these normative data have been collected (a time-consuming process) and made available for a specific evoked potential system with well-defined stimulus and recording parameters, the use of the LIF graph is generally limited and is not in widespread clinical use.

Other Time-Domain Techniques

Averaging, Adding, and Subtracting Waveforms

Many commercial systems have features that allow clinicians to combine two or more waveforms from the same patient in the same recording session. For example, prior to waveform measurements, repeated recordings of the same response can be averaged together. Although not appropriate or even recommended, for some AEPs (e.g., ECochG and ABR), averaging repeated waveforms has the effect of doubling the number of stimulus presentations in the final average. For example, if two response waveforms were collected with 1000 stimulus presentations each, then averaging both into one waveform will increase the total stimulus presentation number to 2000. In turn, this can increase the overall SNR of the averaged response. This technique is advocated for use with the speech-evoked brainstem response (known as BioMARK, Biological Marker of Auditory Processing).

Adding waveforms is another technique that may be used. Instead of averaging one or more waveforms, some AEPs call for summing waveforms. For example, the derived-band ABR (also called stacked ABR [SABR]) has separate waveforms collected from discrete frequency regions of the cochlea using clicks and different high-pass masking noise filter cutoffs. In stacked ABR, there is a prolongation of wave V latency at lower (apical) frequency regions of the cochlea. After marking each wave V and temporally aligning them, the waves are summed together. Because there are some commonalities in the waveform morphology around wave V, the stacked ABR will give the appearance of a very large amplitude V. Using this clever technique, any abnormal amplitude reduction in the stacked ABR may detect tumors smaller than 1 cm.

Finally, there may be times when subtracting waveforms may be needed. For example, when wave I of the ABR is missing, relative latencies I–III and I–V cannot be calculated. If a two-channel ABR has been recorded with reference electrodes on the ears, subtracting the contralateral waveform from the ipsilateral waveform may help to resolve wave I.

The reason this technique sometimes works is because the subtracted waveform emulates an ABR that has been collected with a one-channel horizontal montage. When this technique does not work, and wave I is needed for analysis and interpretation, an ECochG recorded with an ear canal or tympanic membrane (TM) electrode may be needed (Eggermont, Don, and Brackmann, 1980). Another AEP that uses subtraction is the mismatch negativity (MMN). Although the MMN is not in mainstream clinical use, subtracting a waveform response averaged to one stimulus from a waveform response to a stimulus that differs from the first may yield a region of negativity from the auditory system that is able to effectively discriminate the two on a neurophysiologic level.

> **Pearl**
>
> Used appropriately and with stimuli of rarefaction and condensation polarity (not alternating), adding and subtracting ABR waveforms in the analysis can be useful in ECochG and ABR recordings to resolve or eliminate the cochlear microphonic.

Collecting Normative Data

Because of its high dependence on latency measures in neurodiagnoses, the ABR, more than any other AEP, is likely to have published normative data, and clinics are strongly encouraged to collect their own local norms even if two different clinics may have the same equipment. Even LIF normative data should be collected that is age specific. The collection of normative data is relatively easy to do, but it can be time consuming. For the sake of brevity, we will discuss the collection of normative data on young adults with audiologically confirmed normal hearing and no known history of neurologic impairment:

1. Recruit 10 to 20 subjects, preferably balanced in gender, or you may collect gender-specific norms.

2. Set up your neurodiagnostic click–ABR protocol as you plan to use in your clinic (e.g., filter settings, intensity, gain, and transducer type).

3. Collect clean and repeatable ABRs from each subject.

4. Minimally, mark waves I, III, and V, and transfer all latency values, including I–III, III–V, and I–V interwave latencies, to a spreadsheet.

5. Calculate the numerical average of each latency measurement across subjects, and record the values on a normative data sheet that you plan to use. These are mean values that will as a general rule be ~1.5, 3.5, 5.5, 2, 2, and 4 msec for each of the I, III, and V absolute and I–III, III–V, and I–V relative measurements, respectively. Realize, however, that your values may be different from the values indicated by the general rule.

6. The calculation of the SD is complex but not hard to do. The SD value will need to be obtained for each of the absolute and relative latencies. The formula can be found in any statistics textbook or online and derived by hand. Alternatively, the SD can be calculated within a spreadsheet program such as Excel, or there may be an online statistical calculator that can derive this for you. In either case, you will need to take the SD value (which is 1 SD) and multiply it by 2. Next, you will need to obtain two values for your normative data. First, subtract the 2 SD value from the mean (e.g., wave I) that you obtained in step 5. Record this value on your normative data sheet. Second, add 2 SD to the mean that you obtained in step 5. Record this value also. What you should now have are the minimum and maximum limits of what would statistically be considered normal for that one latency measurement. Now repeat this process for all other latency measurements. Although 2 SD is commonly used, there have been reports of other SD values used, such as 2.5 or 3. A SD value of 2 might be considered "conservative" in that more patients may have an abnormality (not a guarantee), whereas a 3 SD value might be considered "liberal," allowing more patients to pass (also not a guarantee).

The process of collecting normative data can be time consuming, but in the long run it will be worthwhile. If time permits, you could also do a biologic calibration of each stimulus you plan to use with the available equipment (e.g., clicks and tone bursts) to determine whether 0 dB nHL (normal hearing level) on the monitor screen is at or close to the numerical average of the biologic threshold of 0 dB in your subjects. Information on how to conduct a biologic calibration is provided in Chapter 22.

Analysis Techniques during Signal Averaging

Although waveform interpretation can be done offline, monitoring the evoked potential as it is being recorded is an important skill to develop. Beginning clinicians will often wait until the averaging is completed before they determine whether or not the recorded waveform is clean. This is not advised, and critical clinical time can be wasted. Instead, beginning clinicians would benefit from some early exposure to the AEP of interest to formulate a template in their minds of what a clean waveform should look like. If this is not possible, an ideal waveform, or representative normal waveform, could be posted on a nearby wall for reference. In any case, major deviations from the template or representative waveform can be caught early, which may signal a technical error. However, rather than just looking at the waveform as it is being averaged, clinicians should be glancing occasionally at the patient, at the rate of artifact rejections, and the ongoing EEG (if displayed on the screen). This type of analysis depends heavily on human judgment and experience and will become more difficult during threshold estimation procedures when the response may be barely detectable above the background EEG activity.

To improve detection of responses, particularly during threshold estimation procedures, reliance on a statistical approach during the averaging process may be considered. Although background EEG is assumed to be random and may be more or less constant throughout a recording, other activity can be recorded that is not the desired response. These other noise sources may include electromagnetic sources of activity in the room and muscular activity from the patient (movement of facial or body muscles, swallowing, breathing, and tensing neck muscles). These additional sources of noise are likely to change in magnitude during the course of the recording. Objective techniques such as Fsp and point-optimized variance ratio (POVR) come in handy here. The Fsp technique is based on the commonly known statistical F-test, in which the numerator includes the variance of signal-plus-noise information from the ongoing averaged recording, and the denominator includes the variance of the noise-only information (Don, Elberling, and Waring, 1984; Sininger, 1993). When the Fsp feature is activated, a number will be shown on the screen that indicates the probability of a present signal. When the Fsp value is high (e.g., a criterion Fsp > 3.1), there is greater confidence that a signal is present and vice versa. As an example, an Fsp of 3.1 might provide 99% probability of a present response, whereas lower Fsp values decrease the probability but do not necessarily indicate its absence. Here, the use of the Fsp objective technique could be supplemental to visual (subjective) detection of a response but not necessarily take the place of the subjective measure. POVR, by contrast, uses a variation of the Fsp and a template-matching scheme (Sininger, Hyde, and Don, 2001). Template matching involves the use of a previously defined target ABR waveform generated from an average of a large number of subjects. Using POVR, objective detection is based in part on the statistical factors related to the SNR, as well as the comparison of the individual ABR to the template ABR. Both Fsp and POVR techniques have been incorporated into commercial newborn screening equipment, and Fsp can also be used for threshold estimation. More information on Fsp and POVR can be found in Chapters 6 and 13.

◆ Analysis in the Frequency Domain: Auditory Steady-State Response

Recall that the ASSR is an AEP that is better analyzed in the frequency domain. This is the case because the responses can mimic or follow spectral and envelope features of a stimulus, and latency measurements are not performed in the time domain. As indicated previously, the instrumentation involved in recording ASSRs is essentially the same as for all other AEPs, particularly transducers, differential amplification, filtering, and signal averaging. In addition, the placement of electrodes is not unlike ABR, with few minor modifications. However, for ASSRs to be analyzed in frequency domain, the EEG must still be time-locked to the modulation frequency of the stimulus, although the ASSR modulation frequency will have some phase delay (or latency) relative to the onset of the stimulus modulation frequency. The resultant averages are analyzed using FFT from which amplitude and phase measures can be obtained by looking for an ASSR that emulates the modulation frequency of the stimulus. For the ASSR to be considered present, it must reach levels that distinguish it from the background noise activity (e.g., SNR), and the phase of the ASSR must have a sufficiently strong coherence (e.g., statistical agreement) with the modulation frequency of the stimulus. The exact

mathematical approach for analyzing the ASSR may vary somewhat among different clinical evoked potential systems, and many are automated. However, the role of the clinician is still critical. As with AEPs in the time domain, clinicians must monitor the patient and the ongoing recording for any potential issues with SNR and number of stimulus presentations required. In terms of monitoring the patient, clinicians should be watching to be certain that physiologic and myogenic noise is kept to a minimum and that transducers and electrodes are still in place. In terms of monitoring the ongoing recordings, clinicians may have access to one or more analysis windows on their screen.

Figure 3.7 shows an example stimulus and ASSR recording (a), and several different analysis windows that may be accessible to the clinician. Windows (b) and (c) show the ongoing response spectral (FFT) analysis. In such windows, the clinician should be able to see a "spike" at or near the stimulus modulation frequency, which should be higher in amplitude compared to background noise activity. The difference between windows (b) and (c) is the range of frequencies

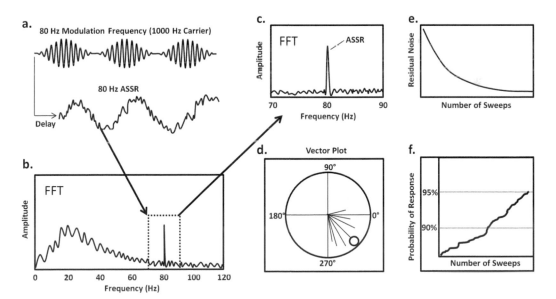

Fig. 3.7 Example stimulus and auditory steady-state response, along with one of several possible analysis windows. See text for description.

represented in the FFT. The wider range shows the larger amplitude EEG energy. Window (d) might be the ongoing amplitude and/or phase analysis depicted in a vector plot. In this vector plot, there is a circle representing phases in degrees. Several vector lines will be portrayed on the circle radiating outward. The more grouped or clustered the vector lines are around a common phase (vector with the open circle) suggests that the response is present. On the other hand, vector lines that appear to be randomly distributed around the circle suggest that there is no response detected. Windows (e) and (f) may also be available to a clinician to provide real-time analysis of residual noise in the ongoing average and the statistical probability of a response. As the number of sweeps (or averages samples) increases, it would be ideal for residual noise to decrease over time and for the probability of a present response increases over time. Taken together, there are numerous ways in which the computer (or the clinician) can make some judgments about whether or not a response is present. Chapters 8 and 15 offer more literature background, potential uses, and current clinical applications for ASSR.

Pitfall

Although many ASSR systems are automated, it remains critical that clinicians continuously monitor the patient and the ongoing recordings using the analysis processes with their clinical system. Judgments may still need to be made about the adequacy of the number of stimulus presentations, the probability of present stimulus response, and phase and spectral analyses, if available. The types of analysis monitoring will depend on the specific and unique features of each clinical system, and clinicians should strive to understand each and every parameter that is on their screen.

Special Consideration

Experts in threshold estimation using AEPs do not currently recommend that ASSR be used in isolation but that it should be supplemented with other measures such as otoacoustic emissions and ABR, as well as age-appropriate audiometric measures.

References

Don, M., Elberling, C., & Waring, M. (1984). Objective detection of averaged auditory brainstem responses. *Scandinavian Audiology, 13*(4), 219–228. PubMed

Eggermont, J. J., Don, M., & Brackmann, D. E. (1980). Electrocochleography and auditory brainstem electric responses in patients with pontine angle tumors. *Annals of Otology, Rhinology, and Laryngology, 89*(Suppl 75), 1–19. PubMed

Galambos, R., & Hecox, K. E. (1978). Clinical applications of the auditory brain stem response. *Otolaryngologic Clinics of North America, 11*(3), 709–722. PubMed

Krishnan, A. (2007). Frequency following responses. In R. F. Burkard, M. Don, & J. J. Eggermont (Eds.), *Auditory evoked potentials: Basic principles and clinical applications* (pp. 313-333). Philadelphia: Lippincott Williams & Wilkins.

Lopes da Silva, F. H. (1976). Sampling, conversion and measurement of bioelectrical phenomena. In F. H. Lopes da Silva (Ed.), *Handbook of electroencephalography and Clinical Neurophysiology*, Vol. 4A, Amsterdam: Elsevier.

Mizrahi, E. M., Maulsby, R. L., & Frost, J. D., Jr (1983). Improved wave V resolution by dual-channel brain stem auditory evoked potential recording. *Electroencephalography and clinical neurophysiology, 55*(1), 105–107. PubMed

Purcell, D. W., & Dajani, H. (2008). The stimulus-response relationship in auditory steady-state response testing. In G. Rance (Ed.), *Auditory steady-state response: Generation, recording and clinical applications* (pp. 55-82). San Diego: Plural Publishing.

Russo, N., Nicol, T., Musacchia, G., & Kraus, N. (2004). Brainstem responses to speech syllables. *Clinical Neurophysiology, 115*(9), 2021–2030. PubMed

Sininger, Y. S. (1993). Auditory brain stem response for objective measures of hearing. *Ear and Hearing, 14*(1), 23–30. PubMed

Sininger, Y., Hyde, M., & Don, M. (2001). U.S. Patent No. 6,196,977 B. Washington, DC: U.S. Patent and Trademark Office.

Chapter 4

Fundamental Principles of Neuroanatomy and Neurophysiology Related to Auditory Evoked Potentials

Samuel R. Atcherson and Sheryl S. Shoemaker

The auditory system is highly complex. It initially captures airborne acoustic signals and converts them ultimately to a neural code that the brain can use. Much of what becomes neurally encoded is a signal that is filtered through the mechanics of the basilar membrane of the cochlea and the cochlear amplifier (i.e., outer cell hairs). Beyond the cochlea, the ability to generate perceptual images of sounds rests on the capacity of both the peripheral and central auditory systems to process this information rapidly and efficiently. In addition, the brain must be able to identify and recognize patterns embedded in ongoing acoustical signals and integrate such information with other areas of the brain. Uniquely, auditory evoked potentials (AEPs) can provide a temporal (time) window into the auditory system, along with some of its many processes, structures, and generating sources. Specifically, they can provide information on the order of millisecond time units about maturation, aging, plasticity, and neurologically impaired or altered auditory structures.

Some fundamental and practical information is presented in this chapter that is considered important for clinicians to know regarding the anatomical and physiologic origins of AEPs. Having this understanding should prime clinicians to anticipate both anatomical and physiologic factors that affect AEPs and as a result allow them to make more informed decisions. In addition, having a working knowledge of basic instrumentation, hearing science, and anatomy and physiology of the peripheral and central auditory systems is a prerequisite for the understanding of AEPs. Because of space limitations, an exhaustive treatment of all topics related to the generation of AEPs cannot realistically be covered within the confines of this chapter. We will touch on anatomy and physiology as they relate to AEPs associated with the auditory system and the processing of acoustic signals, but the assumed anatomical generator sources of each AEP is covered in corresponding chapters of this textbook. Although important to the study of the auditory nervous system, anatomy- and physiology-related information derived from brain-mapping techniques (topographic or tomographic) and dipole source modeling will not be discussed here. Readers who desire a more advanced treatment of neuroscience, neurophysiology, anatomy, and physiology will need to consult other references (e.g., Burkhard, Don, and Eggermont, 2007; Møller, 2006; Musiek and Baran, 2007; Picton, 2011; Rees and Palmer, 2010).

◆ General Neurophysiology Concepts

As a first step, we know that scalp-recorded AEPs must originate from the activity of neurons and any other cells that produce or interact with the movement of electrical charges (i.e., ions) through and within their cellular membranes. What we also know about AEPs has been inferred through (1) simultaneous comparison studies of recordings directly at the source (on a nerve or nucleus) and on the scalp surface; (2) the study of abnormal auditory systems (e.g., lesions); (3) purposeful disrupting of structures, processes, or pathways (e.g., chemical or sectioning) in otherwise normal auditory systems (typically in laboratory animals); and (4) sophisticated interpretations and interpolations of active sources from within and on the surface of the head using multiple recording channels. What we observe in the voltage recordings at the scalp cannot and should not necessarily be taken as a direct electrophysiologic-to-anatomical correspondence. To make this point clear, consider that some AEPs look absolutely nothing like the stimuli with which they were evoked (e.g., auditory brainstem response [ABR]). Others seem to follow the stimulus waveform or its envelope in a steady-state fashion (e.g., cochlear microphonic [CM] and frequency-following response [FFR]). Still others seem to sustain their voltage (positive or negative) like a direct current (e.g., summating potential [SP] and contingent negative variation). What is the basis for these differences? More importantly, how can we use any of this information clinically? Although we have come a long way in understanding AEPs and have enjoyed the use of AEPs clinically for several decades, we are still probably only near the tip of the iceberg. This means that AEPs and their influencing factors will remain an exciting and wonderfully enigmatic mystery for years to come. Below are some general neurophysiologic concepts that every clinician should know.

Basic Neuronal Anatomy and Physiology

Neurons (or nerve cells) are electrically excitable cells within the central nervous system (CNS) capable of generating action potentials (APs, also known as electrical impulses, spikes, or discharges). APs are short-lasting, all-or-none, neuroelectric events that form the means of neuron-to-neuron communication for the entire CNS and also form the means of communication from nerves to muscle fibers for contraction and muscle tone. Neurons are important to each of the five senses, and they play a role in physical, regulatory, and mental faculties, such as attention, memory, and learning. Each neuron consists of three basic parts: cell body, dendrite, and axon. Dendrites tend to have many short processes that project away from the cell body. These dendritic processes receive afferent input and transmit information to the cell body. If there is sufficient excitation within the neuron, the cell body will produce an AP in an area where the axon meets the cell body called the axon hillock. The AP is then conducted through the axon. If the axon is myelinated (i.e., insulated sectionally along the axon), the conduction velocity of the AP is increased as the AP is regenerated and "jumps" at the nodes of Ranvier (i.e., nonmyelinated spots along the axon). At the ends of the axons are terminals where either excitatory or inhibitory neurotransmitters are released into the spaces between adjacent neurons called synapses and can then be picked up by dendrites of other neurons.

> **Pearl**
>
> There are ~10 trillion neurons present at birth, and ~200,000 of these are lost per day over the course of one's lifetime. Neurons do not undergo cell division, and they cannot be replaced once lost or severely damaged.

At rest, neurons attempt to maintain a certain charge across its bilipid cell membrane called the membrane potential. The extracellular composition (outside the neuron) is comprised principally of sodium ions (Na^+), but it also contains negatively charged chloride ions (Cl^-). The intracellular composition (inside the neuron) is comprised principally of potassium ions (K^+), as well as large negatively charged anions (A^-). The resting membrane potential is around -70 mV (negative on the inside). During depolarization, some sodium channels will open allowing sodium ions to come into the neuron. As sodium ions enter the neuron, the membrane potential will become more positive and may cause even more sodium channels to open. If the neuron's depolarization threshold is not reached, an AP will not be produced, and the neuron will attempt to return to its resting potential. If the neuron's depolarization threshold is reached, an AP is produced, sodium channels close, and the neuron will then repolarize itself.

Potentials at the Source

Evoked potentials begin with the neuroelectric activity of sensory cells. In the cochlea, these sensory cells are the outer and inner hair cells giving rise to gross cochlear potentials. The outer hair cells are responsible for intensifying basilar membrane movements through electromotility (Brownell, Bader, Bertrand, and de Ribaupierre, 1985), which serves to sharpen auditory tuning curves. Whether sounds are sufficiently intense on their own or basilar membrane displacement is increased by outer hair cells, the inner hair cells will then be able to perform their task of releasing neurotransmitters to the auditory nerve fibers. Not unlike neurons, there are also movements of charged ions in and out of the outer and inner hair cells as they carry out their functions. AEPs that can arise from these hair cells include the CM and the SP. The CM is likely a summed response of a large number of active outer hair cells in the basal region (Sohmer, Kinarti, and Gafni, 1980). The CM follows the stimulus waveform. The SP is likely a summed response of both outer and inner hair cells with possible neural contributions, but it seems to reflect an electrical voltage shift caused by the basilar membrane not moving equally in both directions (Møller, 2006). Both of these potentials can be seen in electrocochleography (ECochG) recordings.

The generation of APs begins with the first-order, auditory nerve fiber neurons that connect to the sensory hair cells. The AP is best appreciated in ECochG recordings as a "compound action potential" or "whole nerve potential" to depict the summed activity of numerous synchronously active auditory nerve fibers in response to abrupt acoustic stimuli. In addition, APs are strongly associated with all or most components of the ABR.

Although APs are traveling all over the CNS, spontaneously or by stimulation, they are often smeared temporally in such a way that they cannot be recorded for AEPs generated at progressively higher levels of the auditory system. Thus, later AEPs are more likely to arise from slow-graded postsynaptic potentials (PSPs). The slow-graded PSPs (excitatory and inhibitory) reflect an extracellular ebb and flow of ions moving in and out of neuron groupings with slower membrane potential changes over a 10–20 msec range and take much longer to decay compared with APs (Longstaff, 2005). In general, neuron groupings that are similarly aligned and synchronously activated are more likely to be recordable from the scalp surface. In contrast, neuron groupings that are not similarly aligned, yet may be synchronously active, may result in a cancellation of voltages for certain AEP components.

Pearl

Evoked potentials with long latencies (>50 msec) through slow-graded PSPs give the impression that it takes a long time for signals to reach the cortex. Realistically, when we consider neural travel time starting with the cochlea, it takes ~20 msec or less for activation of neurons in the primary auditory cortex (Lütkenhöner, Krumbholz, Lammertmann, Seither-Preisler, Steinsträter, and Patterson, 2003). At the level of the primary auditory cortex, the activation of the neurons appears to depend on the physical characteristics of the stimulus. For example, it takes only ~8 to 10 msec for click stimuli (Liegeois-Chauvel, Musolino, and Chauvel, 1991) and ~11 to 12 msec for syllables (Steinschneider, Volkov, Noh, Garell, and Howard, 1999) to reach the auditory cortex.

Dipoles

Until this point, the origin of neuroelectric activity has been discussed primarily from the extracellular region of individual or large groups of excitable cells (e.g., neurons). During depolarization positive ions rush into one region of a neuron (a sink) and cause the extracellular space in that region to become negative. This initial inward flow of positive ions must eventually exit in another region of the neuron (a source), causing the extracellular space in that adjacent region to become positive. As this current flow is generated by the sink and source, a separation of charges at different regions of the neuron is set up. This separation of charges produces what is called a dipole. Conceptually, a dipole looks a lot like a battery with its positive and negative ends. With some exceptions, far-field potentials appear to be best recorded when electrodes are placed on opposite ends of the dipole (Stegeman, Dumitru, King, and Roeleveld, 1997).

Special Consideration

The terms *voltage* and *potential* are essentially synonymous, as they represent a separation of positive and negative charges. The farther apart the charges are, the greater the voltage or potential difference and the greater the electromotive force. The measurement of evoked potentials is performed by measuring the charge at one site on the scalp relative to another site on the scalp, either on the opposite side of the dipole of interest (Stegeman et al, 1997) or on the dipole's zero potential line (i.e., the midpoint between the charges where there is no difference). The potential difference that is measured will generally be reported in microvolts (μV), though sometimes in the smaller nanovolt (nV) range.

Although APs do propagate along neurons, the dipoles they produce during AEP recordings are stationary. In other words, the averaged AP shown on a monitor screen is not representative of the AP as it is moving along a structure like the auditory nerve. Rather, the initial, abrupt synchronous discharge of numerous auditory nerve fibers of the distal auditory nerve (closer to the cochlea) is what gives rise to the AP of the ECochG (or wave I of the ABR). What is actually seen as wave II of the ABR (i.e., the second AP) is the effect of the surrounding tissue on the scalp-recorded AEP as the AP moves along the auditory nerve within the highly resistive internal auditory meatus in the temporal bone and exits to an area of low resistance within the skull (Lueders, Lesser, Hahn, Little, and Klem, 1983; Stegeman, Van Oosterom, and Colon, 1987). **Figure 4.1A** is an illustration of the second stationary dipole associated with the auditory nerve. This second stationary dipole is set up, as there is a region of positivity (the source) associated with the leading edge of the AP and a region of negativity (the sink follows). This stationary dipole is assumed to arise in the proximal region of the auditory nerve as it terminates in the cochlear nucleus. Later waves of the ABR are also thought to originate from AP stationary dipoles from similarly oriented neurons of the auditory brainstem pathway as they undergo changes in anatomical geometry. Because there are other neuron groups in the auditory brainstem in addition to the auditory nerve, the onset of synchronous discharges in progressively later auditory brainstem nuclei and fiber tracts are likely reflected in the other peaks of the ABR. Thus, the volley of positive and negative voltages at the scalp surface (i.e., the different waves of the ABR and their following troughs) will reflect the stationary dipoles caused by the APs at different levels of the lower auditory system.

Unlike APs, which are fast-moving targets, dipoles in the cortex are typically from pyramidal neurons that are oriented perpendicular to the brain surface. The majority of these pyramidal neurons are in layer V of the auditory cortex, and they interact with several other active neurons (e.g., thalamocortical fibers and stellate cells). At this level of the auditory system, PSPs are the dominant source of AEPs. What leads to the positive and negative voltages at the scalp surface will depend on which portions of the dendrite are being depolarized at any given point in time. For example, depolarization of the dendrite near the cell body will form a sink (extracellular negative), whereas the more superficial aspect (near the scalp) of the dendrite will be the source (extracellular positive). **Figure 4.1B** illustrates this scenario in a pyramidal neuron of the cortex. In this scenario, the scalp surface will be positive. In contrast, when the sink is

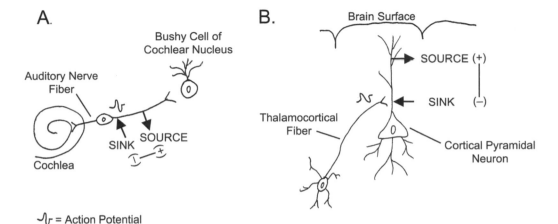

Fig. 4.1 Simple one-neuron dipole examples generated within an auditory nerve fiber of the auditory nerve and a pyramidal neuron of the cortex. Notice the extracellular sinks and sources that give rise to the positive and negative poles of the dipole.

on the superficial dendrite with a deep source, the scalp surface will be negative. It should be noted that interneurons in the cortex, as well as ascending and descending neurons to and from the cortex, can also generate PSPs recordable at the scalp. The basic requirements for recording dipole activity are summarized below.

- A population of similar neurons must be synchronously activated.

- In a population of neurons, certain parts (e.g., axons or dendrites) must be aligned in parallel.

- The greater the number of a population of neurons involved within a nucleus (and across simultaneously and temporally active nuclei), the larger the amplitude.

Near- and Far-Field Potentials

Neural activity can be recorded directly from the surface of cranial nerves, fiber tracts, brainstem nuclei, and the cortical surface, as well as from muscles and organs. It can also be recorded at great distances from the source (e.g., on the scalp or within the ear) through the volume conductor (e.g., the head with brain tissue, cerebrospinal fluid, skull, and scalp). These two types of recordings are referred to as near-field potentials and far-field potentials, respectively. Both are extracellular in nature and depend to a large extent on the size and geometric orientation of the underlying dipole sources. Except for intracranial recordings performed during neurosurgery (Chapter 18), virtually all other AEP recordings are of the far-field type. When neural activity is recorded directly at the source, the voltages recorded can be quite large, and even small movements away from the source can result in dramatic decreases in voltage. When recordings are performed at great distances from the source, the resultant voltages are typically smaller, and small movements away from the initial site may result in little to no voltage change (Stegeman et al, 1997; Wood and Allison, 1981). Whereas near-field potentials tend to reflect activity locally on the desired structure of interest (e.g., exposed auditory nerve or exposed cortical surface), far-field potentials generally reflect neural activity from one or more dipole sources that have time-overlapped activity. Thus, it is difficult to say with any degree of certainty that any AEP component beyond the auditory nerve has a single dipole source.

Because neither near-field nor far-field AEPs reflect activity from a single neuron, the extent to which an AEP can be recorded can depend on the arrangement of the neurons. Neurons that are activated synchronously and are oriented uniformly in a similar direction, such as within a cranial nerve or the dendrites of a nucleus, produces fields that are recordable from the scalp. On the other hand, neurons that are activated synchronously but oriented randomly in different directions produces weak or negligible fields. These two types of fields are known as open and closed fields, respectively (Lorente de No, 1947). The auditory nerve, the lateral lemniscus, and the dendrites of pyramidal neurons in a restricted section of the cortex, for example, all form good open fields. In contrast, the thalamus has nuclei with dendrites arranged non-uniformly and dendrites arranged in a spherical manner, which can lead to an electrically silent, closed field when recorded from the scalp.

◆ Brief Review of the Auditory System

The neuroanatomy of the auditory system begins first with the sensory hair cells in each ear, which have a close relationship with the basilar membrane within the cochlea. Similar to the tonotopic organization of the basilar membrane, the sensory hair cells and associated stereocilia are themselves frequency selective in that they are shorter at the basal end of the cochlea and become progressively longer toward the apical end of the cochlea. The outer hair cells play an important role in amplifying sounds through electromotility, whereas inner cells release excitatory neurotransmitters. When excitatory neurotransmitters are released by the inner hair cells, peripheral auditory nerve fibers making up the auditory branch of the eighth cranial nerve (CN VIII, first-order neurons) produces neural signals (APs) to be sent to the cochlear nucleus complex in the brainstem. The cochlear nucleus is the site where the central auditory nervous system (CANS) begins. Within the brainstem are several bilateral auditory nuclei (cochlear nuclear complex, superior olivary complex, and inferior colliculi) and fiber tracts (acoustic stria and lateral lemniscus) (Moore, 1987; Musiek and Baran, 1986). There are numerous crossovers of fibers called decussations within the brainstem to and from

various nuclei; the first decussation begins at the level of the cochlear nuclei on the way to the superior olives. The inferior colliculi are known to receive ~99% of all synapses before moving farther up in the auditory system (Aitkin and Phillips, 1984). Leaving the inferior colliculi, signals are then sent to the midbrain structures in the thalamus, which are called the medial geniculate bodies. From the medial geniculate, signals course through the internal capsule by way of the auditory radiation (thalamocortical) fibers to the primary auditory cortices in the cerebrum known as Heschl's gyri. Heschl's gyri are located on the supratemporal plane of each temporal lobe (Hickok and Poeppel, 2000; Kaas and Hackett, 2000). Heschl's gyri cannot be seen from the outer surface of the cerebrum, but they can be made visible by prying open the sylvian (lateral) fissure that separates the temporal lobe from the frontal and parietal lobes. The primary auditory cortex is considered to be the site where auditory perception begins. **Figure 4.2** provides an illustration of the ascending auditory pathway from the cochlea to the cortex, including the corpus callosum and general arousal cortex.

Simply perceiving sound is not enough. To give meaning or significance to a sound, additional processing of the neural signal is performed in the secondary (or association) auditory cortex, which involves one or more gyri posterior to Heschl's gyrus called the planum temporale, also located within the temporal lobe. Functionally, however, the auditory cortex appears to be divided into three areas, a core, belt, and parabelt, with each area giving rise to different levels of processing (Hackett, 2008; Kaas and Hackett, 2000). Deep within the lateral fissure underlying the operculum is the insular cortex, which is also considered to have some auditory significance (Bamiou, Musiek, and Luxon, 2003). Another important structure that is related to the auditory system is the isthmus of the corpus callosum. The corpus callosum is a large band of ~200 million myelinated nerve fibers that allows for the exchange of information between the two cerebral hemispheres. Homolateral fibers connect similar regions in both hemispheres, whereas heterolateral fibers connect different loci between the two hemispheres. The isthmus is thought to have connections with the parasylvian regions

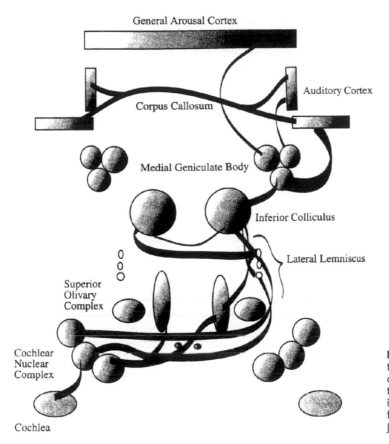

Fig. 4.2 The ascending auditory pathway for low frequencies is shown for one cochlea to the contralateral cortex. The ipsilateral pathway is ignored for clarity. (Courtesy of Herbert Jay Gould, PhD.)

(Aboitiz, Ide, and Olivares, 2002), as well as the fibers from the primary and secondary auditory cortices (superior temporal fibers).

◆ General Principles of the Auditory Nervous System

Synchrony

There are two kinds of synchrony necessary to produce transient AEPs. The first type of synchrony is strongly associated with earlier AEPs, such as the ECochG and ABR. To evoke these two types of AEPs well, a stimulus with a very fast rise time is required, such as a 0.1 msec (or 100 µsec) click. The abrupt rise time associated with the click produces a wide band of energy that can broadly stimulate the cochlea and, in turn, cause numerous auditory nerve fibers to discharge synchronously at the onset of the stimulus. A click stimulus, however, is not perfectly broadband due to 1) the traveling wave delays from the base to the apex in the cochlea and 2) click stimuli do not provide frequency-specific information. To obtain frequency-specific information, short duration tones (called tone bursts) are often used. Because of the requirement of neural synchrony for ECochG and ABR, the rise time for the tone bursts must also be reasonably fast with a total duration of only two to four cycles. With fewer auditory nerve fibers being stimulated by a restricted region of the cochlea when using a tone burst, the AEP recorded with this stimulus tends to be smaller in amplitude than that seen with click stimuli. Thus, AEPs that depend on high neural synchrony are associated with the need for relatively abrupt (transient) stimuli for the purpose of causing numerous neurons (e.g., auditory nerve fibers) to discharge synchronously.

The second kind of synchrony can be appreciated at the level of the auditory cortex. In contrast to earlier AEPs, cortical potentials such as P1, N1, P2, and N2 components do not require the use of stimuli with fast rise times, and they do not require high neural synchrony of peripheral auditory nerve fibers. Although cortical potentials can be evoked using clicks, they can also tolerate longer rise times of up to 80 msec or so (tone burst and speech stimuli). This is not to say, however, that cortical potentials are independent of synchrony. For cortical potentials to be measured, they still require synchrony of neuronal synapses within certain regions of the brain to activate relevant dipoles. Even in the cortex, the large numbers of synchronously activated pyramidal neurons in a region of the brain can produce a large PSP field.

> ### Pearl
>
> The requirement of neural synchrony for earlier potentials, but not for later cortical potentials, can be appreciated in certain cases of auditory neuropathy spectrum disorder (ANSD) where ECochG and ABR may be absent (or grossly distorted), while cortical potentials are more or less present.

Phase Locking

Phase locking is an attribute of neurons to discharge (i.e., generating the AP) by time locking themselves more often to the same phase of a stimulus waveform and less often at other phases. Neurons can phase lock whether the stimulus is a sine wave or a broadband noise, but they generally are based on the neuron's characteristic frequency or frequency response range. Phase locking is first introduced within the auditory system by the peripheral auditory nerve fibers. Realistically, a single auditory nerve fiber may be able to discharge maximally at the rate of only 300 to 500 Hz when one considers the rate of recovery of APs, beyond which they may discharge on the same phase of a sinusoid, but not every phase. When auditory nerve fibers work as a group, they may be able to phase lock together to tonal stimuli up to 2000 Hz, perhaps as high as 5000 Hz. However, the more centrally and rostrally located the neurons are, the proper phase locking becomes (e.g., < 40 Hz). The reason for the decline of phase locking from the lower to higher auditory system, however, is not completely known.

In relation to AEPs, phase locking can generally be appreciated best with auditory steady-state responses (ASSRs; Chapters 8 and 15) and FFRs (Chapter 7). As an example, auditory nerve fibers can produce a post-stimulus time histogram (PSTH) that reveals phase locking to amplitude-modulated signals, not only to the carrier tone, but also its envelope. What a PSTH reveals are the averaged probabilities of neural discharges with increased discharges near a particular phase of a stimulus waveform and progressively fewer discharges away from that particular phase. As seen in **Fig. 4.3**, the 1000-Hz carrier frequency is clearly represented, and the relative time difference between adjacent points where neural discharges are proportionally high is occurring about every 1 msec. Also, as seen in **Fig. 4.3**, the overall pattern of the PSTH appears to repeat itself about every 12 msec, which coincides with the modulation frequency of 80 Hz. The reason the envelope is being represented in the neural code is likely due

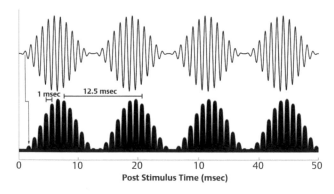

Post Stimulus Time (msec)

Fig. 4.3 Schematic illustration of single auditory nerve fiber responses to an amplitude modulated signal. The waveform at the top of the figure is a 1000 Hz carrier tone modulated at 80 Hz. The bottom of the figure shows the averaged post-stimulus time histogram (PSTH) of a single auditory nerve fiber whose response pattern appears as a half-wave rectification. Notice in the PSTH that phase locking has occurred not only to the envelope (80 Hz), but also to the fine structure (1000 Hz).

to some nonlinearities associated with the fact that only positive amplitudes (a half-wave rectification) are represented by stereocilia movement, receptor potentials, and auditory nerve fiber discharges (Joris, Schreiner, and Rees, 2004; Khanna and Teich, 1989; Lins, Picton, Picton, Champagne, and Durieux-Smith, 1995). In other words, auditory nerve fibers largely discharge only when the basilar membrane moves in one direction (i.e., toward the scala vestibuli). The apparent phase locking to the modulation frequency at intensity levels near threshold makes the ASSR useful as a behavioral threshold estimation tool. It is the modulation frequency that is being evaluated as it is modulating the carrier tone at frequency-specific regions of the cochlea (e.g., 500, 1000, 2000, and 4000 Hz). The modulation frequency that is implemented depends on whether there is interest in evoking responses from cortical (40 Hz) or subcortical (80 Hz) structures (Herdman, Lins, Van Roon, Stapells, Scherg, and Picton, 2002; Kuwada, Anderson, Batra, Fitzpatrick, Teissier, and D'Angelo, 2002; Pethe, Von Specht, Mühler, and Hocke, 2001). The FFR is another type of steady-state response that can reveal phase-locking activity and seems to be well suited to following the stimulus waveform of tones, as well as the fine structure and periodicity pitch associated with steady-state vowels (Hall, 1979; Krishnan, Xu, Gandour, and Cariani, 2004). Because of the frequencies at which phase locking occurs, the FFR is believed to reflect phase locking of the auditory nerve fibers up to neurons in the rostral brainstem.

♦ Peripheral and Central Auditory System Considerations for AEPs

The auditory nerve contains the first-order neurons initiating the propagation of neural activity, nearly mimicking the activity within the cochlea, and throughout the CANS. The signals from the cochlea undergoes parallel and sequential processing on one or both sides of the head (Ehret and Romand, 1997; Phillips, 2007). Most of this processing takes place in a bottom-up fashion. That is, auditory signals are continually processed almost involuntarily

whether or not we are actually paying any attention to them. However, there are some top-down, higher-order cognitive factors that can affect the auditory system. For example, drowsiness and sleep have a significant effect on AEPs, particularly those of thalamic and cortical origin. Although all of these descriptions are overgeneralized, it should be clear to clinicians that any number of factors can affect the auditory system and can and will lead to observable changes in virtually all AEPs.

Special Consideration

Clinicians should always keep in mind that all hearing loss (e.g., sensorineural, conductive, or mixed) has the potential to impact the waveform morphology of AEPs. Some of the change is mediated with intensity reduction or time delay once the stimulus reaches the neural elements. In other cases, impairment of the auditory nerve or central auditory system will cause these changes.

Special Consideration

The auditory system depends quite heavily on the vascular system (blood supply) for nutrients and oxygen to maintain healthy neural function. Disruption, alteration, or even contact with blood can compromise the auditory system in a variety of ways. Although the vascular system is not in and of it itself involved in the generation of evoked potentials, there is a clear, intimate relationship. Thus, clinicians should spend some time learning about vascular anatomy as it relates to the auditory system. The reader is referred to Musiek and Baran (2007) for an excellent discussion of this topic.

Cochlear Mechanics

How cochlear mechanics comes into play with respect to AEPs is somewhat related to the type of stimulus used and certain physical characteristics. Recall that the basilar membrane is a physical structure on which the sensory hair cells of the organ of Corti sit. Along its length are different impedances, with a stiffness gradient that is higher at the base than at the apex. Because of the differences in impedance along the length of the basilar membrane, the inward and outward motion of the stapes produces a traveling wave that moves from the base to the apex, rather than the basilar membrane moving up and down as a unit. The point of maximal displacement along the basilar membrane depends on the stimulus frequency. High frequencies have short traveling wave envelopes that terminate within the basal end, whereas low frequencies have broad traveling wave envelopes that terminate within the apical end. Increasing the stimulus intensity reveals a traveling wave envelope that is shallow toward the base and steep toward the apex. The reason for this asymmetry in the envelope is primarily due to the mass and stiffness gradients of the passive basilar membrane. Because the basal region of the basilar membrane is nearest the stapes, it reacts to virtually all incoming stimuli. In fact, low-frequency stimuli can activate underlying auditory nerve fibers in the basal region (as well as the middle region) when the stimulus is of high intensity.

With abrupt stimuli, such as clicks, the energy reaching the cochlea covers a broad spectrum with the intent of stimulating as many underlying auditory nerve fibers as possible. However, because of the traveling wave, the basal end of the basilar membrane is stimulated first, and the apical end is stimulated a bit later. Although neural synchrony is taking place, the auditory nerve fibers discharge mostly from the basal and middle frequency regions of the cochlea. The discharging of apical auditory nerve fibers is likely out of step temporally with the basal and middle regions and is thought not to be contributing much to the AEPs dependent on neural synchrony. Evidence for this assumption has been demonstrated when the click stimulus is compared with a chirp stimulus. The chirp is designed specifically to temporally align all the neural elements of the auditory nerve by compensating for traveling wave delays (Elberling, Don, Cebulla, and Stürzebecher, 2007). That is, the chirp initially stimulates the apical region of the cochlea before the basal region. By accounting for traveling wave delays associated

with different stimulus frequencies, the basilar membrane and subsequently the underlying auditory nerve fibers are synchronized along their length, with all portions of the cochlea contributing to the AEP. Indeed, the chirp has produced a larger AP in ECochG recordings (Chertoff, Lichtenhan, and Willis, 2010), a larger wave V in ABR recordings (Elberling and Don, 2008), and a larger Na–Pa complex in middle latency response (MLR) recordings (Rupp, Uppenkamp, Gutschalk, Beucker, Patterson, Dau, et al, 2002). In spite of some larger AEP components by chirps, Petoe, Bradley, and Wilson, (2010) have argued that clicks still appear to have greater neural synchrony compared with chirps, as evidenced by the lack of ABR components prior to wave V. More work is needed in this area, particularly in refining the physical characteristics of the chirp, but it is clear that basilar membrane mechanics is playing an important role in shaping the morphology of earlier AEPs.

Pitfall

Although an upward movement of the basilar membrane leads to activation of cochlear hair cells, there is no clear correspondence between rarefaction and condensation polarities on ECochG and ABR latencies. For example, some patients may have earlier waveforms with one polarity versus the other. Also, although it is tempting to conclude that rarefaction polarity will lead to shorter latencies, the mechanics of the cochlea is far too complex to make such a simple assertion.

Monaural Contributions to the Auditory System

As indicated earlier, the cochlear nucleus is the first site in the CNS where signals begin to cross. However, acoustic input to one ear can take one of two paths to the auditory cortices, with an advantage for contralateral over ipsilateral pathways in both latency and strength of the response at the cortex (Fujiki, Jousmaki, and Hari, 2002; Hall and Goldstein, 1968). Rosenzweig (1951) found larger scalp responses for contralateral stimulation compared with ipsilateral stimulation, which may be attributable to the larger number of neural fibers to the contralateral cortex. Scherg and Von Cramon (1986) found larger scalp responses in the hemisphere contralateral to the stimulation for tangential dipole sources. Even AEPs or magnetoencephalographic (MEG) recordings have shown that the contralateral response to monaural stimulation starts earlier and is more sustained than the ipsilateral one (Papanicolaou, Baumann, Rogers, Saydjari, Amparo, and Eisenberg, 1990; Reite, Zimmerman, and Zimmerman, 1981; Romani, Williamson, and Kaufman, 1982). The ABR also appears to reflect monaural input differences, such as in the click-evoked ABR. For example, infants showed interaural latency and amplitude differences with responses to right ear stimulation having earlier and larger responses than those to left ear presentation (Eldredge and Salamy, 1996; Sininger and Cone-Wesson, 2006; Sininger, Cone-Wesson, and Abdala, 1998). Further support for subcortical laterality differences has been demonstrated in the FFR with speech stimuli (/da/) (Hornickel, Skoe, and Kraus, 2009). This stronger contralateral pathway may partly explain the root of laterality in the auditory cortex (e.g., Kimura, 1961; Sidtis, 1982), which is reflected at times in the AEP.

Binaural Interaction in the Auditory System

Normally, we listen with two ears; however, studies comparing monaural and binaural stimulation have revealed interesting findings over the years. Psychoacoustic techniques involving the masking level difference, sound localization, and binaural summation have been used to assess the binaural interaction in the auditory system. Binaural interaction has also been measured through AEPs reflecting activity from the brainstem through the cortex. The binaural interaction component (BIC), or β-wave (e.g., Brantberg, Fransson, Hansson, and Rosenhall, 1999), is a difference wave obtained by mathematical manipulation of three separate AEP recordings: to each ear of stimulation and to binaural stimulation. In the AEP equipment software, the monaural responses are summed (added, not averaged)

together and subtracted from the binaural response (or vice versa). In some studies, the summed monaural response was larger than the binaural response, but in other studies the reverse was found. In either case, where there is a difference between the summed monaural and binaural responses, the subtraction process reveals a waveform that shows activity difference between the two. This suggests a complex interaction of excitation and inhibition is taking place within different levels of the CANS when one or both ears are stimulated. The proposed neural generators include the superior olivary complex (Dobie and Berlin, 1979; Setou, Kurauchi, Tsuzuku, and Kaga, 2001) and lateral nucleus of the superior olivary complex (Ungan and Yagcioglu, 2002) but likely not higher or more rostral than the inferior colliculus (Gardi and Berlin, 1981). However, translating these findings to clinical use has been difficult.

In terms of latency effects, results from click-evoked ABRs have revealed shorter wave IV–V latencies (Brantberg et al, 1999; McPherson and Starr, 1993) and larger overall wave V amplitudes (Jewett, 1970) for the binaurally recorded ABR in comparison to the summed monaural recordings. When tone bursts have been used for binaural recordings, low-frequency stimuli (e.g., 500 and 1000 Hz) have revealed a BIC that resembles the morphology of the FFR (Parthasarathy and Moushegian, 1993). In contrast, tone bursts of higher frequencies (e.g., 2000 Hz) have responses similar to that of BIC responses to click-evoked ABRs.

The BIC has been measured at the level of the cortex but with even greater inhibition levels than that found at the lower levels of the CANS. McPherson and Starr (1993) found that the amplitude of the BIC increases significantly with more rostral AEPs (up to 40% compared with 16% for the brainstem BIC). Also, whereas the peak latency of the BIC for the ABR is ~7 msec (coinciding with the region of waves IV and V), it is ~16 to 32 msec for the MLR (the Pa region) and between 63 and 150 msec for the late latency response (the N1 region). It was concluded in this study that a greater portion of cortical pathways are used for binaural processing as compared with brainstem pathways.

Exogenous versus Endogenous Potentials

Because of the external influence of sound on the auditory system, AEPs are considered to have exogenous characteristics. Whether the AEP is generated in the cochlea or somewhere in the cortex, there are auditory neurons that respond when stimuli have the right set of acoustic parameters necessary to evoke them. For example, some neurons discharge to abrupt stimulus onsets, whereas others may discharge only to time-varying patterns in a modulated stimulus. However, other AEPs are more influenced by factors unrelated to acoustic stimuli. In other words, something other than the stimulus itself is having an influence on the waveform morphology that changes amplitude, latency, or both. AEPs that are affected by internal factors are said to have endogenous characteristics. ECochGs and ABRs are predominantly exogenous; later cortical AEPs are likely to have both exogenous and endogenous characteristics (Chapter 10). Sleep and attention have strong endogenous influences on later AEPs and are briefly discussed below.

Sleep

The effect of sleep on the auditory system is widespread, as evidenced by an entire book written on this topic by Velutti (2008). As one drifts from wakefulness to deep sleep, the spectrum of the electroencephalogram (EEG) changes, with higher thalamocortical oscillations during wakefulness (>15 Hz) and lower oscillations during sleep (1–4 Hz). In general, the slower the oscillations, the larger the EEG amplitude will be. During sleep, the cortex almost becomes disengaged from subcortical structures. The underlying bases of the different states of sleep and wakefulness are mediated by certain neurotransmitters, which alter AP firing patterns (regular firing vs tonic burst firing) in the neurons of the thalamocortical system (Benarroch, 2006). Early AEP components, such as those associated with ECochG, ABR, and the 80-Hz ASSR, generally are not affected by sleep. In addition, these early AEPs can even be elicited, without alteration, while an individual is anesthetized or sedated.

Attention

Generally, attention is a higher-order cognitive process that involves a degree of concentration on something in the environment (e.g., sound) while ignoring other aspects of the environment. There are several different kinds of attention, including orienting, selective, divided, and sustained (Coull, 1998). The neural correlates of different types of attention are generally ascribed to the cortex but can have effects on both cortical and subcortical neurons. Early studies of auditory attention by Picton and colleagues (1971; Picton and Hillyard, 1974) have demonstrated how paying attention to stimuli has a greater effect on cortical AEPs, such as N1–P2 components and little to no effect on earlier evoked potentials, such as the AP of the ECochG, the ABR, and the MLR. In cases of selective attention, however, P2 can become smaller (Hansen and Hillyard, 1980).

◆ Sonomotor Reflexes

Although not directly part of the auditory nervous system, some muscles respond to sound input called sonomotor reflexes. These include the stapedius muscle, postauricular muscle (PAM), the sternocleidomastoid (SCM) muscle, and the extraocular muscles. The stapedius muscle is one of two middle ear muscles involved in the middle ear muscle reflex (MEMR, also called the acoustic reflex). It attaches to the neck of the stapes bone within the middle ear. Innervated by CN VII (facial nerve), the stapedius muscle produces a bilateral, graded response to high-intensity sounds. Generally, the stapedius muscle is not thought to affect AEP measurements, although it might at high intensity levels. The postauricular muscle reflex (PAMR) comprises two or three muscles arising from the mastoid and inserting into the lower portion of the concha. The PAMR can be recorded in the latency range of 12 to 20 msec and significantly interferes with MLR recordings (see Chapter 9). The PAMR is more likely to interfere with MLR when the inverting electrodes are placed near the PAM (earlobe or mastoid), when high intensities (i.e., ≥70 dB nHL [normal hearing level]) are used to elicit a response, or in extremely tense patients.

The SCM and extraocular muscles are sonomotor reflexes associated with the saccule of the inner ear vestibular system (Colebatch, Halmagyi, and Skuse, 1994; Rosengren, McAngus Todd, and Colebatch, 2005). The cochlea and the saccule are in close approximation to the oval window and stapes footplate, so that it should not be too surprising that the otoliths and sensory hair cells of the saccule might be responsive to high-intensity acoustic stimulation. Of interest to

audiologists and other balance specialists is the vestibular evoked myogenic potential (VEMP), which can be a useful test of disorders associated with the vestibular system. Unlike the PAMR, which would be considered a nuisance during some ABR or MLR recordings, the cervical (cVEMP) is a desired electromyographic (EMG) recording of the SCM, whereas the ocular (oVEMP) is recorded from the or extraocular muscles (e.g., inferior oblique and rectus) in response to stimulation of the saccule. The anatomy and physiology of both cVEMP and oVEMP are described in Chapter 11.

References

Aboitiz, F., Ide, A., & Olivares, R. (2002). Corpus callosum morphology in relation to cerebral asymmetries in the postmortem human. In E. Zaidel & M. Iacoboni (Eds.), *The parallel brain: The science of the corpus callosum* (pp. 33–50). Boston: MIT Press.

Aitkin, L. M., & Phillips, S. C. (1984). Is the inferior colliculus an obligatory relay in the cat auditory system? *Neuroscience Letters, 44*(3), 259–264. PubMed

Bamiou, D. E., Musiek, F. E., & Luxon, L. M. (2003). The insula (island of Reil) and its role in auditory processing: Literature review. *Brain Research. Brain Research Reviews, 42*(2), 143–154. PubMed

Benarroch, E. E. (2006). *Basic neurosciences with clinical applications*. Philadelphia: Butterworth Heinemann Elsevier.

Brantberg, K., Fransson, P. A., Hansson, H., & Rosenhall, U. (1999). Measures of the binaural interaction component in human auditory brainstem response using objective detection criteria. *Scandinavian Audiology, 28*(1), 15–26. PubMed

Brownell, W. E., Bader, C. R., Bertrand, D., & de Ribaupierre, Y. (1985). Evoked mechanical responses of isolated cochlear outer hair cells. *Science, 227*(4683), 194–196. PubMed

Burkhard, R. F., Don, M., & Eggermont, J. J. (2007). *Auditory evoked potentials: Basic principles and clinical applications*. Philadelphia: Lippincott Williams & Wilkins.

Chertoff, M., Lichtenhan, J., & Willis, M. (2010). Click- and chirp-evoked human compound action potentials. *Journal of the Acoustical Society of America, 127*(5), 2992–2996. PubMed

Colebatch, J. G., Halmagyi, G. M., & Skuse, N. F. (1994). Myogenic potentials generated by a click-evoked vestibulocollic reflex. *Journal of Neurology, Neurosurgery, and Psychiatry, 57*(2), 190–197. PubMed

Coull, J. T. (1998). Neural correlates of attention and arousal: Insights from electrophysiology, functional neuroimaging and psychopharmacology. *Progress in Neurobiology, 55*(4), 343–361. PubMed

Dobie, R. A., & Berlin, C. I. (1979). Binaural interaction in brainstem-evoked responses. *Archives of Otolaryngology, 105*(7), 391–398. PubMed

Ehret, G., & Romand, R. (1997). *The central auditory system*. New York: Oxford University Press.

Elberling, C., & Don, M. (2008). Auditory brainstem responses to a chirp stimulus designed from derived-band latencies in normal-hearing subjects. *Journal of the Acoustical Society of America, 124*(5), 3022–3037. PubMed

Elberling, C., Don, M., Cebulla, M., & Stürzebecher, E. (2007). Auditory steady-state responses to chirp stimuli based on cochlear traveling wave delay. *Journal of the Acoustical Society of America, 122*(5), 2772–2785. PubMed

Eldredge, L., & Salamy, A. (1996). Functional auditory development in preterm and full term infants. *Early Human Development, 45*(3), 215–228. PubMed

Fujiki, N., Jousmaki, V., & Hari, R. (2002). Neuromagnetic responses to frequency-tagged sounds: A new method to follow inputs from each ear to the human auditory cortex during binaural hearing. *Journal of Neuroscience, 22*(3), RC205. PubMed

Gardi, J. N., & Berlin, C. I. (1981). Binaural interaction components: Their possible origins in guinea pig auditory brainstem response. *Archives of Otolaryngology, 107*(3), 164–168. PubMed

Hackett, T. A. (2008). Anatomical organization of the auditory cortex. *Journal of the American Academy of Audiology, 19*(10), 774–779. PubMed

Hall, J. L., II, & Goldstein, M. H., Jr. (1968). Representation of binaural stimuli by single units in primary auditory cortex of unanesthetized cats. *Journal of the Acoustical Society of America, 43*(3), 456–461. PubMed

Hall, J. W., III. (1979). Auditory brainstem frequency following responses to waveform envelope periodicity. *Science, 205*(4412), 1297–1299. PubMed

Hansen, J. C., & Hillyard, S. A. (1980). Endogenous brain potentials associated with selective auditory attention. *Electroencephalography and Clinical Neurophysiology, 49*(3–4), 277–290. PubMed

Herdman, A. T., Lins, O., Van Roon, P., Stapells, D. R., Scherg, M., & Picton, T. W. (2002). Intracerebral sources of human auditory steady-state responses. *Brain Topography, 15*(2), 69–86. PubMed

Hickok, G., & Poeppel, D. (2000). Towards a functional neuroanatomy of speech perception. *Trends in Cognitive Sciences, 4*(4), 131–138. PubMed

Hornickel, J., Skoe, E., & Kraus, N. (2009). Subcortical laterality of speech encoding. *Audiology and Neuro-Otology, 14*(3), 198–207. PubMed

Jewett, D. L. (1970). Volume-conducted potentials in response to auditory stimuli as detected by averaging in the cat. *Electroencephalography and Clinical Neurophysiology, 28*(6), 609–618. PubMed

Joris, P. X., Schreiner, C. E., & Rees, A. (2004). Neural processing of amplitude-modulated sounds. *Physiological Reviews, 84*(2), 541–577. PubMed

Kaas, J. H., & Hackett, T. A. (2000). Subdivisions of auditory cortex and processing streams in primates. *Proceedings of the National Academy of Sciences USA, 97*(22), 11793–11799. PubMed

Khanna, S. M., & Teich, M. C. (1989). Spectral characteristics of the responses of primary auditory-nerve fibers to amplitude-modulated signals. *Hearing Research, 39*(1–2), 143–157. PubMed

Kimura, D. (1961). Cerebral dominance and the perception of verbal stimuli. *Canadian Journal of Psychology, 15*, 166–171.

Krishnan, A., Xu, Y., Gandour, J. T., & Cariani, P. A. (2004). Human frequency-following response: Representation of pitch contours in Chinese tones. *Hearing Research, 189*(1–2), 1–12. PubMed

Kuwada, S., Anderson, J. S., Batra, R., Fitzpatrick, D. C., Teissier, N., & D'Angelo, W. R. (2002). Sources of the scalp-recorded amplitude-modulation following response. *Journal of the American Academy of Audiology, 13*(4), 188–204. PubMed

Liegeois-Chauvel, C., Musolino, A., & Chauvel, P. (1991). Localization of the primary auditory area in man. *Brain, 114*(Pt 1A), 139–151. PubMed

Lins, O. G., Picton, P. E., Picton, T. W., Champagne, S. C., & Durieux-Smith, A. (1995). Auditory steady-state responses to tones amplitude-modulated at 80-110 Hz. *Journal of the Acoustical Society of America, 97*(5, Pt 1), 3051–3063. PubMed

Longstaff, A. (2005). *Neuroscience* (2nd ed.). New York: Taylor & Francis Group. PubMed

Lorente de No, R. (1947). Action potential of the motoneurons of the hypoglossus nucleus. *Journal of Cellular and Comparative Physiology, 29*(3), 207–287. PubMed

Lueders, H., Lesser, R., Hahn, J., Little, J., & Klem, G. (1983). Subcortical somatosensory evoked potentials to median nerve stimulation. *Brain, 106*(Pt 2), 341–372. PubMed

Lütkenhöner, B., Krumbholz, K., Lammertmann, C., Seither-Preisler, A., Steinsträter, O., & Patterson, R. D. (2003). Localization of primary auditory cortex in humans by magnetoencephalography. *NeuroImage, 18*(1), 58–66. PubMed

McPherson, D. L., & Starr, A. (1993). Binaural interaction in auditory evoked potentials: brainstem, middle- and long-latency components. *Hearing Research, 66*(1), 91–98. PubMed

Møller, A. R. (2006). *Hearing: Anatomy, physiology, and disorders of the auditory system* (2nd ed.). Amsterdam: Academic Press.

Moore, J. K. (1987). The human auditory brain stem: A comparative view. *Hearing Research, 29*(1), 1–32. PubMed

Musiek, F. E., & Baran, J. A. (1986). Neuroanatomy, neurophysiology, and central auditory assessment: 1. Brain stem. *Ear and Hearing, 7*(4), 207–219. PubMed

Musiek, F. E., & Baran, J. A. (2007). *The auditory system: anatomy, physiology, and clinical correlates.* Needham Heights, MA: Allyn & Bacon.

Papanicolaou, A. C., Baumann, S., Rogers, R. L., Saydjari, C., Amparo, E. G., & Eisenberg, H. M. (1990). Localization of auditory response sources using magnetoencephalography and magnetic resonance imaging. *Archives of Neurology, 47*(1), 33–37. PubMed

Parthasarathy, T. K., & Moushegian, G. (1993). Rate, frequency, and intensity effects on early auditory evoked potentials and binaural interaction component in humans. *Journal of the American Academy of Audiology, 4*(4), 229–237. PubMed

Pethe, J., Von Specht, H., Mühler, R., & Hocke, T. (2001). Amplitude modulation following responses in awake and sleeping humans—a comparison for 40 Hz and 80 Hz modulation frequency. *Scandinavian Audiology Supplementum, 52*(52), 152–155. PubMed

Petoe, M. A., Bradley, A. P., & Wilson, W. J. (2010). On chirp stimuli and neural synchrony in the suprathreshold auditory brainstem response. *Journal of the Acoustical Society of America, 128*(1), 235–246. PubMed

Phillips, D. P. (2007). An introduction to central auditory neuroscience. In F. E. Musiek & G. D. Chermak (Eds.). *Handbook of (central) auditory processing disorder: Auditory neuroscience and diagnosis* (Vol. 1, pp. 53–88). San Diego: Plural Publishing.

Picton, T. W. (2011). *Human auditory evoked potentials.* San Diego: Plural Publishing.

Picton, T. W., & Hillyard, S. A. (1974). Human auditory evoked potentials: 2. Effects of attention. *Electroencephalography and Clinical Neurophysiology, 36*(2), 191–199. PubMed

Picton, T. W., Hillyard, S. A., Galambos, R., & Schiff, M. (1971). Human auditory attention: A central or peripheral process? *Science, 173*(994), 351–353. PubMed

Rees, A., & Palmer, A. B. (2010). *The Oxford handbook of auditory science: The auditory brain.* New York: Oxford University Press.

Reite, M., Zimmerman, J. T., & Zimmerman, J. E. (1981). Magnetic auditory evoked fields: Interhemispheric asymmetry. *Electroencephalography and Clinical Neurophysiology, 51*(4), 388–392. PubMed

Romani, G. L., Williamson, S. J., & Kaufman, L. (1982). Tonotopic organization of the human auditory cortex. *Science*, *216*(4552), 1339–1340. PubMed

Rosengren, S. M., McAngus Todd, N. P., & Colebatch, J. G. (2005). Vestibular-evoked extraocular potentials produced by stimulation with bone-conducted sound. *Clinical Neurophysiology*, *116*(8), 1938–1948. PubMed

Rosenzweig, M. R. (1951). Representations of the two ears at the auditory cortex. *American Journal of Physiology*, *167*(1), 147–158. PubMed

Rupp, A., Uppenkamp, S., Gutschalk, A., Beucker, R., Patterson, R. D., Dau, T., et al. (2002). The representation of peripheral neural activity in the middle-latency evoked field of primary auditory cortex in humans(1). *Hearing Research*, *174*(1–2), 19–31. PubMed

Scherg, M., & Von Cramon, D. (1986). Evoked dipole source potentials of the human auditory cortex. *Electroencephalography and Clinical Neurophysiology*, *65*(5), 344–360. PubMed

Setou, M., Kurauchi, T., Tsuzuku, T., & Kaga, K. (2001). Binaural interaction of bone-conducted auditory brainstem responses. *Acta Oto-Laryngologica*, *121*(4), 486–489. PubMed

Sidtis, J. J. (1982). Predicting brain organization from dichotic listening performance: Cortical and subcortical functional asymmetries contribute to perceptual asymmetries. *Brain and Language*, *17*(2), 287–300. PubMed

Sininger, Y. S., & Cone-Wesson, B. (2006). Lateral asymmetry in the ABR of neonates: Evidence and mechanisms. *Hearing Research*, *212*(1-2), 203–211. PubMed

Sininger, Y. S., Cone-Wesson, B., & Abdala, C. (1998). Gender distinctions and lateral asymmetry in the low-level auditory brainstem response of the human neonate. *Hearing Research*, *126*(1–2), 58–66. PubMed

Sohmer, H., Kinarti, R., & Gafni, M. (1980). The source along the basilar membrane of the cochlear microphonic potential recorded by surface electrodes in man. *Electroencephalography and Clinical Neurophysiology*, *49*(5–6), 506–514. PubMed

Stegeman, D. F., Dumitru, D., King, J. C., & Roeleveld, K. (1997). Near- and far-fields: Source characteristics and the conducting medium in neurophysiology. *Journal of Clinical Neurophysiology*, *14*(5), 429–442. PubMed

Stegeman, D. F., Van Oosterom, A., & Colon, E. J. (1987). Far-field evoked potential components induced by a propagating generator: Computational evidence. *Electroencephalography and Clinical Neurophysiology*, *67*(2), 176–187. PubMed

Steinschneider, M., Volkov, I. O., Noh, M. D., Garell, P. C., & Howard, M. A., III (1999). Temporal encoding of the voice onset time phonetic parameter by field potentials recorded directly from human auditory cortex. *Journal of Neurophysiology*, *82*(5), 2346–2357. PubMed

Ungan, P., & Yagcioglu, S. (2002). Origin of the binaural interaction component in wave P4 of the short-latency auditory evoked potentials in the cat: Evaluation of serial depth recordings from the brainstem. *Hearing Research*, *167*(1–2), 81–101. PubMed

Velutti, R. A. (2008). *The auditory system in sleep*. London: Academic Press.

Wood, C. C., & Allison, T. (1981). Interpretation of evoked potentials: A neurophysiological perspective. *Canadian Journal of Psychology*, *35*(2), 113–135. PubMed

Chapter 5

Electrocochleography

Abby R. Nolder, John L. Dornhoffer, and Samuel R. Atcherson

Electrocochleography (ECochG) is one of the earliest described forms of auditory evoked potentials (AEPs). In 1930 the journal *Science* featured the works of Ernest Glen Wever and Charles W. Bray, two Princeton University researchers who were attempting to record the auditory nerve of a cat when they noted that an auditory stimulus presented to the animal's ear could be transmitted through an electrode to a telephone receiver. Subsequent scientists were able to reproduce these observations in other animals and eventually in a human, thus leading to the discovery of what is now known as the cochlear microphonic (CM), one of three major components of the ECochG. In the early 1950s, the other two components, the summating potential (SP; also arising from the cochlea) and the action potential (AP; arising from the auditory nerve), were described in animal models and then extrapolated to human subjects (Tasaki, 1954; Tasaki, Davis, and Eldridge, 1954). By the 1960s, Ruben and colleagues at Johns Hopkins University were recording these measurements intraoperatively on patients undergoing corrective middle ear surgery (Ruben, Bordley, Nager, Sekula, Knickerbocker, and Fisch, 1960; Ruben, Knickerbocker, Sekula, Nager, and Bordley, 1959; Ruben and Walker, 1963). However, routine clinical use of ECochG did not become popular until the 1970s with the discovery of the auditory brainstem response (ABR; Jewett, Romano, and Williston, 1970), which brought renewed attention and interest to virtually all AEPs. More elegant and noninvasive recording techniques have emerged, allowing for more widespread use of AEPs, including ECochG. Today, ECochG is used primarily as a means of evaluating patients suspected of having Meniere disease, a progressive disease that can affect hearing and balance, and as a method of assessing the auditory nerve during otologic surgery. ECochG testing is also sometimes used in clinical studies of cochlear and peripheral neural auditory disorders. This chapter outlines the components of the ECochG, how they are evoked and measured, important factors affecting their acquisition, and some clinical applications.

◆ Electrocochleography as an Auditory Evoked Potential

AEPs are one type of physiologic assessment that can be used to evaluate the patient with suspected hearing or balance problems. An AEP is a voltage "response" within the auditory system (the cochlea, the auditory nerve, or the auditory regions of the brain) that is stimulated, or "evoked," by acoustic stimuli. The stimuli can be in the form of continuous pure tones, transient tone bursts, or broadband clicks. The responses are usually measured by placing electrodes as close to their source as possible (near field) or at some distance from the source (far field). In the case of ECochG, electrodes are placed using one of two approaches: transtympanic (through the tympanic membrane on the cochlear promontory or round window) or extratympanic (within the ear canal). In ECochG, activity arising from the cochlear hair cells in the organ of Corti (CM and SP) and the auditory nerve (AP) is typically measured. **Figure 5.1** shows examples of normal and abnormal click and tone burst ECochGs and the three associated components.

◆ Components of Electrocochleography

The three components of ECochG, (i.e., CM, SP, and AP) are the electrophysiologic manifestation of the chain of events that occur in the cochlea and auditory nerve when a stimulus is presented to the ear of an individual with normal hearing. All three components can typically be recorded within 3 to 4 msec of stimulus presentation. Click- and tone burst–evoked ECochGs are commonly recorded, yet the two

stimuli have slightly different presentations of the three components.

Cochlear Microphonic

The CM is an alternating current (AC) voltage generated by outer hair cells (Wever and Bray, 1930). This component is stimulus-dependent, appearing as a series of peaks and troughs that mirror the waveform, or frequency, of the acoustic stimulus that is presented. It has no latency, as it begins as soon as the stimulus is introduced, and in certain recording setups it can persist as long as the stimulus is present. Increasing the intensity level of the stimulus will produce increased basilar membrane displacement, causing increased CM activity with greater amplitude (Hall, 2007). Because the CM follows the polarity of the stimulus, it is most effectively elicited by single polarity (condensation or rarefaction) stimuli, while alternating polarity stimuli can be used to help cancel out the CM during averaging to avoid obscuring the other components (Peake and Kiang, 1962; Yoshie, 1971). However, according to Peake and Kiang (1962), true CM cancellation with alternating polarity is possible only at lower stimulus intensity levels. At higher stimulus intensity levels, the basilar membrane mechanics will introduce some slight

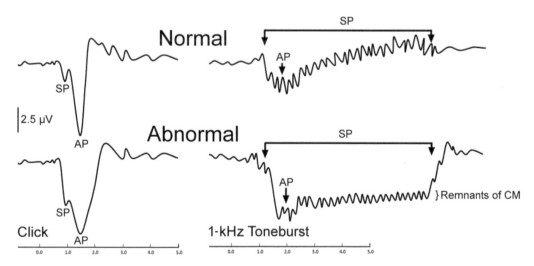

Fig. 5.1 Examples of normal (*top*) and abnormal (*bottom*; endolymphatic hydrops) electrocochleogram (ECochG) recordings Note the summating potential (SP), action potential (AP), and remnants of the cochlear microphonic (CM) with alternating polarity click (*left*) and tone burst (*right*) stimuli. In both click- and tone burst–evoked ECochG recordings, endolymphatic hydrops has the effect of enlarging the SP.

distortions, and remnants of the CM may remain in the recording. Although CM has shown some promise in the evaluation of auditory neuropathy spectrum disorder (ANSD; Berlin, Bordelon, St. John, Wilensky, Hurley, Kluka, et al, 1998), its clinical relevance in diagnosing other hearing and balance disorders is generally limited.

> **Special Consideration**
>
> The CM can be elicited using different stimulus frequencies. However, despite what we might think, the CM arises predominantly from the outer hair cells in the basal end of the cochlea, regardless of what the stimulus frequency is (Sohmer, Kinarti, and Gafni, 1980).

Summating Potential

The second component of the ECochG, SP, is also derived from the cochlea and is thought to represent the net depolarization of the hair cells within the organ of Corti (Brown and Johnson, 2010). More specifically, the SP is a direct current (DC) voltage that is thought to reflect the extracellular activity of the hair cells during acoustic stimulation (Davis, Deatherage, Eldredge, and Smith, 1958). In the ECochG, the SP appears as a unidirectional voltage deflection (usually negative) from baseline (Ferraro and Durrant, 2006). This voltage bias may be attributable to a distortion product caused by the basilar membrane not moving equally in both directions (Møller, 2006). ECochG recordings in response to a click generally produce the SP prior to the AP, whereas long-duration tone burst ECochG produces the SP following the AP (see **Fig. 5.1**). The cochlear transduction processes associated with ECochG may be distorted in patients with endolymphatic hydrops, or Meniere disease, making the SP an important measurement in the evaluation of the patient suspected of having this disorder. This clinical application is addressed in greater detail later in this chapter.

Action Potential

The last component of the ECochG, AP, represents the synchronous firing of thousands of auditory nerve fibers in response to a transient auditory stimulus, such as a click or tone burst (Goldstein and Kiang, 1958). The most important features of the AP in clinical ECochG are amplitude and latency. As with most other AEPs, latency is decreased and amplitude is increased as stimulus intensity is increased. The AP associated with ECochG has a few different names in the literature, which can be confusing. Early near-field ECochG recordings often produced one or more APs in a series (**Fig. 5.2**), and because they were of negative voltage, they were labeled N1, N2, and so on. The terms *whole nerve action potential* and *compound action potential* (CAP) are also used to denote that this ECochG component arises from not one but many (thousands) of auditory nerve fibers. The terms *N1* and *CAP* continue to appear in the literature. Although they are synonymous with the AP of the ECochG, they are not to be confused with the N100 (also called N1) of the cortical potential.

◆ Recording Electrocochleography

The ECochG can be recorded using the transtympanic or extratympanic electrode approach and a combination of broadband clicks and/or tone bursts. Although we provide some discussion of necessary equipment and various recording and stimulus parameters for ECochG, interested readers are directed to Chapter 12 for specific guidance on how to record ECochGs.

Transtympanic versus Extratympanic ECochG

Placement of electrodes for ECochG is very important because the magnitude and quality of the responses depend directly on the distance from the response generators, the cochlea, and the auditory nerve. The highest quality responses are measured when a needle electrode is placed through the tympanic membrane (transtympanic approach) directly onto the promontory of the cochlea (Aran and Le Bert, 1968; Yoshie, Ohashi, and Suzuki, 1967). As one can imagine, this method is more invasive, can be uncomfortable for the patient, and may be difficult for the

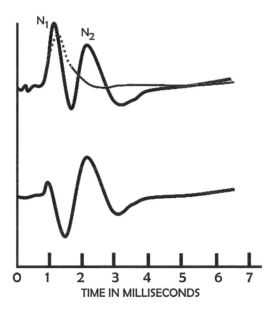

Fig. 5.2 Components N1 and N2 seen in rat round window recordings. The top two traces are recordings from the round window with the cochlear nucleus intact (*solid line*) and after the cochlear nucleus is removed (*dashed line*). The bottom trace is the difference between those two recordings. Negative polarity is up. AP, action Potential; SP, summating potential. (*From Møller* (*1983*). On the origin of the compound action potentials (N1, N2) of the cochlea of the rat. *Experimental Neurology*, 80, 633–644, with permission.)

average audiologist to administer without assistance from a medical professional because of the need for local anesthetic. For these reasons, the extratympanic method appears to be more widely used in the United States. This method involves placing an electrode as close to the tympanic membrane (TM) as possible, either in the ear canal wall or resting on the TM itself, the latter of which may be referred to as a tympanic or TM electrode approach (Ferraro and Ferguson, 1989; Ruth and Lambert, 1989). The Tymptrode, designed by Ferraro (1997, 2003), is a modified version described by Stypulkowski and Staller (1987) and is an extratympanic electrode that consists of an electrode wire with a foam rubber tip impregnated with conductive gel that gently rests on the TM. Ruth and Lambert (1989) have indicated that the TM electrode will yield ECochG recording as good as, if not better than, extratympanic electrodes placed more laterally in the ear canal.

Another commonly used extratympanic electrode is the TIPtrode, which is a gold foil–covered insert earphone foam tip that serves as the extratympanic electrode within the ear canal, as well as the sound delivery port. The TIPtrode does not require placement on the TM and therefore is often more comfortable for the patient. The ease of insert probably makes this extratympanic electrode a stronger preference for audiologists. However, clinicians should consider the TM electrode, as it will produce waveforms more comparable to transtympanic electrodes (Ferraro, Thedinger, Mediavilla, and Blackwell, 1994) while producing ECochG results that are the same as, if not better than, ear canal extratympanic electrodes (Ruth and Lambert, 1989).

Electrode Montage

Because the recording site of interest for the ECochG is either transtympanic or extratympanic, this electrode will serve as the active (or noninverting) electrode. The reference (inverting) electrode is usually placed on the contralateral (or opposite) ear on either the earlobe or the mastoid. The ground is usually placed on the forehead. This electrode montage will produce the classic AP-down (usually negative) polarity seen in **Fig. 5.1**. To achieve an AP-up polarity, the evoked potential system may allow the scale to be inverted (the AP will still be negative), or the active and reference electrodes can be swapped out in the electrode box. Given that different evoked potential systems have different labeling schemes for electrodes, **Table 5.1** offers some clarification.

Recording Parameters

The instrumentation involved in recording ECochGs is not unlike that used for single-channel ABR, with some exceptions. The analysis time window is usually set for ~5 msec to view only the ECochG components. Some clinicians,

however, prefer to set the analysis time window to 10 msec to visualize the ABR in addition to the ECochG. Realize, however, that if a transtympanic or extratympanic electrode is used, the AP (or wave I of the ABR) will likely be larger than is typical. Related to the analysis time window is the number of sampling points, which can usually be set to 256 or 512 points and yield 5-msec time window sampling rates of 51,200 to 102,400 samples per second, which is more than sufficient for the spectrum of the ECochG. The filters are generally set for 10 to 3000 Hz for both clicks and tone bursts, although higher-low-pass cutoffs (e.g., 5000 Hz) may be required for higher-stimulus frequency tone bursts to visualize the CM. The amplification (or gain) will depend on whether the transtympanic or extratympanic electrode is used and may even depend on whether the TM electrode or TIPtrode is used. Amplification factors of ~75,000 times are sufficient for most recordings, although 25,000 or 50,000 times may be expected for transtympanic electrodes and up to 100,000 times for TIPtrodes. The actual number of stimulus presentations (or sweeps) required for averaging will also depend on the type of electrode used. In general, as few as 100 stimuli may be all that is needed for transtympanic recordings, whereas as many as 2000 stimuli may be required for TIPtrode recordings. Adherence to well-established protocols is helpful for most recording parameters, but others will depend on clinical judgment through some trial and error.

Stimulus Parameters

Stimuli with abrupt onset, short duration, and broad spectra are most effective in producing the ECochG components. Therefore, broadband high-intensity clicks (0.1 msec pulses) are the most commonly used acoustic stimulus. The stimuli should be intense enough to evoke a

Table 5.1 Electrode Montage and Labeling Conventions

Ipsilateral Ear	Contralateral Ear	Forehead
Active	Reference	Ground (or common)
Noninverting	Inverting	Ground (or common)
Positive (+)	Negative (−)	Ground (or common)
Input 1	Input 2	Ground (or common)

well-defined SP–AP complex, especially when using ECochG to help diagnose Meniere disease. Tonal stimuli can also be used, usually in the form of tone bursts at 500, 1000, and 2000 Hz, which are common and even advocated (Gibson, 2009). Longer tone burst durations are helpful to better visualize the SP (e.g., Dauman, Aran, Charlet de Sauvage, and Portmann, 1988) and fast stimulus rise times are still necessary to evoke the AP by neural synchronization across auditory nerve fibers. Stimulus polarity is an important factor in recording ECochG. Stimulus artifact and the CM component can obscure the SP and AP, which are critical in clinical ECochG, especially when evaluating the patient with Meniere disease. Both stimulus artifact and CM can be overcome by using alternating polarity stimuli (Peake and Kiang, 1962; Yoshie, 1971). When assessing ANSD, it would be preferable to use both single-polarity stimuli (usually clicks); when the two recordings are overlaid, the CM component for the two polarities will be mirror images of one another (e.g., Berlin et al, 1998).

Except when there is interest in assessing thresholds or studying the behavior of various ECochG components, a high-level intensity is almost always used with ECochG. Depending on calibration variables, as well as the output limits of the transducers, it is not uncommon to present stimuli as high as 95 dB. Although the AP will remain fairly stable and visible at lower intensity levels, the SP amplitude will likely get smaller with decreases in intensity.

In terms of neural adaptation and stimulation rate, there is always a trade-off between the rate of stimulus presentations and the morphology of the AEP. In the case of ECochG, a slow rate (usually ≤7.1/s) is desirable for a large AP. But if the SP is of greater clinical interest, faster stimulus rates that diminish the AP while leaving the SP relatively intact are permissible (Eggermont and Odenthal, 1974).

Finally, the choice of transducer has some degree of importance. Although virtually any type of transducer could be used, there are several distinct advantages to using tubal insert earphones. The tubing allows for a time delay (0.8–0.9 msec) separation between any electromagnetic, stimulus-related artifact and the ECochG components. Even though insert earphones help to delay the response relative to the stimulus artifact, long-duration stimuli

(e.g., tone bursts) for CM recordings may still be affected. Therefore, mu-metal shielding of the transducer may still be necessary (Riazi and Ferraro, 2008). In the absence of mu-metal shielding, clinicians can verify the lack of stimulus artifact by conducting a "dry run" recording with the tubing clamped (using one or more large binder clips or clothes pins). There should be no response and no evidence of the stimulus within the waveform. The insert earphone tip can serve to hold the electrode in place (or dually serve as the extratympanic electrode).

◆ Subject Effects and Special Considerations

Success with ECochG requires patient education, appropriate electrode placement, and expert interpretation. Patient education is necessary to ensure the patient's comfort during the test. Electrode placement can be done safely and without much discomfort using the extratympanic technique described earlier. Patient factors, such as gender, age, and degree of hearing impairment, can all affect the interpretation of the ECochG. These factors have not been as widely investigated for ECochG as for other AEPs (e.g., ABR); nonetheless, they should all be considered when performing ECochG testing. Although ECochG can be successfully recorded from infants and young children, it often requires a level of sedation; therefore, it is usually reserved for cooperative adults. The aging adult poses a special challenge given that older individuals often have a high-frequency hearing loss (presbycusis) that alters the ECochG (Oku and Hasegewa, 1997). These individuals usually show an increase in latency and reduction in amplitude of the ECochG components. With advancing age the AP amplitude decreases relative to the SP amplitude, causing an increased SP/AP ratio (Chatrian, Wirch, Edwards, Turella, Kaufman, and Snyder, 1985). Thus, both age and hearing loss may need to be considered when interpreting the ECochG for clinical use, especially when evaluating the patient suspected of having Meniere disease. Although largely abandoned today in favor of ABR or nuclear imaging techniques (e.g., magnetic resonance imaging [MRI]), patients with retrocochlear pathology (e.g., vestibular schwannomas or cerebellopontine angle tumors) may show an altered or absent AP component, depending on the location and size of the tumor (Eggermont, Don, and Brackmann, 1980).

♦ Clinical Applications

The clinical uses of ECochG include (1) assessing hearing thresholds; (2) monitoring the status of the auditory nerve during otologic surgery; (3) identifying wave I of the ABR, which corresponds to N1 or AP of the ECochG; (4) aiding in the assessment, diagnosis, and monitoring of Meniere disease or endolymphatic hydrops; and (5) identifying patients, usually children, with ANSD. The assessment of hearing thresholds using ECochG has largely been replaced by ABR and auditory steady-state responses (ASSRs), so it is not covered further here. Because the ECochG is resistant to the effects of anesthesia, it is useful in the operating room. Interested readers are referred to Chapter 18 for some practical discussion of ECochG in the operating room. Because of the closer proximity of the recording electrode to the inner ear with ECochG, there is a potentially useful advantage in enhancing wave I amplitude for use with ABR measurements. The remaining clinical applications for Meniere disease and ANSD as auditory disorders of the peripheral ear are discussed in greater detail below.

Pearl

Wave I of the ABR is a useful diagnostic marker for measuring neural conduction time, particularly the wave I–V interpeak latency. When hearing loss or a retrocochlear pathology precludes the recording of wave I, some minor adjustments to the recording parameter, including adding an electrode in the ear canal, may help to enhance wave I by virtue of recording the AP component. Once the AP latency is measured, it can be substituted for the missing wave I latency (Eggermont et al, 1980).

Auditory Neuropathy Spectrum Disorder

Although still new, the use of ECochG for cases of ANSD shows some promise. The classic clinical presentation of ANSD is usually associated with normal (or near normal) otoacoustic emissions (OAEs) and abnormal or absent ABRs (Starr, McPherson, Patterson, Don, Luxford, Shannon, et al, 1991; Starr, Picton, Sininger, Hood, and Berlin, 1996). For unknown reasons, some patients lose their OAEs over time (Deltenre, Mansbach, Bozet, Christiaens, Barthelemy, Paulissen, et al, 1999; Starr, Sininger, Nguyen, Michalewski, Oba, and Abdala, 2001), and some ABR recordings show abnormally long and persistent CMs in spite of the use of click stimuli (Berlin et al, 1998). The difficulty in the diagnosis of ANSD stems from the lack of a test measure that will differentially diagnose whether the disorder is caused by neuropathy of the auditory nerve (postsynaptic) or by inner hair cell and/or synaptic dysfunction (presynaptic). However, employing transtympanic and extratympanic electrodes, investigators have used ECochG to try to better understand the presynaptic (CM and SP) and postsynaptic (AP) contributions to ANSD (Lu, Zhang, Wen, Ji, Chen, Xi, et al, 2008; Santarelli, Starr, Michalewski, and Arslan, 2008). In some patients with ANSD, the SP and AP are present but small, with low SP/AP ratios. In other patients with ANSD, the AP is absent, but the CM and SP may remain. Manipulating intensity and/or rate parameters may help to differentiate the possible contributions of ANSD in individual patients, potentially making ECochG, not ABR, the most appropriate tool. More recently, it appears that ECochG may assist in differentiating the pre- versus postsynaptic types of ANSD using round window electrodes (McMahon, Patuzzi, Gibson, and Sanli, 2008). McMahon and colleagues were able to demonstrate using ECochG that patients who exhibited an SP followed by a dendritic potential (DP; possible clue to faulty voltage-gated channels in the auditory nerve) had a dysfunction of the auditory nerve (i.e., postsynaptic). Patients with SPs, present or absent APs, and no DPs had a presynaptic dysfunction. Thus, it was not entirely surprising to the authors that ANSD patients with the presynaptic disorder produced normal electrically evoked ABR (EABR) waveforms following cochlear implantation.

Meniere Disease

The French physician Prosper Ménière, who first attributed vertigo to inner ear causes, described Meniere disease nearly a century and a half ago (Ménière, 1861). The disease is a progressive disorder characterized by recurrent episodic vertigo, tinnitus, aural fullness, and fluctuating hearing loss. Although the exact pathophysiology of this disease has not been completely elucidated, it is thought to be caused by increased endolymphatic pressure within the scala media (Brown and Johnson, 2010). This increased endolymphatic pressure, also called hydrops, affects the normal vibration of the basilar membrane. **Table 5.2** shows the four classic symptoms associated with Meniere disease, which can vary somewhat among patients. Patients with Meniere disease often show abnormally enlarged SP amplitudes, possibly as a result of the distortion of basilar membrane movement caused by the increased endolymphatic pressure. The amplitude of the AP is compared with the SP to form the SP/AP ratio, which, if enlarged, is a positive finding for Meniere disease (Coats, 1981; Dornhoffer, 1998; Dornhoffer and Arenberg, 1993; Ferraro, Arenberg, and Hassanein, 1985). Although ECochG has shown great promise in the diagnosis of this disorder, the sensitivity and specificity of the test have been questioned. The episodic nature of Meniere disease and the recording electrode of choice (i.e., transtympanic vs extratympanic) pose special challenges in diagnosis using ECochG. Ferraro et al (1985) found positive (i.e., enlarged) SP/AP ratios in greater than 90% of patients with active symptoms (aural fullness and hearing loss); however, other studies have shown enlarged SP/AP ratios in only 60 to 70% of the patients with Meniere disease at any given time (Campbell, Harker, and Abbas, 1992; Dornhoffer, 1998; Ge and Shea, 2002; Kim, Kumar, Battista, and Wiet, 2005). In addition to the enlarged SP/AP ratio, the width (or broadening) of the AP may be a clinically useful finding because 70% of 2140 patients followed during a 10-year period from the same clinic exhibited this finding (Ge and Shea, 2002). According to a meta-analysis of 20 papers by Wuyts and colleagues (Wuyts, Van de Heyning, Van Spaendonck, and Molenberghs, 1997), normal ears had SP/AP ratios less than, 0.30 whether transtympanic or extratympanic electrodes were used. However, diagnostic criteria for a positive SP/AP ratio, determined from patients with endolymphatic hydrops, was slightly different for the two electrode types, at greater than 0.35 for transtympanic and greater than 0.42 for extratympanic. Although these diagnostic criteria can be borrowed, it is always ideal to collect local normative data, given the different types of electrodes, stimulus and recording parameters, and analysis techniques that can be used. Additional research and improvements in recording technique are needed to improve the sensitivity and specificity of the test, but ECochG remains one of the most promising diagnostic tools for the audiologist and otolaryngologist assessing the patient with suspected Meniere disease.

Table 5.2 Symptoms of Meniere Disease

Below are symptoms typically seen in patients with Meniere disease. They usually exhibit one or two symptoms but could have all symptoms; however, some may be asymptomatic, which does not necessarily preclude diagnosis.

VERTIGO: This is the most distressing symptom of Meniere disease. The vertigo can last from 10 minutes to many hours. It may be associated with nausea and vomiting. After the vertigo has subsided, most patients have imbalance for 1 or 2 days until returning to normal.

HEARING LOSS: In Meniere disease, hearing loss usually fluctuates. In most cases where there is hearing loss, it is unilateral, but in rare instances, a person can have a bilateral hearing loss. Typically, the hearing loss is in the low frequencies. If left untreated, hearing loss can become permanent.

AURAL FULLNESS can occur before or during an attack. It will usually resolve when the attack has resolved.

TINNITUS is usually a result of the hearing loss. It is typically described as a seashell sound or a low-tone buzzing.

Source: Adapted from the Prosper Meniere Society (http://www.prospermeniere.com).

◆ Summary

Despite some challenges with respect to ease of administration, interpretation, and clinical use, ECochG remains an important tool for the audiologist and the electrophysiologic assessment of the patient with hearing and balance problems. Practical applications of the ECochG in the clinic and the operating room can be reviewed in Chapters 12 and 18.

References

Aran, J. M., & Le Bert, G. (1968). Les responses nerveuse cochleaires chex l'homme, image du fonctionnement de l'oreille et nouveau test d'audiometrie objectif. *Revue de Laryngologie–Otologie–Rhinologie, 89*(7), 361–365. PubMed

Berlin, C. I., Bordelon, J., St. John, P., Wilensky, D., Hurley, A., Kluka, E., et al. (1998). Reversing click polarity may uncover auditory neuropathy in infants. *Ear and Hearing, 19*(1), 37–47. PubMed

Bonucci, A. S., & Hyppolito, M. A. (2009). Comparison of the use of tympanic and extratympanic electrodes for electrocochleography. *Laryngoscope, 119*(3), 563–566. PubMed

Brown, C., & Johnson, T. A. (2010). Electrophysiologic assessment of hearing. In P. W. Flint (Ed.), *Cumming's otolaryngology head and neck surgery*, 1094-1915 (5th ed.). Philadelphia: Mosby Elsevier.

Campbell, K. C., Harker, L. A., & Abbas, P. J. (1992). Interpretation of electrocochleography in Ménière's disease and normal subjects. *Annals of Otology, Rhinology, and Laryngology, 101*(6), 496–500. PubMed

Chatrian, G. E., Wirch, A. L., Edwards, K. H., Turella, G. S., Kaufman, M. A., & Snyder, J. M. (1985). Cochlear summating potential to broadband clicks detected from the human external auditory meatus: A study of subjects with normal hearing for age. *Ear and Hearing, 6*(3), 130–138. PubMed

Coats, A. C. (1981). The summating potential and Meniere's disease: 1. Summating potential amplitude in Meniere and non-Meniere ears. *Archives of Otolaryngology—Head and Neck Surgery, 107*(4), 199–208. PubMed

Dauman, R., Aran, J. M., Charlet de Sauvage, R., & Portmann, M. (1988). Clinical significance of the summating potential in Ménière's disease. *American Journal of Otology, 9*(1), 31–38. PubMed

Davis, H., Deatherage, B. H., Eldredge, D. H., & Smith, C. A. (1958). Summating potentials of the cochlea. *American Journal of Physiology, 195*(2), 251–261. PubMed

Deltenre, P., Mansbach, A. L., Bozet, C., Christiaens, F., Barthelemy, P., Paulissen, D., et al. (1999). Auditory neuropathy with preserved cochlear microphonics and secondary loss of otoacoustic emissions. *Audiology, 38*(4), 187–195. PubMed

Dornhoffer, J. L. (1998). Diagnosis of cochlear Ménière's disease with electrocochleography. *Journal for Oto-Rhino-Laryngology and Its Related Specialties, 60*(6), 301–305. PubMed

Dornhoffer, J. L., & Arenberg, I. K. (1993). Diagnosis of vestibular Ménière's disease with electrocochleography. *American Journal of Otology, 14*(2), 161–164. PubMed

Eggermont, J. J., Don, M., & Brackmann, D. E. (1980). Electrocochleography and auditory brainstem electric responses in patients with pontine angle tumors. *Annals of Otology, Rhinology, and Laryngology, 89*(6), 1–19. PubMed

Eggermont, J. J., & Odenthal, D. W. (1974). Electrophysiological investigation of the human cochlea: Recruitment, masking and adaptation. *Audiology, 13*(1), 1–22. PubMed

Ferraro, J. A. (1997). *Laboratory exercises in auditory evoked potentials.* San Diego: Singular Publishing.

Ferraro, J. A. (2003). Clinical electrocochleography: Overview of theories, techniques, and applications. *Audiology Online.* Retrieved from http://www.audiologyonlinc.com/articles/article_detail.asp?article_id=452

Ferraro, J. A., Arenberg, I. K., & Hassanein, R. S. (1985). Electrocochleography and symptoms of inner ear dysfunction. *Archives of Otolaryngology, 111*(2), 71–74. PubMed

Ferraro, J. A., & Durrant, J. D. (2006). Electrocochleography in the evaluation of patients with Ménière's disease/endolymphatic hydrops. *Journal of the American Academy of Audiology, 17*(1), 45–68. PubMed

Ferraro, J. A., & Ferguson, R. (1989). Tympanic ECochG and conventional ABR: A combined approach for the identification of wave I and the I–V interwave interval. *Ear and Hearing, 10*(3), 161–166. PubMed

Ferraro, J. A., Thedinger, B. S., Mediavilla, S. J., & Blackwell, W. L. (1994). Human summating potential to tone bursts: Observations on tympanic membrane versus promontory recordings in the same patients. *Journal of the American Academy of Audiology, 5*(1), 24–29. PubMed

Ge, X., & Shea, J. J., Jr. (2002). Transtympanic electrocochleography: A 10-year experience. *Otology and Neurotology, 23*(5), 799–805. PubMed

Gibson, W. P. (2009). A comparison of two methods of using transtympanic electrocochleography for the diagnosis of Meniere's disease: Click summating potential/action potential ratio measurements and tone burst summating potential measurements. *Acta Oto-Laryngologica Supplementum, 129*(560), 38–42. PubMed

Goldstein, M. H., & Kiang, N. Y. S. (1958). Synchrony of neural activity in electric responses evoked by transient acoustic stimuli. *Journal of the Acoustical Society of America, 30*(2), 107–114.

Hall, J. W. (2007). *New handbook of auditory evoked responses.* Needham Heights, MA: Allyn & Bacon.

Jewett, D. L., Romano, M. N., & Williston, J. S. (1970, Mar). Human auditory evoked potentials: Possible brain stem components detected on the scalp. *Science, 167*(924), 1517–1518. PubMed

Kim, H. H., Kumar, A., Battista, R. A., & Wiet, R. J. (2005). Electrocochleography in patients with Meniere's disease. *American Journal of Otology, 26*(2), 128–131. PubMed

Lu, Y., Zhang, Q., Wen, Y., Ji, F., Chen, A., Xi, X., et al. (2008). The SP-AP compound wave in patients with auditory neuropathy. *Acta Oto-Laryngologica, 128*(8), 896–900. PubMed

McMahon, C. M., Patuzzi, R. B., Gibson, W. P., & Sanli, H. (2008). Frequency-specific electrocochleography indicates that presynaptic and postsynaptic mechanisms of auditory neuropathy exist. *Ear and Hearing, 29*(3), 314–325. PubMed

Ménière, P. (1861). Pathologic auriculaire: Mémoire sur les lésions de l'oreille interne donnant lieu à des symptoms de congestion cérébrale applectiforme. *Gazette Medicale de Paris, 16,* 88–89.

Møller, A. R. (1983). On the origin of the compound action potentials (N1, N2) of the cochlea of the rat. *Experimental Neurology, 80*(3), 633–644.

Møller, A. R. (2006). *Hearing: Anatomy, physiology, and disorders of the auditory system* (2nd ed.). London: Academic Press.

Oku, T., & Hasegawa, M. (1997). The influence of aging on auditory brainstem response and electrocochleography in the elderly. *Journal for Oto-Rhino-Laryngology and Its Related Specialties, 59*(3), 141–146. PubMed

Peake, W. T., & Kiang, N. Y. S. (1962, January). Cochlear responses to condensation and rarefaction clicks. *Biophysical Journal, 2,* 23–34. PubMed

Riazi, M., & Ferraro, J. A. (2008). Observations on mastoid versus ear canal recorded cochlear microphonic in newborns and adults. *Journal of the American Academy of Audiology, 19*(1), 46–55. PubMed

Ruben, R. J., Bordley, J. E., Nager, G. T., Sekula, J., Knickerbocker, G. G., & Fisch, U. (1960, June). Human cochlea responses to sound stimuli. *Annals of Otology, Rhinology, and Laryngology, 69,* 459–479. PubMed

Ruben, R. J., Knickerbocker, G. G., Sekula, J., Nager, G. T., & Bordley, J. E. (1959). Cochlear microphonics in man: A preliminary report. *Laryngoscope, 69*(6), 665–671. PubMed

Ruben, R. J., & Walker, A. E. (1963, November). The VIIIth nerve action potential in Ménière's disease. *Laryngoscope, 73,* 1456–1464. PubMed

Ruth, R. A., & Lambert, P. R. (1989). Comparison of tympanic membrane to promontory electrode recordings of electrocochleographic responses in patients with Ménière's disease. *Otolaryngology–Head and Neck Surgery, 100*(6), 546–552. PubMed

Santarelli, R., Starr, A., Michalewski, H. J., & Arslan, E. (2008). Neural and receptor cochlear potentials obtained by transtympanic electrocochleography in auditory neuropathy. *Clinical Neurophysiology, 119*(5), 1028–1041. PubMed

Sohmer, H., Kinarti, R., & Gafni, M. (1980). The source along the basilar membrane of the cochlear microphonic potential recorded by surface electrodes in man. *Electroencephalography and Clinical Neurophysiology, 49*(5–6), 506–514. PubMed

Starr, A., McPherson, D., Patterson, J., Don, M., Luxford, W., Shannon, R., et al. (1991, June). Absence of both auditory evoked potentials and auditory percepts dependent on timing cues. *Brain, 114*(Pt 3), 1157–1180. PubMed

Starr, A., Picton, T. W., Sininger, Y., Hood, L. J., & Berlin, C. I. (1996, June). Auditory neuropathy. *Brain, 119*(Pt 3), 741–753. PubMed

Starr, A., Sininger, Y., Nguyen, T., Michalewski, H. J., Oba, S., & Abdala, C. (2001). Cochlear receptor (microphonic and summating potentials, otoacoustic emissions) and auditory pathway (auditory brain stem potentials) activity in auditory neuropathy. *Ear and Hearing, 22*(2), 91–99. PubMed

Stypulkowski, P. H., & Staller, S. J. (1987). Clinical evaluation of a new ECoG recording electrode. *Ear and Hearing, 8*(5), 304–310. PubMed

Tasaki, I. (1954). Nerve impulses in individual auditory nerve fibers of guinea pig. *Journal of Neurophysiology, 17*(2), 97–122. PubMed

Tasaki, I., Davis, H., & Eldridge, D. H. (1954). Exploration of cochlear potentials in guinea pigs with a microelectrode. *Journal of the Acoustical Society of America, 26*(2), 765–773.

Wever, E.G., & Bray, C.W. (1930). Auditory nerve impulses. *Science, 17*(1834), 215.

Wuyts, F. L., Van de Heyning, P. H., Van Spaendonck, M. P., & Molenberghs, G. (1997). A review of electrocochleography: Instrumentation settings and meta-analysis of criteria for diagnosis of endolymphatic hydrops. *Acta Oto-Laryngologica Supplementum, 526,* 14–20. PubMed

Yoshie, N. (1971, November). Clinical cochlear response audiometry by means of an average response computer: Non-surgical technique and clinical use. *Revue de Laryngologie–Otologie–Rhinologie, 92*(Suppl), 646–672. PubMed

Yoshie, N., Ohashi, T., & Suzuki, T. (1967). Non-surgical recording of auditory nerve action potentials in man. *Laryngoscope, 77*(1), 76–85. PubMed

Chapter 6

The Auditory Brainstem Response

Samuel R. Atcherson

The auditory brainstem response (ABR) is probably the most widely used auditory evoked potential (AEP) with clinical applications in estimating behavioral thresholds in infants (and difficult-to-test patients) and in detecting neurologic abnormalities of the eighth cranial nerve (CN VIII, auditory nerve) and brainstem. It has also been one of the most widely studied of all AEPs because of its ease of setup, good test–retest reliability, and generally quick administration, particularly with cooperative patients. The published literature of ABRs, both past and present, could easily fill an entire book or volume of books. Because of space limitations, this chapter provides a general overview and focus mainly on the normative aspects of the ABR. Where appropriate, a discussion will be provided on key clinical effects of the ABR. Other sections of this textbook offer more relevant information of a narrower and more practical scope. These include portions of Chapter 13 on the use of the ABR in early identification and intervention programs, Chapter 14 on ABR threshold estimation, Chapter 15 on the use of the ABR in evaluating retrocochlear disease and auditory neuropathy spectrum disorder (ANSD), and some portions of Chapter 17 on the use of both click- and speech-evoked ABRs for evaluating central auditory disorders.

◆ Brief History

The ABR is known by other names, such as the brainstem evoked response (BSER), the brainstem auditory evoked response (BAER), and the brainstem auditory evoked potential (BAEP). The earliest published recording of the human ABR was presented by Sohmer and Feinmesser (1967), who described the responses as cochlear action potentials. However, it was Jewett and colleagues (1970; Jewett and Williston, 1971) who correctly described the sequence of ABR waveform components as responses arising from the auditory nerve and various auditory brainstem structures. The ABR collectively is considered a far-field, early exogenous potential, often grouped with electrocochleography (ECochG) for its short latencies within 10 msec of stimulus onset. Indeed, the compound action potential (CAP) of the ECochG is essentially one and the same with wave I of the ABR. As with all exogenous potentials, the ABR is highly influenced by changes in the stimulus parameters. For example, decreasing the intensity level can drastically reduce the overall amplitudes of all waves and correspondingly increase their latencies. A 100-µsec duration click stimulus with abrupt rise time will produce the largest ABR amplitudes and the shortest latencies, whereas slower-rising tone burst envelopes will produce somewhat smaller ABR amplitudes and increased latencies. Finally, frequency-specific tone bursts (500 Hz vs 4000 Hz) will appreciably stimulate different regions of the cochlea such that the effect of the longer travel time from the base to the apex of the cochlea can be observed in the recordings as well. Without a doubt, various pathologies will differentially affect the ABR morphology, sometimes in very predictable ways, whereas others may not.

◆ Description

Waveform Morphology

The classic "textbook" ABR is evoked by a 100-µs click of moderately high intensity level yielding several positive-to-negative waves within 10 msec after stimulus onset. The individual waves are commonly labeled using Roman numerals. Waves I, III, and V are clinically most useful for neurodiagnostic purposes, and wave V is most useful clinically when estimating behavioral thresholds. Waves II and IV are sometimes visible and can be marked. **Figure 6.1** shows two click-evoked ABR waveforms at two different intensity levels (40 and 80 dB nHL [normal hearing level]) and two different rates (17.7 and 57.7/s). At moderately high intensity levels (e.g., 80 dB nHL), the ABR shows a full complement of waves. As a general rule, waves I, III, and V have mean latencies at ~1.5, 3.5, and 5.5 msec, respectively, and interpeak latencies of ~2 msec for I–III and III–V and 4 msec for I–V. As intensity is lowered, wave V appears to "linger," thus illustrating its clinical usefulness in estimating behavioral thresholds in infants and other difficult-to-test patients. When the rate is increased from 17.7/s to 57.7/s, the ABR can still show the full complement of waves, but with some amplitude reductions as well as slight prolongation of latencies. Within the 0 to 1 msec time frame, there appears to be some small activity, which when compared using different click stimulus polarities might reveal a small yet visible

cochlear microphonic (CM). This is not to be confused with a possible stimulus artifact that can also appear in this same time frame when using supra-aural headphones that offer no time delay between the stimulus artifact and the neural signal (i.e., the ABR). The amplitude of the ABR can range from 0.1 to 1 µV, and the amplitudes among the different waves and overall waveform morphology can vary considerably from person to person with normal hearing. The ABR also has a reasonably short maturational time course, but its various peaks undergo changes in amplitude and latency at different rates in the first few years of life, and it does not become adultlike until around 3 years of age (Fria and Doyle, 1984; Hecox and Burkard, 1982; Salamy, 1984).

The ABR, like any acoustical or electrical signal, can be spectrally analyzed and broken up into its constituent frequencies. At higher intensity levels, the ABR contains a larger spectral peak at 200 Hz and two smaller spectral peaks at 500 and 1000 Hz (Malinoff and Spivak, 1990; Sininger, 1995). When the ABR waveform is viewed in the time domain, the 500- and 1000-Hz waves appear to be riding on top of the lower 200-Hz wave. This is significant because changes in the recording bandpass filter will alter the waveform morphology of the ABR. Any time the intensity level of the stimulus is lowered, the spectral energy of the ABR will also be lowered (Spivak, 1993). In contrast to the adultlike ABR, the infant and toddler ABR has slightly greater low-frequency energy (Katbamna, Metz, Bennett, and Dokler, 1996; Spivak, 1993). Comparisons of ABR spectra of younger and older adults have also shown an increase of low-frequency energy with advancing age (Spivak and Malinoff, 1990). **Figure 6.2** shows age-related effects up to 3 years of age.

Neural Generators

In spite of the name, the neural generators (or sources) of the ABR involve structures within the brainstem and the auditory nerve. Several different techniques by multiple investigators over the years have led to some very consistent findings as well as ongoing debate. Based on a scholarly synthesis of his

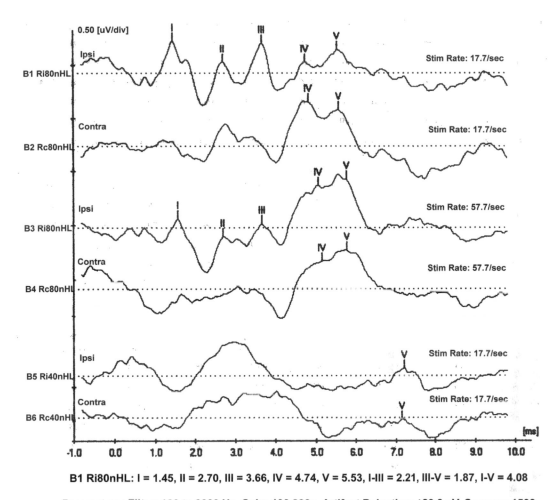

B1 Ri80nHL: I = 1.45, II = 2.70, III = 3.66, IV = 4.74, V = 5.53, I-III = 2.21, III-V = 1.87, I-V = 4.08

Parameters: Filter: 100 to 3000 Hz, Gain: 100,000x, Artifact Rejection: ±23.8 µV, Sweeps: 1500

Fig. 6.1 Normal two-channel adult human auditory brainstem response to click stimuli at two different intensity levels and two different stimulation rates. Absolute and relative latencies, as well as some of the stimulus and recording parameters, are shown below the time axis for the 80-dB nHL (normal hearing level) ipsilateral waveform at the 17.7/s stimulation rate.

own work and the work of others, Møller (2006) concluded that wave I arises from the distal portion of the auditory nerve (within the inner ear), wave II from the proximal portion of the auditory nerve (brainstem termination), wave III from the cochlear nucleus, wave IV from midline brainstem structures (perhaps acoustic stria, trapezoid bodies, and the superior olivary complex), and wave V from the termination of the lateral lemniscus within the inferior colliculus on the contralateral side. Beyond waves I and II, which are largely restricted to the auditory nerve,

waves III through V likely have more than one anatomical contributor, given the complexity of the auditory brainstem and parallel ipsilateral and contralateral pathways with multiple decussations (crossovers).

Viewed in another way, the various peaks of the ABR are likely produced by action potentials forming stationary dipoles (Chapter 4) based on their travel from the inner ear synapse to the inferior colliculus. Scherg and von Cramon (1985) developed a setup that would allow them to estimate the approximate orientation and strength of dipoles associated with

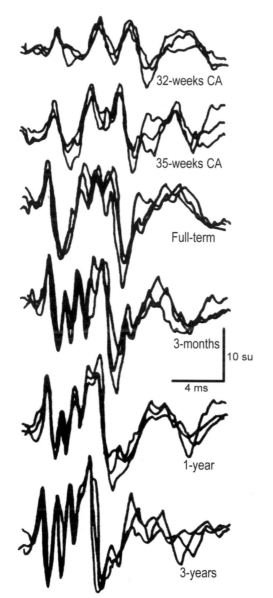

Fig. 6.2 Normal maturation of the auditory brainstem response from 32 weeks' conceptional age to 3 years of age. (From Salamy (1984). Maturation of the auditory brainstem response from birth through early childhood. *Journal of Clinical Neurophysiology, 1,* 293–329, with permission.)

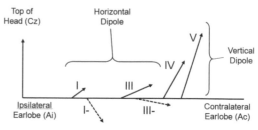

Fig. 6.3 Two-dimensional dipoles of the ABR. (From Scherg, M., & von Cramon, D. (1985). A new interpretation of the generators of BAEP waves IV: Results of a spatio-temporal dipole model. *Electroencephalography and Clinical Neurophysiology, 62,* 290–299, with permission).

acoustic stria crossing over from the ipsilateral cochlear nucleus to the contralateral superior colliculus. The more vertical orientations of waves IV and V seem to be in agreement with the alignment of the superior olivary complex and inferior colliculus between which the lateral lemniscus runs vertically. The collective horizontal and vertical dipoles become important in understanding the influence of electrode placement on the ABR waveform morphology. Specifically, certain electrode arrays will enhance certain waves while attenuating others. For example, placing the noninverting electrode on one ear and the inverting (reference) electrode on the other ear for a horizontal montage can enhance wave I amplitude while attenuating wave V amplitude. Conversely, placing the noninverting electrode on the forehead and the inverting (reference) electrode at the base of the neck on a vertebra will enhance wave V amplitude while attenuating wave I amplitude.

◆ Effects of Various Stimulus and Recording Parameters on the Auditory Brainstem Response

Stimulus Types

The ABR can be evoked by virtually any stimulus that is abrupt in nature, such as 100-μsec clicks (resembling a square pulse)

four peaks (I, III, IV, and V) and two troughs (I and III) (**Fig. 6.3**). The horizontal orientations of peaks I and III (and their following troughs) appear to support the horizontal arrangement of the auditory nerve fibers, as well as the with an essentially instantaneous onset, tone bursts with rise times of a few milliseconds, and even gaps in broadband noise with fall times of a few milliseconds. The abruptness of these various stimuli causes a synchronous discharge of numerous auditory nerve fibers (Chapter 4). Clicks presented to the ears by way of transducers are said to broadly stimulate the cochlea because of their instantaneous rise causing a spectral splattering of frequencies. Although clicks have energy across a wide range of frequencies, the ABR seems to favor the click frequency region from 1000 to 4000 Hz. That is, when the click is still in its electrical form, it has a main lobe of spectral energy that spans to ~10,000 Hz, at which point it creates its first spectral zero. This span of spectral energy makes it ideal for broadly stimulating the cochlea. However, when the click is in an acoustic form coming out of a transducer, the spectral energy changes somewhat and has one or more spectral peaks around 2000 to 4000 Hz. This explains, in part, the tendency for the click-evoked ABR to be sensitive to sensorineural hearing loss ~4000 Hz audiometric frequency and is argued by some to be a valid estimate of high-frequency sensitivity (Gorga, Johnson, Kaminski, Beauchaine, Garner, and Neely, 2006). ER-3A tubal insert earphones have the advantage of delaying the onset of the click and separating it in time from the stimulus artifact, but its spectral output remains the same. Any spectral differences for acoustic clicks produced by supra-aural earphones (e.g., TDH-49) and insert earphones are most likely due to different couplers in which they are measured (e.g., Van Campen, Sammeth, Hall, and Peek, 1992).

In addition to click stimuli, tone bursts also widely used. Tone bursts used with the ABR are short-duration sinusoids, usually no more than ~4 to 5 cycles long at typical octave audiometric frequencies from 500 to 4000 Hz. This will provide stimulus durations of 10 msec for a 500 Hz tone burst and 1.25 msec for a 4000 Hz tone burst. The brevity of tone burst stimuli in ABR recordings is necessary for the ABR's dependency on neural synchrony. With such brief stimuli, however, they will appear clicklike with sudden onset and will require an envelope (or gating function) to gradually ramp the tone burst on and then off to minimize spectral splatter and provide some degree of frequency specificity. Gorga and Thornton (1989) provide an excellent discussion and examples of gating functions on short-duration tones. The two most commonly used tone burst gating functions are linear (also called Bartlett) and Blackman, as evidenced by the work of some major infant hearing programs (e.g., British Columbia Early Hearing Program, 2008; Gorga et al, 2006).

Polarity

Stimuli used for evoking the ABR can be presented in one of two polarities (or phases): condensation or rarefaction. Although the latencies do not change much with the different polarities, the waveform morphology may change in the same individual and produce different waveform morphologies in different individuals. Fowler, Bauch, and Olsen (2002) compared click-evoked ABR with both polarities using insert earphones and did not find any significant polarity-related differences in patients seen for unilateral acoustic neuromas. However, significant differences may appear with TDH-type headphones (e.g., de Lima, Alvarenga, Foelkel, Monteiro, and Agostinho, 2008). For low-frequency tone bursts, there is a clear effect of stimulus polarity on absolute latency (Fowler, 1992; Orlando and Folsom, 1995). In some cases, low-frequency tone bursts presented using a single polarity (i.e., rarefaction or condensation) may produce a stimulus-related artifact within the ABR recording. One way to counteract the stimulus artifact is to present the stimuli using an alternating polarity. An ABR threshold case in Chapter 14 demonstrates the use of alternating polarity using a 500 Hz tone burst. However, alternating polarity is not recommended for diagnosing ANSD where the presence of an abnormally large, oftentimes ringing CM would be canceled out. Instead, separate recordings using rarefaction only and condensation only polarities are required, unless the system's software has the ability to store both polarity recordings in separate buffers (Chapter 16). The advantage of this software feature is that the alternating polarity recording can later be split into rarefaction and condensation recordings.

Intensity

As described earlier in this chapter, the ABR will express its full complement of waves at moderately high intensity levels and can show up to seven waves in some cases. For neurodiagnostic purposes, intensity levels ~70 to 90 dB nHL are not uncommon. The reason for these relatively high intensity levels is to produce the largest amplitude and shortest latency waves possible. High intensities have the effect of maximally stimulating numerous auditory nerve fibers (i.e., high neural synchrony). When it is desirable to estimate behavioral thresholds on an audiogram, decreasing intensity level will subsequently cause a reduction of wave amplitudes and prolong latencies. When decreasing the intensity level, the earlier waves (e.g., waves I and III) tend to drop out first, and wave V will often remain and prolong in latency when all other waves have disappeared (Hecox and Galambos, 1974; Pratt and Sohmer, 1976). A noticeable effect of reducing the intensity on the ABR is that the spectrum will also shift to the lower frequencies.

Stimulation Rate

The general rule with stimulation rate is that there can be no more than one stimulus presented in the same analysis time window, or else overlapped and time-shifted responses will be averaged. For example, if a 10-msec window is used, then click stimuli could be presented 1 every 10-msec, or 100/s. At such a high rate, however, neural adaptation occurs that results in smaller waveforms and prolongation of waves (Eggermont and Odenthal, 1974). In conventional ABR recordings, stimuli are generally presented at rates ~10 to 40/s, usually with odd and decimal numbers (e.g., 27.7/s) to avoid multiples of the 60-Hz line noise. In some neurodiagnostic protocols (particularly for vestibular schwannoma detection), both low- and high-rate click presentations are used, with the latter being used to "stress" the auditory system and see how well it performs (e.g., **Fig. 6.1**). Whether the high-rate addition to the protocol adds another neurodiagnostic criterion is a matter of some continued speculation (Burkard and Don, 2007) because most ABRs are likely to miss tumors smaller than 1 cm and will depend on which groups of auditory nerve fibers are affected as well as the type of disorder (e.g., vestibular schwannoma vs multiple sclerosis). However, Ackley and colleagues (2006) reported a unilateral "cookie bite" hearing loss in single case study in which the initial stimulation rate of 31.1/s yielded normal ABRs bilaterally. When doubling the stimulation rate to 61.1/s, a clear asymmetry emerged in the absolute wave V between ears. Magnetic resonance imaging (MRI) later confirmed a small 6 × 10-mm vestibular schwannoma, which was later surgically removed.

Transducer Types and Artifact

The ABR can be recorded using either supraaural or insert (tubal) earphones (Van Campen et al, 1992). The rubber tube of the insert earphone introduces a 0.8- to 0.9-msec acoustic delay between the transducer box and the foam insert that is coupled to the patient's ear. The purpose of this acoustic delay is to separate in time the stimulus-related artifact produced by the transducer and the desired ABR. Another advantage of the insert earphones for ABR is the increased interaural attenuation (Killion, Wilber, and Gudmunsen, 1985; Munro and Agnew, 1999), which may help to prevent the need for contralateral masking (Beauchaine, Kaminski, and Gorga, 1987). One disadvantage of the insert earphones is that the sound pressure level differences are greater between infant and adult ears when compared with circumaural and supra-aural earphones (Voss and Herrmann, 2005). This is an especially important concern for pure-tone threshold estimation when calibration standards are based on the thresholds of adults with normal hearing (see Chapter 22). The most common insert earphones (e.g., ER-3A) are manufactured by Etymotic Research Inc. (Elk Grove, Village, IL) and have been distributed by Aearo Corporation E-A-R Auditory Systems (Indianapolis, IN) under the names E-A-RTone 3A.

The bone oscillator is often underused in ABR recordings, particularly in estimating frequency-specific thresholds in the pediatric population for diagnostic and hearing aid fitting purposes. The underuse of the bone oscillator has a variety of different reasons: (1) not knowing how or when to use it, (2) much lower output limits compared with an air conduction transducer, (3) concerns about calibration, (4) concerns about head placement and fitting, (5) stimulus-related artifact and waveform distortion (at presentation levels > 30 dB nHL), and (6) need for contralateral masking for ear-specific information. These various concerns are understandable; however, bone-conduction ABR can still provide invaluable information. Hooks and Weber (1984) were among the first to compare air (TDH-49; Telephonics Corporation, Hunington, NY) and bone conduction (Radioear Corporation B-70A, New Eagle, PA) ABRs in infants (premature). One of the most striking findings of this study is that a greater proportion of these infants had a recordable ABR at 30 and 45 dB nHL for bone conduction compared with air conduction. Small and Stapells (2003) demonstrated that the properly calibrated B-71 bone oscillator could be used with short-duration tone bursts up to 51 dB nHL at 500 Hz and ~61 to 63 dB nHL at 1000, 2000, and 4000 Hz with alternating polarity. Beyond these levels, a stimulus artifact

may be observable. Work by Small, Hatton, and Stapells (2007) on the auditory steady-state response (ASSR) suggests that assistants (clinicians or technicians) can be trained to apply the proper amount of coupling force on the bone oscillator using an elastic band (a facial band) or by handheld placement. Another potentially important finding in the Small et al (2007) study is that leaving the insert earphones in an infant while conducting evoked potential bone-conduction measurements (which usually produces an occlusion effect in adults) will not cause substantial changes in infants. Finally, contralateral masking is rarely employed, but it may be used when there is suspicion of a difference of 60 dB or greater in hearing sensitivity between ears (see Contralateral Masking section).

Monaural versus Binaural Presentation

Ear-specific (monaural) information is often desired for most ABR clinical applications. The advantage to obtaining ear-specific information is to assess the ipsilateral peripheral auditory system (cochlea and auditory nerve) up to the cochlear nuclei independently. If there is unilateral hearing loss, unilateral acoustic tumor, or unilateral auditory ANSD, ear-specific ABRs will likely produce clear and robust asymmetries. Unilateral peripheral disorders typically will also affect structures beyond the ipsilateral cochlear nucleus as can be seen in later ABR components. The presentation of the same stimulus to both ears simultaneously could be used to assess binaural interaction. For example, when clicks are presented bilaterally, the resultant ABR is the binaural interaction component (BIC) (Brantberg, Fransson, Hansson, and Rosenhall, 1999). The BIC is a difference wave obtained by recording two monaural click-evoked ABRs and then one that is binaural. The two monaural ABRs are summed (not averaged) and then subtracted from the binaural ABR. Activity seen in BIC (usually in the time range of 4–8 msec) indicates presence of the BIC. Abnormal BICs have been reported in brainstem pathology, as well as in children suspected of having auditory processing disorders (Delb, Strauss, Hohenberg, and Plinkert, 2003; Gopal and Pierel, 1999). Recently, there has been a growing interest in a modified fast-rate, binaural ABR for use in neurologic intensive care units (not neonatal intensive care unit) for the monitoring of ischemia, herniation, and increased intracranial pressure (Stone, Calderon-Arnulphi, Watson, Patel, Mander, Suss, et al, 2009). However, there are no published data to date on the sensitivity and specificity of this modified technique in patient populations.

Contralateral Masking

A common assumption is that contralateral masking is unnecessary when using insert earphones because of larger interaural attenuation values compared with supra-aural headphones. However, although there is a greater interaural attenuation for insert earphones, they do not completely eliminate the need for contralateral masking (Van Campen, Sammeth, and Peek, 1990). For most patients, this is probably true, and contralateral masking will not be required. However, if there is significant asymmetry between ears, contralateral masking may be warranted. The general rule is to employ contralateral masking anytime you think a signal will cross over. Clinicians may have the advantage of knowing the audiometric degree and configuration prior to the ABR test, and this is helpful. However, if the clinician is blind to the sensitivity of each ear, the situation becomes a bit more complex. When there is no *a priori* knowledge of audiometric degree and configuration, clinicians will often be compelled to determine which of the ears is the poorer of the two, and ABR is one way of making this determination. If there is profound or total unilateral hearing loss, stimulus levels as high as 95 dB nHL may effectively cross over, and the resultant ABR generated by the nontest ear will show a false ABR with abnormal latencies due to the time delay of crossing over the head. This is a sure sign that contralateral masking is needed. If, however, the stimulation of the poorer test ear shows a wave I with expected latency, then it can be assumed that crossover has not occurred. Because the interaural attenuation of insert earphones is ~65 dB and greater, presenting contralateral masking in the nontest ear 50 to 60 dB below the click intensity level in the test ear will generally be all that is needed, whether or not it is warranted. However, it is not recommended that contralateral

masking levels ever exceed 50 dB nHL to avoid potential central masking effects on the ABR. Munro and Agnew (1999) compared the insert earphone and supra-aural earphone and found that the insert earphone produced on average 15 to 20 dB greater interaural attention compared with the TDH-39. However, they still recommended insert earphone contralateral masking when the nontest earphone air-conduction threshold exceeded the bone conduction threshold of the same ear by 55 dB HL or more.

Typical Setup

With few exceptions, ABR parameters are largely fixed as the result of years of research study and clinical use and are already well described in Chapters 14 and 15. Clinicians should note at least three major differences between the neurodiagnostic and threshold estimation protocols. First, it is recommended to extend the analysis time window to greater than 10 msec for threshold estimation. How much to extend the analysis time will depend in part on the evoked potential system and in part on clinical preference and protocols. Analysis time windows of 15, 20, or 25 msec are often used. For neurodiagnostic purposes, a 10-msec analysis time window is usually sufficient. The second major difference is lowering the high-pass filter setting (or low-frequency cutoff) from 100 to 30 Hz for threshold estimation. Recall earlier that infants have lower-spectrum ABRs, and decreasing intensity will produce smaller ABRs that also shift to a lower-spectrum. Because the presence or absence of wave V is sought during threshold estimation, some clinicians will also lower the low-pass filter (or high-frequency cutoff) from 3000 Hz to 1500 Hz. Finally, slower stimulation rates (e.g., 11.1/s) are often desired for neurodiagnostic protocols to maximize synchrony and reduce neural habituation, whereas faster stimulation rates (e.g., 31.1/s) are often used for threshold estimations as a way to save time without considerable degradation of the waveform.

Electrode Montage

As indicated earlier, the principal ABR neural generators have certain spatial orientations and directions that often dictate the placement of electrodes. Specifically, waves I and III seem to have generators in a more horizontal arrangement, whereas wave V has a more vertical arrangement. The most common clinical placement for a one-channel ABR setup involves a high forehead placement (Fz) for the noninverting electrode and earlobe or mastoid of the stimulation ear for the inverting (reference) electrode. The ground electrode placement is a matter of preference, but it is usually placed on the contralateral ear or the lower forehead. With a one-channel montage, the clinician may need to be sure to switch the inverting and ground electrodes on the electrode headbox, depending on which ear is being stimulated.

It is customary to use a two-channel ABR setup, with a noninverting electrode on the high forehead (Fz), an inverting (reference) electrode on each earlobe or mastoid, and a ground electrode on the lower forehead. Many clinicians seem to prefer this electrode montage for at least two basic reasons: it eliminates the need to switch electrodes on the electrode headbox, and it provides the opportunity to record simultaneously both ipsilateral and contralateral ABRs to help resolve fused IV/V complexes (**Fig. 6.1**). The two-channel setup is also ideal for bone conduction ABR measurements.

Pearl

The contralateral ABR recording in a two-channel setup can be useful for neurodiagnostic purposes to assist with wave V identification in the ipsilateral recording when there is a wave IV/V complex. In many cases, the contralateral recording shows a clear split between waves IV and V, but it should have the same latencies as the ipsilateral recording (except for a missing wave I in the contralateral recording).

Although not a change in electrode montage, an ear canal reference electrode has been advocated by some for wave I enhancement (Bauch and Olsen, 1990; Brantberg, 1996; Ferraro and Ferguson, 1989). More recently, Gaddam and Ferraro (2008) suggested the use of an ear canal reference site with a modified (shortened)

TIPtrode. In this study of 45 infants, the ear canal reference produced a larger wave I, making it easier to detect wave I and calculate the I–V interwave interval. However, wave V amplitude was slightly smaller with the ear canal reference compared with the mastoid. Atcherson, Lim, Moore, and Minaya (2012) studied the effect of ear canal, earlobe, and mastoid references on the ABR in 20 young adults. Using a consistent placement at the first ear canal bend, there were no statistical differences in amplitude or latency. However, it was clear that some subjects had enhanced wave I amplitudes with an ear canal reference, and that more subjects might also have had the same results with a deeper ear canal placement. Furthermore, these authors, as well as Gaddam and Ferraro (2008), suggest that an ear canal reference takes no more time than it takes to prepare the earlobe or mastoid, yet it offers a potentially distinct neurodiagnostic advantage when implemented appropriately and consistently.

◆ Measurement Parameters

Overall Waveform Morphology

In spite of identical stimulus and recording parameters and setups, there is great interindividual variability of ABR waveform morphology, even among patients with normal hearing and intact auditory nervous systems. These interindividual differences may be due to some differences in physical anatomy and size. Some patients are physically quieter (motor and breathing activities) than others, which will affect signal-to-noise ratios (SNRs) during the averaging process. There can even be differences between ears in the same patient (**Fig. 6.4**).

Latency

Although there is interindividual variability, including waveform morphology, absolute and relative latency measures of the ABR are the most useful for neurodiagnostic applications. Latency prolongations that arise are due to neuronal slowing (injury, compression, or obstruction) and/or poor neural synchrony, including hearing loss (Eggermont, Don,

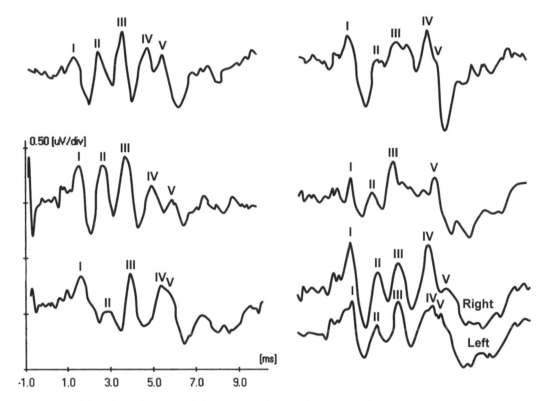

Fig. 6.4 Variability of waveform morphology in normal adults. All waveforms were collected with a Bio-Logic Navigator Pro (Natus Medical Inc., Mundelein, IL), with the same stimulation and recording parameters. The pair of waves in the bottom right-hand corner represent the ipsilateral waveforms from the right and left ears of the same person, but with different wave IV and V patterns.

and Brackmann, 1980; Musiek and Gollegly, 1985). Given that abnormal latency prolongations are what we often look for in the analysis and interpretation of ABRs, absolute latencies (time of peak appearance relative to stimulus onset), interwave (interpeak) (IWI) latencies (relative differences between subsequent peaks), and wave V interaural latency differences (ILDs or IT5) are the most commonly reported information. **Table 6.1** shows the most common latency criteria (or indices) used in neurodiagnostic ABR.

Amplitude

Amplitude measures for ABR are often the least useful because of their sensitivity to SNR conditions and the artifact rejection process. When SNRs are optimal, amplitudes are more likely to be constant during the ongoing averaging process. When they are poor, there can be drastic changes in amplitude during the

ongoing averaging process. Although absolute peak and peak-to-trough measures can be easily obtained for any of the prominent ABR waves for general normative comparison, the wave V-to-I (or V/I) amplitude ratio may have some neurodiagnostic significance (Musiek, Kibbe, Rackliffe, and Weider, 1984; Musiek, McCormick, and Hurley, 1996). The mathematical calculation is to divide wave V amplitude by wave I amplitude. That is, if waves V and I are equal, there will be a ratio of 1. If wave V is smaller than I, then the ratio will be less than 1. Typically, wave V is larger than wave I, so a significantly smaller wave V is suspect for retrocochlear lesion, but not always. A criterion of 0.75 or less has been recommended for abnormal V/I amplitude ratio (Musiek, McCormick, and Hurley, 1996). Additional information is available in **Table 6.1**.

The other most common use of ABR amplitude, without actually observing the precise amplitude value, is the tracking of various

Table 6.1 Commonly Used Neurodiagnostic Criteria for Auditory Brainstem Response

	Clinical Utility	Comments
Monaural		
Absolute latencies for waves I, III, and V	• Measurement of latency at peak relative to stimulus onset • Wave V latency may be the most useful • 1.5, 3.5, and 5.5 msec, respectively, for waves I, III, and V are commonly used, but gender-specific local norms are ideal • Any absolute latency that exceeds 2 standard deviations is considered diagnostically significant	• Take into account time delay of insert earphones compared with TDH headphones • Wave I usually unaffected by vestibular schwannomas, but can be diminished or absent in the presence of hearing loss • Though debatable, may need to consider prolongations of wave V caused by cochlear hearing loss
Interwave (interpeak) latency interval (IWI) for waves I–III, III–V, and I–V	• Calculate difference between subsequent waves • 2 msec for I–III and III–V and 4 msec for I–V are commonly used, but gender-specific local norms are ideal • Any IWI that exceeds 2 standard deviations is considered diagnostically significant	• Generally better diagnostically than absolute latencies • Depends on wave I presence (which may be absent in cochlear hearing loss)
V/I amplitude ratio	• Divide wave V amplitude by wave I amplitude • <0.75 is considered diagnostically significant	• Amplitudes can be variable and unreliable • Wave IV/V complexes can be problematic
Binaural		
Interaural latency difference (interaural latency differences or IT5) for wave V	• Calculating difference in wave V latency between ears • 0.2 to 0.4 msec is considered diagnostically significant (see Chapter 16)	• Differences in intensity between right and left earphone placements could complicate measurement • Presence of hearing loss (cochlear or conductive) could complicate measurement • Selters and Brackmann (1977) correction for hearing loss could be used

waves with each decrease in intensity for threshold estimation purposes. As the threshold is approached, wave V is often the last of the ABR complex to remain visible in the recordings. However, Bush, Jones, and Shinn (2008) conducted a pilot study to determine the feasibility and utility of comparing the click-evoked ABR threshold with a behavioral threshold as another neurodiagnostic criterion. In seven patients with MRI-confirmed vestibular schwannomas, all had an ABR-behavioral threshold difference of 30 dB or higher (mean threshold of 41.4 dB) in the diseased ear; the opposite, normal ear had a threshold difference less than 30 dB (mean threshold of 15.8 dB). Whereas other neurodiagnostic criteria fell short, identifying only five of seven patients with the vestibular schwannoma, the threshold difference approach had 100% sensitivity. Although this is a promising neurodiagnostic criterion, the evidence base is lacking at this time.

Special Consideration

The use of locally collected normative data, as opposed to published normative data, is encouraged. The basic reasons for this are that no two commercial systems are ever exactly alike (even if they are the same model) and because of potential differences in earphone/headphone combinations. Instructions on how to collect local norms are available in Chapter 3.

◆ Subject Effects

Maturation and Aging Effects

As indicated earlier, maturation has a significant effect on overall morphology of the ABR, particularly for patients younger than 2 to 3 years of age. Each peak of the ABR has a slightly different maturational time course, and infant ABRs are characteristically lower in spectral content compared with mature brainstems (Katbamna et al, 1996; Spivak, 1993). With advancing age in older adults, anatomical, physiologic, and functional changes have always been speculated to result in longer click-evoked latencies, but the data are generally mixed (cf., Costa, Benna, Bianco, Ferrero, and Bergamasco, 1990; Rowe, 1978). When high stimulation rates are used (Burkard and Sims, 2001) or gaps-in-noise stimulus are implemented (Poth, Boettcher, Mills, and Dubno, 2001), the effects of aging on the ABR can be seen more readily.

Gender

Men, especially older men, are more likely to show prolongations in the ABR, but this may be due in large part to the presence of high-frequency hearing loss. Lourenço, Oliveira, Umemura, Vargas, Lopes Kde, and Pontes Júnior (2008) retrospectively analyzed 403 patients across the life span (younger than 1 year to older than 70 years) and found that there were no obvious gender differences for interwave intervals, but male patients tended to have longer wave I, III, and V absolute latencies. One often overlooked gender-specific factor is the effect of the menstrual cycle (Al-Mana, Ceranic, Djahanbakhch, and Luxon, 2010; Elkind-Hirsch, Stoner, Stach, and Jerger, 1992), menopause (Wharton and Church, 1990), and pregnancy (Egeli and Gürel, 1997; Tandon, Misra, and Tandon, 1990) on the latencies of the ABR. Although there are some reported effects of two main hormones (estrogen and progesterone), the results are largely mixed, but they may have clinical significance for neurodiagnostic purposes.

Hearing Sensitivity

The effect of hearing sensitivity on the ABR is an important clinical consideration, but it also creates difficulties in the analysis and interpretation. Hearing losses have the effect of reducing the perceived intensity level of the stimulus, which we would assume would cause a prolongation of all or most waves of the ABR as if the clinician were decreasing the physical intensity level. The reality, however, is that this is not always the case. For instance, a patient with a low-frequency hearing loss could have a normal ABR because of the bias of click stimulus energy to the basal end of the cochlea (Don, Eggermont, and Brackmann, 1979). A patient with a moderate to severe sensorineural hearing loss could also have a normal ABR with all absolute and relative latencies within the normative range. A person with a rapidly sloping, high-frequency sensorineural hearing loss (normal lows) could produce an ABR whose wave V is prolonged, giving an impression that an acoustic tumor (e.g., vestibular schwannoma) is causing this shift (which may invariably be true with further testing). When audiometric pure-tone averages are or greater ~70 dB HL (hearing level), it is not uncommon to have absent ABRs. When the threshold at 2000 Hz is not greater than 40 dB HL, and the three frequency audiometric average is not greater than 50 dB HL, it has been reported that 80% of ABRs can be normal (Bauch and Olsen, 1988). Sensorineural hearing loss can really become a problem when one is trying to determine whether there is a unilateral acoustic tumor in the presence of hearing loss. Selters and Brackmann (1977) have suggested a technique to correct for hearing loss by subtracting 0.1 msec for every 10 dB of hearing greater than 50 dB at 4 kHz. This technique can be used with the wave V ILD (or IT5) neurodiagnostic criterion, but it is generally not recommended clinically unless there is a chance that the unilateral tumor is greater than 1 cm (Don and Kwong, 2009). Further discussion about the use of correction factors for hearing loss is offered in Chapter 16.

◆ Useful and Promising Applications

The ease of setup, good test–retest reliability, and general speed of data collection for the ABR make it one of the most desirable AEPs in widespread clinical use. However, these observations will generally only be true with optimal recording conditions, a high stimulus intensity level, a very quiet and cooperative patient, and no poorly understood or evasive neurologic disorders. When conditions are not optimal, or when there are situations when the conventional ABR will not be effective, alternative strategies become important. Advances in computing and digital signal processing have made it possible to optimize the use of the ABR where conventional techniques fall short. Many of the applications described as follows are introduced in Chapters 2 and 3 and may be used with other AEPs. Here we describe the impact of these applications for the ABR.

Waveform Enhancement without Increasing Recording Time

Although not commonplace in all clinically commercial systems, we are seeing more and more interest and development in the use of weighted averaging techniques (e.g., bayesian estimation and Kalman filtering). Weighted averaging, for ABR, offers a way to increase the SNR and potentially decrease recording time. Weighted averaging in its basic form seeks to give more mathematical weight to quieter sweeps and less to noisier sweeps for a cleaner, final averaged ABR. Maximum length sequence (MLS) is another technique that has been around (Eysholdt and Schreiner, 1982) for a while and has been explored with ABR. This technique offers a way to present click stimuli at very fast rates >500/s and not be constrained by the time window limitation (cannot present multiple stimuli in the same time window) or habituation (which can occur at stimulation rates between 50 and 100/s). Although MLS seems promising for ABR, Burkard (1994) indicates that it may not be any more time efficient or as robust as the conventional method. Nevertheless, there is still interest in the technique for infants (e.g., Li, Chen, Wilkinson, and Jiang, 2011).

Objective Detection Techniques

Although evoked potentials are considered objective measures, the reality is that for most AEPs, especially ABR, there is still subjective influence on the part of the clinician, and any confidence that is placed in

one's recordings is only as good as the quality of the recordings obtained. An objective technique incorporated into several commercially available systems is a mathematical procedure called Fsp (where sp means a single latency point). This technique is based on the commonly known statistical F-test, in which the numerator includes the variance of signal-plus-noise information from the ongoing averaged recording, and the denominator includes the variance of the noise-only information (Don, Elberling, and Waring, 1984; Sininger, 1993). When the Fsp value is high (e.g., a criterion Fsp >3.1), there is greater confidence that a signal is present and vice versa. Used for ABR threshold detection or newborn hearing screening, the Fsp technique enhances the objectivity of the ABR test and may even allow for shorter recording times by requiring fewer stimulus presentations. **Figure 6.5** illustrates the use of the click-evoked ABR Fsp technique in an adult with normal hearing. Notice at 10 dB the discrepancy in the Fsp values (objective measure) for repeated runs (e.g., 3.17 vs. 0.61), yet wave V is clearly present with both runs (subjective measure). The discrepancy may be related to differences in SNR between the two runs, and presenting more stimuli might have yielded an improved Fsp value. Another technique that uses a variation of the Fsp and a template-matching scheme is the point-optimized variance ratio (POVR) measure (Sininger, Hyde, and Don, 2001). Template matching involves the use of a target ABR waveform generated from an average of a large number of subjects. Using POVR, objective detection will be based in part on the statistical factors related to the SNR, as well as the comparison of the individual ABR to the template ABR. This is ideal for newborn hearing screening devices, and an example of the ABR template for infants can be found in Chapter 13.

> ### Pearl
>
> Objective detection techniques such as Fsp and POVR make it possible for technicians and other health professionals to participate in newborn hearing screening initiatives without undue cost and resource issues.

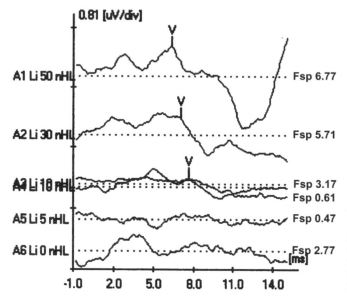

Fig. 6.5 Use of the Fsp technique as an objective detection technique for auditory brainstem response threshold estimation. See text discussion for discrepancy at 10 dB nHL.

Special Stimuli

Derived-Band and Chirp Responses

The derived-band ABR technique involves presenting a click at systematically lower high-pass noise cutoffs and subtracting certain waveforms from each other to derive frequency-specific ABRs (i.e., stimulating discrete groups of auditory nerve fibers). The derived-band ABRs show progressively longer wave V latencies that correspond to traveling wave delays. Stacked ABR is a technique that uses derived-band ABRs but uses them in a way to estimate total auditory fiber nerve activity (Don, Kwong, Tanaka, Brackmann, and Nelson, 2005). The way Stacked ABR works is to mark wave V for each derived-band ABR, artificially time-shift all the ABRs so that the wave Vs line up, and finally sum all the ABRs. The resultant Stacked ABR has been shown to be sensitive to acoustic tumors (vestibular schwannomas) 1 cm or smaller, where traditional click-evoked ABRs were likely to miss them. Several problems with Stacked ABR are (1) it takes a long time (even if automated), requiring multiple ABR recordings; (2) simultaneous presentation of the band of noise and click stimuli may cause patient discomfort; and (3) a combination of the stimulus and inability of the patient to relax may cause post-auricular muscle reflex, which can contaminate the ABR recordings. Using a reverse-engineered process based on derived-band ABRs, Elberling

and colleagues (Elberling and Don, 2008; Elberling, Don, Cebulla, and Stürzebecher, 2007) created a short-duration stimulus that quickly changes in frequency from low to high to meet the requirement of neural synchrony of a large group of fibers and does so by taking traveling wave velocity into account. This new stimulus, called a chirp, may prove to be useful for tumor detection and is a more time- and cost-effective solution to immediate and automatic initial referral for MRI. The developers of the Stacked ABR and Chirp strongly recommend the use of the ER-2 insert earphones (Etymotic Research Inc., Elk Grove Village, IL) for its broader and flatter frequency response compared to the traditional ER-3A.

> **Pitfall**
>
> Although Stacked and chirp-evoked ABRs are neurodiagnostic measures, they are at best a screening tool for possible MRI referral.

Speech-evoked Responses

Dr. Nina Kraus and her colleagues and students (current and former) in the Auditory Neuroscience Laboratory at Northwestern

University have spent considerable time, effort, and resources in studying ABR and accompanying fast Fourier transformation (FFR) to a consonant–vowel speech syllable /da/ (Johnson, Nicol, and Kraus, 2005; Skoe and Kraus, 2010). The work has converged on the development of the BioMARK (Biological Marker of Auditory Processing). Potential clinical applications of this type of ABR/FFR include diagnosis and remediation of children with auditory, language, and/or learning problems with an underlying auditory deficit. Some clinical experiences with the BioMARK are described in Chapter 17.

References

Ackley, R. S., Herzberger-Kimball, L., Burns, S., & Balew, S. D. (2006). Auditory brainstem response testing: stimulus rate revisited. Retrieved from http://www.audiologyonline.com/articles/article_detail.asp?article_id=1719.

Al-Mana, D., Ceranic, B., Djahanbakhch, O., & Luxon, L. M. (2010). Alteration in auditory function during the ovarian cycle. *Hearing Research*, 268(1–2), 114–122. PubMed

Atcherson, S.R., Lim, T.J., Moore, P.C, & Minaya, C.P. (2012). Comparison of auditory brainstem response peak measures using ear lobe, mastoid, and custom ear canal reference electrodes. *Audiology Research*, 2:e3(1), 8-11.

Bauch, C. D., & Olsen, W. O. (1988). Auditory brainstem responses as a function of average hearing sensitivity for 2,000-4,000 Hz. *Audiology*, 27(3), 156–163. PubMed

Bauch, C. D., & Olsen, W. O. (1990). Comparison of ABR amplitudes with TIPtrode and mastoid electrodes. *Ear and Hearing*, 11(6), 463–467. PubMed

Beauchaine, K. A., Kaminski, J. R., & Gorga, M. P. (1987). Comparison of Beyer DT48 and etymotic insert earphones: auditory brain stem response measurements. *Ear and Hearing*, 8(5), 292–297. PubMed

Brantberg, K. (1996). Easily applied ear canal electrodes improve the diagnostic potential of auditory brainstem response. *Scandinavian Audiology*, 25(3), 147–152. PubMed

Brantberg, K., Fransson, P. A., Hansson, H., & Rosenhall, U. (1999). Measures of the binaural interaction component in human auditory brainstem response using objective detection criteria. *Scandinavian Audiology*, 28(1), 15–26. PubMed

British Columbia Early Hearing Program (2008). *Diagnostic audiology protocol*. Accessed February 19, 2011, from http://www.phsa.ca/NR/rdonlyres/06D79FEB-D187-43-E9-91E4-8C09959F38D8/40115/aDAAGProtocols1.pdf.

Burkard, R. (1994). The use of maximum length sequences to obtain brainstem auditory evoked responses at rapid rates of stimulation. *American Journal of Audiology*, 3(3), 16–20.

Burkard, R. F., & Don, M. (2007). The auditory brainstem response. In R. F. Burkard, M. Don, & J. J. Eggermont (Eds.), *Auditory evoked potentials: Basic principles and clinical applications*. Philadelphia, PA: Lippincott Williams & Wilkins.

Burkard, R. F., & Sims, D. (2001). The human auditory brainstem response to high click rates: aging effects. *American Journal of Audiology*, 10(2), 53–61. PubMed

Bush, M. L., Jones, R. O., & Shinn, J. B. (2008). Auditory brainstem response threshold differences in patients with vestibular schwannoma: A new diagnostic index. *Ear, Nose, and Throat Journal*, 87(8), 458–462. PubMed

Costa, P., Benna, P., Bianco, C., Ferrero, P., & Bergamasco, B. (1990). Aging effects on brainstem auditory evoked potentials. *Electromyography and Clinical Neurophysiology*, 30(8), 495–500. PubMed

Delb, W., Strauss, D. J., Hohenberg, G., & Plinkert, P. K. (2003). The binaural interaction component (BIC) in children with central auditory processing disorders (CAPD). *International Journal of Audiology*, 42(7), 401–412. PubMed

de Lima, J. P., Alvarenga, Kde. F., Foelkel, T. P., Monteiro, C. Z., & Agostinho, R. S. (2008). Polarity stimulation effects on brainstem auditory evoked potentials. *Revista Brasileira de Otorrinolaringologia*, 74(5), 725–730. PubMed

Don, M., Eggermont, J. J., & Brackmann, D. E. (1979). Reconstruction of the audiogram using brain stem responses and high-pass noise masking. *Annals of Otology, Rhinology and Laryngology. Supplement*, 3(Pt 2, Suppl 57) 1–20. PubMed

Don, M., Elberling, C., & Waring, M. (1984). Objective detection of averaged auditory brainstem responses. *Scandinavian Audiology*, 13(4), 219–228. PubMed

Don, M., & Kwong, B. (2009). Auditory brainstem response: differential diagnosis. In J. Katz, L. Medwetsky, R. Burkard, & L. Hood (Eds.), *Handbook of clinical audiology*. Philadelphia, PA: Lippincott Williams & Wilkins.

Don, M., Kwong, B., Tanaka, C., Brackmann, D. E., & Nelson, R. A. (2005). The stacked ABR: A sensitive and specific screening tool for detecting small acoustic tumors. *Audiology & Neuro-Otology*, 10(5), 274–290. PubMed

Egeli, E., & Gürel, S. A. (1997). The aspect of the ABR in pregnancy. *Turkish Archives of Laryngology*, 37(1–2), 11–14.

Eggermont, J., Don, M., & Brackmann, D. (1980). Electrocochleography and auditory brain stem electric responses in patients with pontine angle tumors. *Annals of Otology, Rhinology, and Laryngology*, 89(Suppl 75), 1–19.

Eggermont, J. J., & Odenthal, D. W. (1974). Electrophysiological investigation of the human cochlea: Recruitment, masking and adaptation. *Audiology*, 13(1), 1–22. PubMed

Elberling, C., & Don, M. (2008). Auditory brainstem responses to a chirp stimulus designed from derived-band latencies in normal-hearing subjects. *Journal of the Acoustical Society of America, 124*(5), 3022–3037. PubMed

Elberling, C., Don, M., Cebulla, M., & Stürzebecher, E. (2007). Auditory steady-state responses to chirp stimuli based on cochlear traveling wave delay. *Journal of the Acoustical Society of America, 122*(5), 2772–2785. PubMed

Elkind-Hirsch, K. E., Stoner, W. R., Stach, B. A., & Jerger, J. F. (1992). Estrogen influences auditory brainstem responses during the normal menstrual cycle. *Hearing Research, 60*(2), 143–148. PubMed

Eysholdt, U., & Schreiner, C. (1982). Maximum length sequences—a fast method for measuring brain-stem-evoked responses. *Audiology, 21*(3), 242–250. PubMed

Ferraro, J. A., & Ferguson, R. (1989). Tympanic ECochG and conventional ABR: A combined approach for the identification of wave I and the I–V interwave interval. *Ear and Hearing, 10*(3), 161–166. PubMed

Fowler, C. G. (1992). Effects of stimulus phase on the normal auditory brainstem response. *Journal of Speech and Hearing Research, 35*(1), 167–174. PubMed

Fowler, C. G., Bauch, C. D., & Olsen, W. O. (2002). Diagnostic implications of stimulus polarity effects on the auditory brainstem response. *Journal of the American Academy of Audiology, 13*(2), 72–82. PubMed

Fria, T. J., & Doyle, W. J. (1984). Maturation of the auditory brain stem response (ABR): additional perspectives. *Ear and Hearing, 5*(6), 361–365. PubMed

Gaddam, A., & Ferraro, J. A. (2008). ABR recordings in newborns using an ear canal electrode. *International Journal of Audiology, 47*(8), 499–504. PubMed

Gopal, K. V., & Pierel, K. (1999). Binaural interaction component in children at risk for central auditory processing disorders. *Scandinavian Audiology, 28*(2), 77–84. PubMed

Gorga, M. P., Johnson, T. A., Kaminski, J. R., Beauchaine, K. L., Garner, C. A., & Neely, S. T. (2006). Using a combination of click- and tone burst-evoked auditory brain stem response measurements to estimate pure-tone thresholds. *Ear and Hearing, 27*(1), 60–74. PubMed

Gorga, M. P., & Thornton, A. R. (1989). The choice of stimuli for ABR measurements. *Ear and Hearing, 10*(4), 217–230. PubMed

Hecox, K., & Burkard, R. (1982). Developmental dependencies of the human brainstem auditory evoked response. *Annals of the New York Academy of Sciences, 388* (June), 538–556. PubMed

Hecox, K., & Galambos, R. (1974). Brain stem auditory evoked responses in human infants and adults. *Archives of Otolaryngology, 99*(1), 30–33. PubMed

Hooks, R. G., & Weber, B. A. (1984). Auditory brain stem responses of premature infants to bone-conducted stimuli: A feasibility study. *Ear and Hearing, 5*(1), 42–46. PubMed

Jewett, D. L., Romano, M. N., & Williston, J. S. (1970). Human auditory evoked potentials: Possible brain stem components detected on the scalp. *Science, 167*(924), 1517–1518. PubMed

Jewett, D. L., & Williston, J. S. (1971). Auditory-evoked far fields averaged from the scalp of humans. *Brain, 94*(4), 681–696. PubMed

Johnson, K. L., Nicol, T. G., & Kraus, N. (2005). Brain stem response to speech: A biological marker of auditory processing. *Ear and Hearing, 26*(5), 424–434. PubMed

Katbamna, B., Metz, D. A., Bennett, S. L., & Dokler, P. A. (1996). Effects of electrode montage on the spectral composition of the infant auditory brainstem response. *Journal of the American Academy of Audiology, 7*(4), 269–273. PubMed

Killion, M. C., Wilber, L. A., & Gudmunsen, G. I. (1985). Insert earphones for more interaural attenuation. *Hearing Instruments, 36*(2), 34–36.

Li, Z. H., Chen, C., Wilkinson, A. R., & Jiang, Z. D. (2011). Maximum length sequence brainstem auditory evoked response in low-risk late preterm babies. *Journal of Maternal-Fetal and Neonatal Medicine, 24*(3), 536–540. PubMed

Lourenço, E. A., Oliveira, M. H., Umemura, A., Vargas, A. L., Lopes Kde, C., & Pontes Júnior, A. V. (2008). Evoked response audiometry according to gender and age: Findings and usefulness. *Brazilian Journal of Otorhinolaryngology, 74*(4), 545–551. PubMed

Malinoff, R. L., & Spivak, L. G. (1990). Effect of stimulus parameters on auditory brainstem response spectral analysis. *Audiology, 29*(1), 21–28. PubMed

Møller, A. R. (2006). *Hearing: Anatomy, physiology, and disorders of the auditory system* (2nd ed.). Amsterdam: Academic Press.

Munro, K. J., & Agnew, N. (1999). A comparison of interaural attenuation with the Etymotic ER-3A insert earphone and the Telephonics TDH-39 supra-aural earphone. *British Journal of Audiology, 33*(4), 259–262. PubMed

Musiek, F. E., & Gollegly, K. M. (1985). ABR in eighth nerve and low brainstem lesions. In Jacobson, J.T. (Ed.), *The Auditory Brainstem Response.* San Diego: College Hill Press, pp. 181–202.

Musiek, F. E., Kibbe, K., Rackliffe, L., & Weider, D. J. (1984). The auditory brain stem response I–V amplitude ratio in normal, cochlear, and retrocochlear ears. *Ear and Hearing, 5*(1), 52–55. PubMed

Musiek, F. E., McCormick, C. A., & Hurley, R. M. (1996). Hit and false-alarm rates of selected ABR indices in differentiating cochlear disorders from acoustic tumors. *American Journal of Audiology, 5*(1), 90–96.

Orlando, M. S., & Folsom, R. C. (1995). The effects of reversing the polarity of frequency-limited single-cycle stimuli on the human auditory brain stem response. *Ear and Hearing, 16*(3), 311–320. PubMed

Poth, E. A., Boettcher, F. A., Mills, J. H., & Dubno, J. R. (2001). Auditory brainstem responses in younger and older adults for broadband noises separated by a silent gap. *Hearing Research, 161*(1–2), 81–86. PubMed

Pratt, H., & Sohmer, H. (1976, May). Intensity and rate functions of cochlear and brainstem evoked responses to click stimuli in man. *Archives of Oto-Rhino-Laryngology, 212*(2), 85–92. PubMed

Rowe, M. J., III. (1978). Normal variability of the brain-stem auditory evoked response in young and old adult subjects. *Electroencephalography and Clinical Neurophysiology, 44*(4), 459–470. PubMed

Salamy, A. (1984). Maturation of the auditory brainstem response from birth through early childhood. *Journal of Clinical Neurophysiology, 1*(3), 293–329. PubMed

Scherg, M., & von Cramon, D. (1985). A new interpretation of the generators of BAEP waves I-V: Results of a spatio-temporal dipole model. *Electroencephalography and Clinical Neurophysiology, 62*(4), 290–299. PubMed

Selters, W. A., & Brackmann, D. E. (1977). Acoustic tumor detection with brain stem electric response audiometry. *Archives of Otolaryngology, 103*(4), 181–187. PubMed

Sininger, Y. S. (1993). Auditory brain stem response for objective measures of hearing. *Ear and Hearing, 14*(1), 23–30. PubMed

Sininger, Y. S. (1995). Filtering and spectral characteristics of averaged auditory brain-stem response and background noise in infants. *Journal of the Acoustical Society of America, 98*(4), 2048, 2055.

Sininger, Y., Hyde, M., & Don, M. (2001). U.S. Patent No. 6,196,977 B. Washington, DC: U.S. Patent and Trademark Office.

Skoe, E., & Kraus, N. (2010). Auditory brain stem response to complex sounds: A tutorial. *Ear and Hearing, 31*(3), 302–324. PubMed

Small, S. A., Hatton, J. L., & Stapells, D. R. (2007). Effects of bone oscillator coupling method, placement location, and occlusion on bone-conduction auditory steady-state responses in infants. *Ear and Hearing, 28*(1), 83–98. PubMed

Small, S. A., & Stapells, D. R. (2003). Normal brief-tone bone-conduction behavioral thresholds using the B-71 transducer: three occlusion conditions. *Journal of the American Academy of Audiology, 14*(10), 556–562. PubMed

Sohmer, H., & Feinmesser, M. (1967). Cochlear action potentials recorded from the external ear in man. *Annals of Otology, Rhinology, and Laryngology, 76*(2), 427–435. PubMed

Spivak, L. G. (1993). Spectral composition of infant auditory brainstem responses: Implications for filtering. *Audiology, 32*(3), 185–194. PubMed

Spivak, L. G., & Malinoff, R. (1990). Spectral differences in the ABRs of old and young subjects. *Ear and Hearing, 11*(5), 351–358. PubMed

Stone, J. L., Calderon-Arnulphi, M., Watson, K. S., Patel, K., Mander, N. S., Suss, N., et al. (2009). Brainstem auditory evoked potentials—a review and modified studies in healthy subjects. *Journal of Clinical Neurophysiology, 26*(3), 167–175. PubMed

Tandon, O. P., Misra, R., & Tandon, I. (1990). Brainstem auditory evoked potentials (BAEPs) in pregnant women. *Indian Journal of Physiology and Pharmacology, 34*(1), 42–44. PubMed

Van Campen, L. E., Sammeth, C. A., Hall, J. W. III, & Peek, B. F. (1992). Comparison of Etymotic insert and TDH supra-aural earphones in auditory brainstem response measurement. *Journal of the American Academy of Audiology, 3*(5), 315–323. PubMed

Van Campen, L. E., Sammeth, C. A., & Peek, B. F. (1990). Interaural attenuation using etymotic ER-3A insert earphones in auditory brain stem response testing. *Ear and Hearing, 11*(1), 66–69. PubMed

Voss, S. E., & Herrmann, B. S. (2005). How does the sound pressure generated by circumaural, supra-aural, and insert earphones differ for adult and infant ears? *Ear and Hearing, 26*(6), 636–650. PubMed

Wilber, L. A., Kruger, B., & Killion, M. C. (1988). Reference thresholds for the ER-3A insert earphone. *Journal of the Acoustical Society of America, 83*(2), 669–676. PubMed

Wharton, J. A., & Church, G. T. (1990). Influence of menopause on the auditory brainstem response. *Audiology, 29*(4), 196–201. PubMed

Chapter 7

Frequency-Following Responses

Shaum Bhagat

An interesting property of some auditory neurons involves their tendency to fire action potentials on one phase of the acoustic waveform at low frequencies of stimulation. This property, known as phase locking, is illustrated best by examining period histograms that reveal the number of times a neuron will fire an action potential in a given period of time. For example, a period histogram may reveal that in response to a 100- Hz tone, a neuron tends to discharge action potentials on one phase of the stimulus waveform at 10-msec intervals. In this case, the timing of most of the neural discharges coincides with the period of the tone; the neuron's discharges appear to "follow" the frequency of the tone. The ability of auditory neurons to encode spectral information is limited mainly by their location and the frequency of the tone. Auditory neurons in caudal locations, such as the auditory nerve and cochlear nucleus, exhibit better phase-locking ability than neurons in more rostral locations, such as the medial geniculate body and auditory cortex. Neurons also generate better phase-locked responses to low-frequency tones than to high-frequency tones. If a signal tone is presented to an ear, low-voltage changes related to the tone are produced in the electroencephalogram (EEG) waveform. Because single auditory neurons have the capability to phase lock their discharges at low frequencies, it is not surprising that spectral information

may be found in the auditory evoked potential (AEP) waveform reflecting the phase-locked activity of an ensemble of neurons. Frequency-following responses (FFRs) are scalp-recorded potentials that exhibit positive and negative voltage peaks that mimic the cycle-by-cycle variations in sound pressure of low-frequency tones. The original description of FFRs in an animal model was provided by Worden and Marsh (1968), and the existence of FFRs in humans was confirmed in later studies (Gerken, Moushegian, Stillman, and Rupert, 1975; Moushegian, Rupert, and Stillman, 1973). Initial interest in the FFR concerned its use as a frequency-specific method to estimate hearing thresholds. However, subsequent discoveries indicating that the FFR could be recorded only for low-frequency tones presented at suprathreshold levels limited its use as an audiometric tool (Davis and Hirsh, 1976; De Boer, Machiels, and Kruidenier, 1977). Consequently, the use of FFRs in clinical applications was abandoned for several decades. However, recent research showing that FFRs can be used to document neural correlates of cochlear nonlinearities and can provide an indication of neural processing of speech sounds has rekindled interest in using the FFR in the clinic. The purpose of this chapter is to introduce the reader to the basic properties of the FFR and to highlight its emerging role as an indicator of the neural processing of complex sounds.

◆ Basic Properties of the Frequency-Following Response

The analysis of AEPs in the time domain typically involves the description of the amplitude and latency of specific waveform peaks. Frequency-domain analysis of AEPs can provide additional information that is not evident in the AEP waveform, including the amplitude and phase of particular frequency components. The benefits of frequency-domain analysis are readily apparent for AEPs that encode frequency information, such as the FFR. When evoked by a signal tone, the acquired FFR waveform is periodic, and spectral analysis of the waveform reveals a prominent peak at the signal frequency (**Fig. 7.1**).

Given the fact that the FFR waveform is similar to the signal waveform, a considerable amount of effort was spent on establishing the neurogenic origins of the FFR. The ability to rule out nonneural contributions to the generation of the FFR contributed to its acceptance as a valid measure of the neural processing of the spectral content of the signal.

Origins of the FFR

In humans, identification of the generators of the FFR has been inferred from studies that have examined the latency of the response, effects of lesions on the response, or the electrode montage used to record the FFR. Examination of response latencies has revealed two main sources that contribute to the FFR waveform. The first source exhibits a latency of ~6 to 8 msec, which is consistent with an origin within the rostral brainstem based on basilar membrane travel times and synaptic delays. The second source has a latency of ~1 msec, suggesting that the response reflects a contribution from the cochlear microphonic (CM; Batra, Kuwada, and Maher, 1986; Sohmer, Pratt, and Kinarti, 1977). Like the FFR, the CM is an electrical waveform that follows the frequency of the signal tone, but it is generated by preneural elements (outer hair cells). Evidence suggests that FFRs evoked by tones lower than 1000 Hz may be generated by both sources, but the CM dominates FFRs evoked by tones near 1000 Hz (Batra et al, 1986). The results

of studies examining the effects of specific lesions in the auditory system support multiple sources contributing to the FFR. In patients with known neurologic impairment who had absent waves IV and V of the auditory brainstem response (ABR), the short-latency FFR component was intact, and the long-latency FFR component was missing (Sohmer et al, 1977; Yamada, Marsh, and Handler, 1982). Because neurons in structures caudal to the rostral brainstem are capable of exhibiting phase-locked responses, other sources may contribute to the FFR waveform. The electrode montage used to record the FFR waveform can determine which source dominates the recording. Galbraith, Bagasan, and Sulahian (2001) recorded FFRs simultaneously with three horizontal electrode arrays and one vertical electrode array. They found that the latency of the FFR recorded in the vertical channel suggested a central brainstem origin, whereas the latency of the FFR in the horizontal channels was consistent with an origin in the auditory nerve.

Signal Effects on the FFR

As an exogenous response, the FFR is heavily dependent on signal parameters. Indeed, under the right conditions, signal artifact may masquerade as the FFR itself. This occurs when the recording electrodes act as antennas and record the electrical waveform of the signal that is being transduced by the supra-aural or insert earphones used to deliver the signal into the ear canal of the individual being tested. The astute clinician will recognize signal artifact immediately, as an artifactual FFR has no latency, and its amplitude is usually several orders of magnitude larger than the typical physiologic FFR response. To prevent signal artifact from contaminating the FFR waveform, electrically and magnetically shielded earphones are often used to deliver the signal. These transducers help to prevent the recording electrodes from detecting the signal as it is being presented.

Another concern involves limiting the contribution of the CM to the FFR waveform. If the FFR is to provide an index of neural processing of the signal, elimination or reduction of the CM is required. In the past, FFR recordings were obtained with signals that alternated in polarity, and then the FFR waveform acquired with one signal polarity was added to the FFR

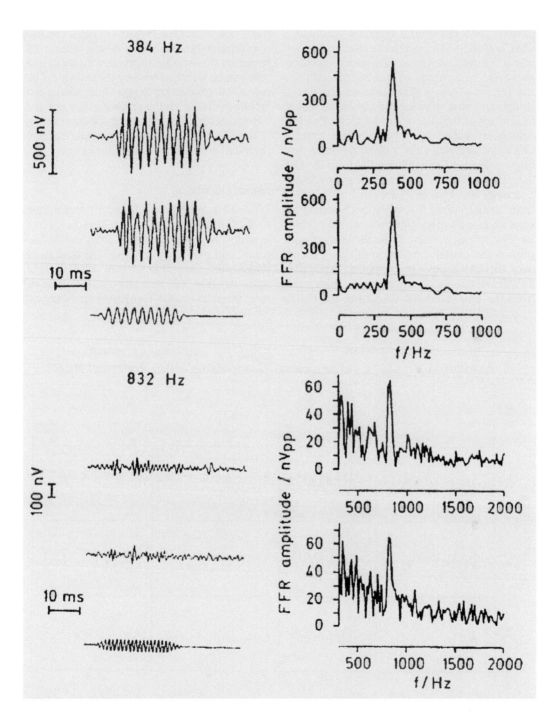

Fig. 7.1 Replicated frequency-following response (FFR) waveforms (*left panels*) and spectra (*right panels*) recorded from one individual for signals presented at 384 and 832 Hz. The acoustic signal is shown in the lower left of each panel.   (From Hoormann, J., Falkenstein, M., Hohnsbein, J., & Blanke, L. (1992). The human frequency-following response (FFR): Normal variability and relation to the click-evoked brainstem response. *Hearing Research*, 59(2), 179–188, with permission.)

waveform obtained with the opposing signal polarity. Because the CM follows the signal polarity, and the neural response essentially does not, the CM theoretically is canceled out when the two waveforms are added together. However, as a result of waveform addition, the FFR waveform is distorted and contains a component that is twice the signal frequency as a result of the lack of cancellation of neural responses evoked by opposite-phase signals. Chimento and Schreiner (1990) designed another technique to remove the CM from the FFR waveform without distorting it. They employed a strategy of subtracting a forward-masked FFR from an unmasked FFR when both responses were acquired with signals of the same polarity. This strategy assumes that the masker suppresses the neural component of the FFR, and only the CM component remains. When the forward-masked FFR waveform is subtracted from the unmasked FFR waveform, the CM is

eliminated, and the residual waveform contains the neural FFR component. A limitation of this technique is that the forward-masked FFR may not completely suppress the neural component, requiring an increase in masker intensity that may not be tolerated well by the individual being tested. In addition to preventing signal artifact from obscuring the FFR waveform and manipulating the signal to reduce the contribution of the CM, other aspects of the signal can have profound effects on the FFR waveform.

Signal Duration

FFRs can be evoked by either continuous tones or short-duration tone bursts. Tone bursts have a wider acoustic spectrum than continuous tones, and tone burst–evoked FFRs have larger amplitudes than FFRs evoked with continuous tones (**Fig. 7.2**). The effect of gating on the tone burst may also contribute to FFRs with

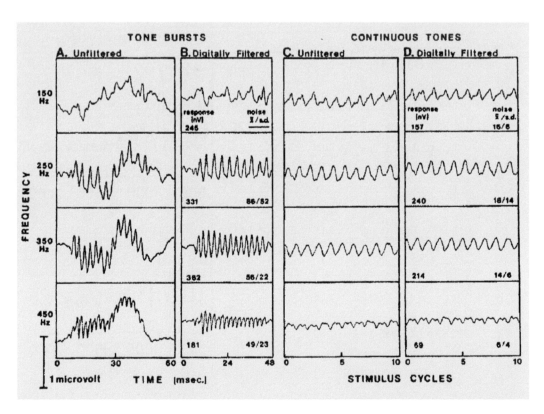

Fig. 7.2 FFR waveforms acquired with tone bursts at 150, 250, 350, and 450 Hz **(A)** before digital filtering and **(B)** after digital filtering. FFR waveforms acquired at the same frequencies with continuous tones are shown **(C)** before digital filtering and **(D)** after digital filtering. FFR amplitudes (in nanovolts) and noise floor estimates are displayed in panels **(B)** and **(D)**. (From Batra, R., Kuwada, S., & Maher, V. L. (1986). The frequency-following response to continuous tones in humans. *Hearing Research*, 21(2), 167–177, with permission.)

larger amplitudes, as the tone burst–evoked FFR waveform consists of a transient response to the onset of the burst, as well as a sustained response to the burst frequency. In contrast, the FFR evoked by a continuous tone reflects a steady-state response that is free of transients (Batra et al, 1986). The response to the onset of the burst can be reduced by increasing the rise/fall time of the signal. It is recommended that constant signal duration of at least four signal cycles be implemented when comparing FFRs obtained at different signal frequencies to allow adequate comparisons of response amplitude (Hoormann, Falkenstein, Hohnsbein, and Blanke, 1992).

Signal Frequency

The FFR amplitude is highly dependent on the signal frequency. In adults with normal hearing, the FFR amplitude increases from ~100 to 250 Hz, reaches a peak, then rapidly declines above 400 Hz, with the smallest-amplitude FFRs evident for signals between 600 and 800 Hz (**Fig. 7.3**). Peak FFR amplitudes generally occur for signals near 320 Hz (Batra et al,

1986; Hoormann et al, 1992). FFRs evoked by signals greater than 1000 Hz can be difficult to detect when the response is recorded using a vertical electrode montage.

The decline in FFR amplitude with increasing signal frequency is believed to be related to a reduction in the phase-locking ability of brainstem neurons to encode higher frequencies. Previous work examining the effects of signal frequency on the FFR has mostly used the vertical electrode montage to record the response. However, robust FFRs can be recorded to signal frequencies up to 950 Hz when the response is recorded with a horizontal electrode montage (**Fig. 7.4**). When using a horizontal electrode montage, the location of the electrodes is closer to FFR generators in the auditory nerve (Galbraith, Threadgill, Hemsley, Salour, Songdej, Ton, et al, 2000). It is believed that auditory nerve neurons exhibit better phase-locking ability at higher signal frequencies than brainstem neurons. Thus, recording FFRs with the horizontal electrode montage can extend the range of signal frequencies capable of evoking the FFR as high as 2500 Hz.

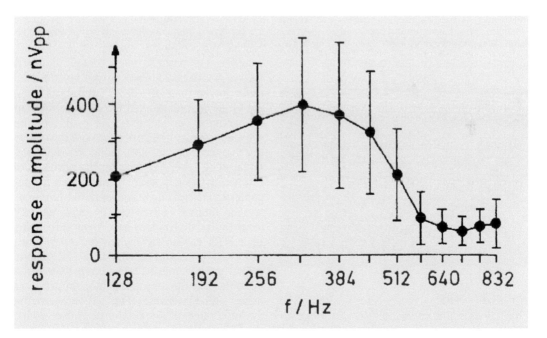

Fig. 7.3 Average FFR amplitudes from 14 individuals are plotted as a function of signal frequency. Error bars represent standard deviations. (From Hoormann, J., Falkenstein, M., Hohnsbein, J., & Blanke, L. (1992). The human frequency-following response (FFR): Normal variability and relation to the click-evoked brainstem response. *Hearing Research*, *59*(2), 179–188, with permission.)

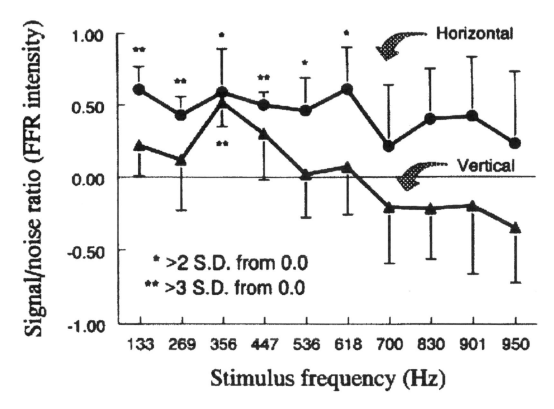

Fig. 7.4 Average FFR signal-to-noise ratios across signal frequency for horizontal electrode montage recordings (*circles*) and vertical electrode montage recordings (*triangles*). Error bars represent one standard deviation. Asterisks represent departures from the zero line by two (*) or three (**) standard deviations. (From Galbraith, G. C., Threadgill, M. R., Hemsley, J., Salour, K., Songdej, N., Ton, J., et al. (2000). Putative measure of peripheral and brainstem frequency-following in humans. *Neuroscience Letters*, 292(2), 123–127, with permission.)

Pearl

FFR can be measured using either a vertical or a horizontal electrode montage. The most appropriate montage depends on the signal frequency. A vertical montage is advantageous when measuring the response to a high low-frequency tone (<1000 Hz), whereas a horizontal montage provides the ability to record FFR to higher (up to 2500 Hz) frequencies.

Signal Intensity

The lowest signal intensity that can evoke an FFR in an individual is known as the FFR threshold. FFR thresholds can vary across individuals, but moderate signal levels are usually required to evoke the FFR at threshold. FFRs evoked by tones lower than 40 dB SL (sensation level) are often difficult to distinguish from random EEG activity. The fact that FFRs could only be evoked by signal intensities considerably above the threshold of audibility led to the FFR being replaced by other AEP tests for the purposes of estimating the audiogram in individuals not capable of participating in conventional audiometry (e.g., infants). FFRs evoked by low-frequency tones (300–500 Hz) may have lower thresholds than FFRs evoked by higher-frequency tones (600–800 Hz). Above threshold, the FFR exhibits growth with increasing signal intensity, and the periodicity of the response is more apparent at higher signal intensities (**Fig. 7.5**). However, the dynamic range of signal intensities over which the FFR amplitude increases is limited to 20 dB at 350 Hz and 10 dB at 500 Hz (Batra et al, 1986). Signal intensity levels greater than 70 dB SL can cause a reduction in the FFR amplitude.

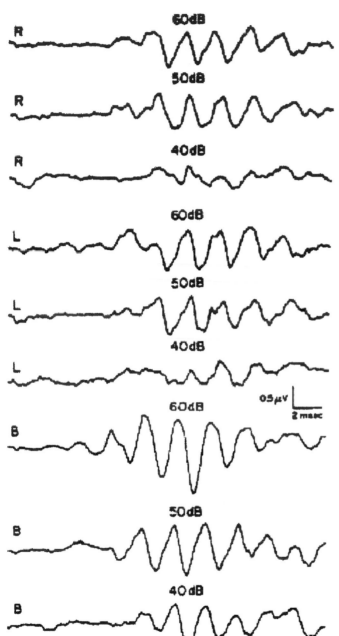

Fig. 7.5 FFR waveforms recorded to right monaural (R), left monaural (L), and binaural (B) stimulation at 500 Hz at 40 to 60 dB intensity levels. (From Ballachanda, B. B., & Moushegian, G. (2000). Frequency-following response: Effects of interaural time and intensity differences. Journal of the American Academy of Audiology, 11(1), 1–11, with permission.)

Recording the FFR

As with other AEPs, recording of the FFR waveform entails signal presentation; detection of the response with scalp electrodes; digitizing of the response; and amplification, averaging, and filtering of the response waveform. Unlike most AEPs, quantification of the FFR amplitude is benefited by examining the spectrum of the FFR waveform. This entails submitting the waveform for fast Fourier transform (FFT) analysis. The decisions of which ear to stimulate, where to place the electrodes, selection of the number of averages, and the filter settings all can affect the quality of the recording. In addition, to ensure the quality of the FFR recording, measures should be taken to rule out the contribution of signal artifacts.

Monaural versus Binaural Stimulation

FFRs can be evoked by either monaural or binaural stimulation. Usually, when examining one ear at a time, the signal tone is presented monaurally. In some individuals, asymmetries exist between right and left ear responses (Ballachanda, Rupert, and Moushegian, 1994). That is, FFR amplitudes in a given individual may be larger when the signals are presented to the right ear. In another individual, FFR amplitudes may be larger when the signal is presented to the left ear. These apparent ear differences may also interact with signal intensity to produce unique patterns of asymmetries in a given individual. The FFR can also be acquired with binaural stimulation by presenting the signal tone to both ears at once. Under these conditions, the binaural FFR amplitude is larger than the monaural FFR amplitude. However, it is less than twice the monaural FFR amplitude, indicating that the binaural FFR is not the simple sum of two monaural FFR responses (Ballachanda and Moushegian, 2000).

Electrode Placement

The most basic electrode montage for recording the FFR involves the use of a noninverting electrode, inverting electrode, and ground electrode. In a vertical electrode montage, the noninverting electrode is placed at the vertex, the inverting electrode is placed on the ipsilateral earlobe/mastoid, and the ground electrode is usually placed on the forehead. If it is suspected that the CM is contaminating the recording (the latency of the response is substantially < 6 msec), the inverting electrode may be placed on the contralateral earlobe/mastoid to reduce the contribution of the CM to the recording. Alternatively, the inverting electrode may be placed on a cervical location. A horizontal electrode montage may be selected to extend the frequency range of signals capable of evoking the FFR (**Fig. 7.6**). This entails placing the noninverting electrode on the ipsilateral earlobe/mastoid and placing

the inverting electrode on the contralateral earlobe/mastoid, with the ground electrode remaining in the same location as for the vertical electrode montage. If gold foil electrodes are available, these may be placed in the ear canals to achieve the horizontal electrode montage.

Recording Parameters

Recording the FFR waveform acquired with single tones requires instrumentation that can amplify, digitize, average, and filter the FFR waveform. Depending on signal and acquisition parameters, typical FFR amplitudes can range from tens to hundreds of nanovolts. To adequately detect this miniscule electrical activity in the midst of much larger random EEG electrical activity, the gain on the amplifier should amplify the electrical response at least 100,000 to 200,000 times. The sampling rate should be configured with knowledge that the dominant frequency in the FFR response occurs at the signal frequency. The FFR waveform may also contain significant energy at the second and third harmonics of the signal frequency, and the sampling rate on the A/D converter should be set high enough to adequately sample these FFR components. To improve the FFR signal-to-noise ratio (SNR), the FFR waveform should be averaged, with 1000 to 2000 signal sweeps typically required to obtain a quality waveform. More averages may be required for FFRs acquired with higher frequency signals. The FFR waveform acquired with tone burst signals is usually averaged over a time window equal to the duration of the signal, plus an additional 10 to 20 msec. The elongated time window allows for the response latency and the fact that the initial response occurs to the onset of the burst, and the sustained response to the signal frequency follows several cycles later. The acquired FFR waveform should be bandpass filtered, again with knowledge that the filter should encompass the dominant frequency components of the acquired FFR waveform. Because FFRs are typically not acquired with signals lower than 50 Hz or greater than 3000 Hz, bandpass filter settings of 30 to 3000 Hz are usually adequate. Following the acquisition of the FFR waveform, it is usually submitted for FFT analysis offline. Inspection of the magnitude spectrum allows for the quantification of the Fourier component

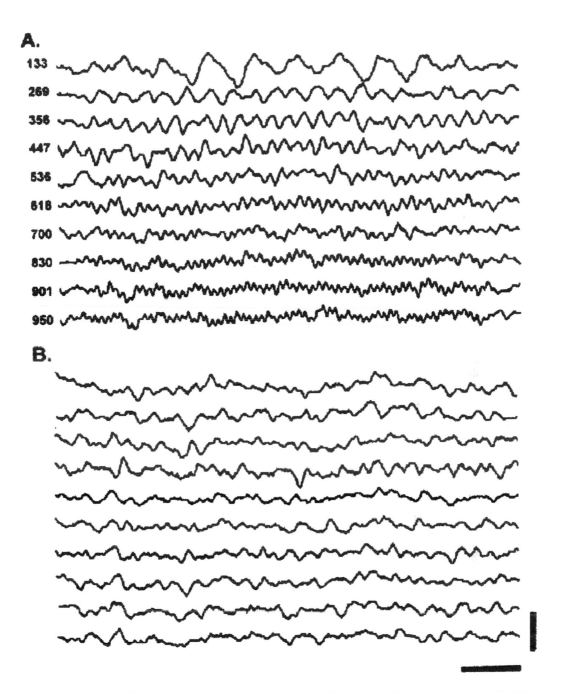

A.

133
269
356
447
536
618
700
830
901
950

B.

Fig. 7.6 Frequency-following responses waveforms acquired from one individual across signal frequencies from 133 to 950 Hz for **(A)** the horizontal electrode montage and **(B)** the vertical electrode montage. The horizontal bar equals 10 msec, and the vertical bar equals 0.5 µV. (From Galbraith, G. C., Threadgill, M. R., Hemsley, J., Salour, K., Songdej, N., Ton, J., et al. (2000) *Neuroscience Letters* 292;124, with permission.)

corresponding to the signal frequency. The typical signal and response acquisition parameters required for recording FFRs with single tones are summarized in **Table 7.1**. An additional step of ruling out signal artifact is required in the case of FFR recordings to ensure

Table 7.1 Typical Parameters for Recording Frequency-Following Responses to Single Tones

Recording Parameter	Requirements
Signal	Tone or tone burst
Number of channels	One to three
Differential amplifier gain	100,000 to 200,000
Bandpass filter	30 to 3000 Hz
Analysis time	Signal duration*
Number of averages	1000 to 2000
Artifact rejection	On

* An additional 10 to 20 msec is required.

that the acquired response is physiologic. This entails recording control FFR waveforms to compare with FFR waveforms acquired with the signal being presented to the listener's ear. To record control waveforms, the positioning of the transducer, location of the electrodes, and recording parameters should be identical to conditions when the response is being recorded with actual signals. To check for electromagnetic artifact from the recording instrumentation, the transducers should be unplugged from their connections. Signal artifact emanating from the transducers should be checked by clamping off the transducer tubing. During recording of the control waveforms, the individual being tested obviously should not hear the signal. Therefore, if the control and signal FFR waveforms are different, with the signal waveform resembling the typical FFR response, and the control waveform exhibiting random morphology unrelated to the signal, signal artifact can be ruled out. However, if the control and signal waveforms are similar or identical, both recordings likely reflect signal artifact. Additional measures must then be undertaken (e.g., changing the transducers) to ensure quality FFR recordings.

♦ Frequency-Following Response Correlates of Cochlear Nonlinearities

When two tones are presented simultaneously to an ear, the healthy cochlea processes the incoming signals nonlinearly, resulting in the creation of intermodulation distortion products. Some of this distortion escapes from the cochlea and is expressed acoustically in the ear canal as distortion-product otoacoustic emissions (DPOAEs). Cochlear distortion also evokes neural activity that ostensibly leads to the perception of aural combination tones that can be heard for certain two-tone signal combinations. The two-tone signals are referred to as the primary tones, $f1$ and $f2$, with $f2$ occurring at a higher frequency than $f1$. The distortion products occur at mathematical combinations of the primaries; the most prominent of these are the cubic difference tone (CDT) that occurs at $2f1-f2$ and the quadratic difference tone (QDT) that occurs at $f2-f1$. Apart from perceptual studies, evidence that the CDT and QDT distortion products evoke their own neural activity comes from studies that have investigated the averaged FFR waveform acquired with two-tone signals. Rickman, Chertoff, and Hecox (1991) reported that two-tone FFR waveforms obtained from electrodes placed on the scalp of adults with normal hearing were complex, and FFT analysis of the waveforms revealed spectral peaks at the $f1$ and $f2$ frequencies. Spectral peaks were also identified at the CDT and QDT distortion-product frequencies (**Fig. 7.7**).

The presence of these distortion-product FFRs (dp-FFRs) suggested that neurons at the level of the auditory nerve or brainstem were phase locking their discharges at the CDT and QDT frequencies. Several studies have replicated these findings, indicating that dp-FFRs are evident for low-frequency primary tones in individuals with normal hearing (Bhagat and Champlin, 2004; Elsisy and Krishnan, 2008; Krishnan, 1999; Pandya and Krishnan, 2004; Purcell, John, and Picton, 2003). Additional knowledge concerning the effects of primary-tone frequency, primary-tone ($f2/f1$) ratio, contralateral noise, and primary-tone level on dp-FFRs has been acquired that has both supported the conjecture concerning the cochlear origin of some of these responses and enabled comparisons with DPOAEs.

Primary-Tone Frequency

At $f1$ frequencies in the range of 500 to 800 Hz in adults with normal hearing, the dp-FFR at the QDT frequency is larger than at the

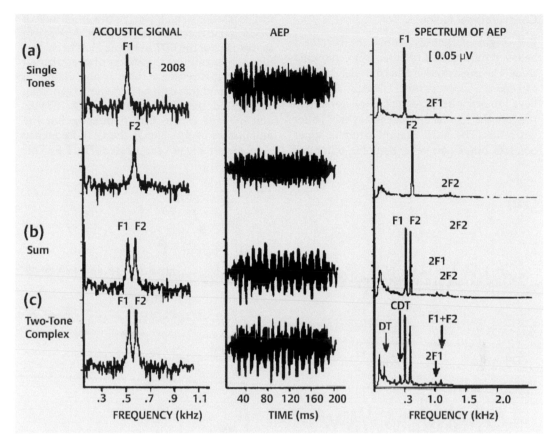

Fig. 7.7 Acoustic signals, FFR waveforms, and FFR spectra acquired from an individual are displayed for **(A)** single tones, **(B)** summed responses, and **(C)** the two-tone complex. The distortion-product frequency-following responses (dp-FFRs) at the cubic difference tone (CDT) and quadratic difference tone (QDT) frequencies are only evident for the two-tone complex condition. (From Rickman, M. D., Chertoff, M. E., & Hecox, K. E. (1991) Electrophysiological evidence of nonlinear distortion products to two-tone stimuli. *Journal of the Acoustical Society of America*, 89(6), 2818–2826, with permission.)

CDT frequency (Bhagat and Champlin, 2004; Rickman et al, 1991). The dp-FFR amplitude at the QDT frequency decreases, and the dp-FFR amplitude at the CDT frequency is largely unaffected by raising the $f1$ frequency from 510 to 800 Hz (Rickman et al, 1991). The dp-FFRs are generally less robust for $f1$ frequencies greater than 1000 Hz, and to date dp-FFRs have been recorded up to $f1 = 1400$ Hz at the CDT frequency and up to $f1 = 3515$ Hz at the QDT frequency (Pandya and Krishnan, 2004; Purcell et al, 2003). The reduction in dp-FFR amplitudes for primary-tone frequencies greater than 1000 Hz may be partially attributed to a decline in phase-locking ability at higher frequencies seen in brainstem neurons.

Primary-Tone (f_2/f_1) Ratio

Similar to DPOAEs, the amplitude of the dp-FFR at the CDT frequency depends on the $f2/f1$ ratio. An increase in amplitude is observed as the ratio is increased from 1.16 to 1.46. The peak amplitude for dp-FFRs at the CDT frequency occurs at a $f2/f1$ ratio between 1.36 and 1.46 (Rickman et al, 1991). This suggests that the degree of primary-tone interaction along the basilar membrane within the cochlea influences the generation of CDT distortion products that initiate phase-locked neuronal discharges. In contrast, the amplitude of dp-FFRs at the QDT frequency is not dependent on the $f2/f1$ ratio (Rickman et al, 1991).

Contralateral Noise

The origin of DPOAEs within the cochlea is believed to be linked to outer hair cell oscillations. The presentation of a contralateral noise can cause a suppression of DPOAEs. This is believed to occur because the contralateral noise triggers the medial olivocochlear (MOC) efferent reflex. The MOC efferent neurons hyperpolarize outer hair cells, damping outer hair cell oscillations and lowering the amplitude of DPOAEs. Further evidence of a cochlear origin for dp-FFRs at the CDT frequency has been provided by examining the effects of contralateral noise on this response. Bhagat and Champlin (2004) found that contralateral noise generally suppressed the amplitudes of both DPOAEs and dp-FFRs at the CDT frequency, but the amplitudes of dp-FFRs at the QDT frequency were essentially not suppressed (**Fig. 7.8**). This

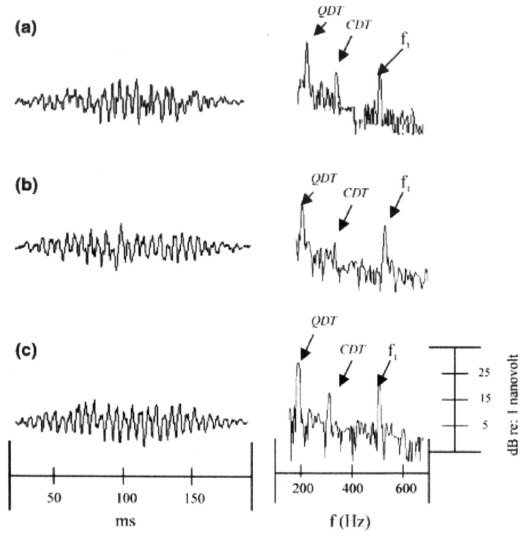

Fig. 7.8 Three consecutive dp-FFR measurements from one individual. The primary tones were at f_1 = 500 Hz and f_2 = 690 Hz. The dp-FFR waveforms are depicted in the left panels, and spectra are depicted in the right panels. Waveforms in **(A)** and **(C)** were acquired without contralateral noise. The waveform in **(B)** was acquired with contralateral noise at 60 dB SPL (sound pressure level). The dp-FFR at the CDT frequency was suppressed by the contralateral noise. (From Bhagat, S. P., & Champlin, C. A. (2004). Evaluation of distortion products by the human auditory system. *Hearing Research*, *193*(1–2), 51–67, with permission.)

suggested that activation of the MOC efferent reflex inhibited CDT distortion products generated within the cochlea, which led to a decrease in the phase-locked neuronal discharges responsible for the appearance of the dp-FFR in the averaged waveform. The lack of effect on the dp-FFR at the QDT frequency suggested that this response may not arise solely from a cochlear nonlinearity.

Primary-Tone Level

Evidence indicating that dp-FFRs at the CDT frequency may arise from a cochlear nonlinearity has also been provided by studies that have examined the growth of the response with increasing primary-tone level. Pandya and Krishnan (2004) found that dp-FFR input-output functions in three primary-tone regions less than 2000 Hz were compressive, whereas more linear growth was found for FFRs phase-locked to the $f1$ and $f2$ frequencies. The amplitudes of the dp-FFRs were smaller than FFRs that were phase-locked to the $f1$ frequency for primary-tone levels from 65 to 95 dB SPL (sound pressure level). However, dp-FFR responses could often be identified at the lowest primary-tone level. The growth functions for dp-FFRs at the CDT frequency were qualitatively similar to the type of compressive growth functions exhibited by DPOAEs. Elsisy and Krishnan (2008) made direct comparisons between DPOAE and dp-FFR growth patterns by simultaneously recording both responses together. They measured growth functions at the same CDT frequency (388 Hz) for primary tones presented from 40 to 70 dB HL. Both responses exhibited nonlinear growth, but the dp-FFR functions were more compressive than the DPOAE functions. In addition, dp-FFRs could be identified at lower primary-tone levels compared with DPOAEs. This suggested that measuring dp-FFRs could be a viable alternative to DPOAEs in examining cochlear nonlinearities at low frequencies.

Recommendations for Recording Distortion-Product Frequency-Following Responses

Clinicians interested in recording dp-FFRs will find that the procedure and instrumentation are similar to what is needed to record

conventional FFRs to single tones, with certain exceptions. A transducer capable of presenting two tones simultaneously is obviously required. I prefer that the electrical waveforms of each primary tone be transduced separately and mixed acoustically in the ear canal by the transducer. It is also preferable that the transducer have electrical and magnetic shielding, which can be accomplished by placing shielding materials (such as mu-metal) on the transducer itself and on its cables. Because any transducer can generate distortion itself, the purity of the pure-tone signals should be checked. This can be accomplished by turning on the primary-tone signals, placing the transducer in an acoustic coupler, connecting the coupler to the microphone of a sound-level meter, and sending the output from the sound-level meter to a spectrum analyzer. Ideally, any harmonic or intermodulation distortion products identified should be at least 60 dB below the level of the primary tones. This significantly increases the likelihood that any distortion products present in the averaged FFR waveform originated from distortion occurring in the ear, rather than distortion coming from the transducer. If the primaries are tone bursts, the duration of the tone bursts can affect the time required to average the FFR waveform. Although short-duration tone bursts (~50 msec) can shorten the time required to acquire the waveform, I prefer to use longer duration tone bursts (~200 msec). Longer tone bursts evoke more robust dp-FFRs at the CDT and QDT frequencies (**Fig. 7.9**). As with conventional FFRs, it is important to rule out the contribution of signal artifact by recording control waveforms. Control waveforms can be recorded by unplugging the transducers and clamping transducer tubing, as was recommended for conventional FFR recordings. The recording instrumentation can introduce electromagnetic intermodulation distortion; therefore, it is important to determine that the averaged FFR waveform containing distortion products is "clean" and free of distortional artifact (**Fig. 7.10**).

The dp-FFR waveform is typically acquired using the same recording parameters as conventional FFRs. Given that dp-FFRs are smaller in amplitude than FFRs evoked by signal tones, the electrical waveform recorded by the electrodes may be increased up to 300,000 times by the

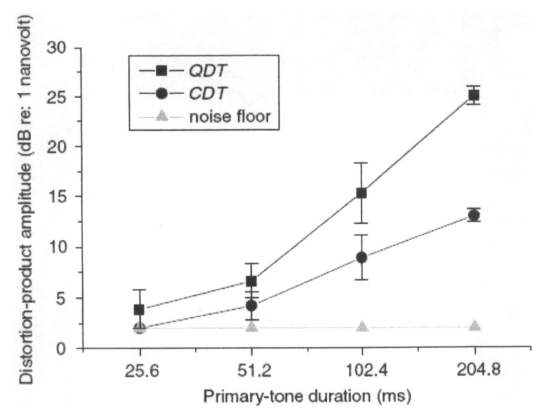

Fig. 7.9 Average dp-FFR amplitudes at the quadratic difference tone (QDT) frequency (*squares*) and cubic difference tone (CDT) frequency (*circles*) are shown for four primary-tone durations. Error bars represent one standard error. Noise floor estimates (*triangles*) at each duration are also depicted. (From Bhagat, S. P., & Champlin, C. A. (2004). Evaluation of distortion products by the human auditory system. *Hearing Research, 193*(1–2), 51–67, with permission.)

amplifier to accommodate detection of smaller responses. A larger number of averages may also be used to enhance the SNR of the dp-FFR waveform. The typical signal and response acquisition parameters required for recording dp-FFRs are summarized in **Table 7.2**.

Pearl

Use of mu-metal shielding of transducers will help to minimize stimulus-related artifact. In the absence of mu-metal shielding, it is important to consider "dry runs" with insert earphone tubing clamped and/or earphones unplugged to that ensure your recording is the desired response waveform rather than signal artifact.

Clinical Applications of Distortion-Product Frequency-Following Responses

Previous work investigating dp-FFRs has focused on examining the response in adults with normal hearing. The dp-FFR has untapped potential as a diagnostic test that may be used to supplement information provided by DPOAE tests. Because DPOAE levels are often at or below the level of the noise floor for primary tones lower than 1000 Hz, the dp-FFR test potentially offers a better means to examine cochlear function at low frequencies. Currently, clinical dp-FFR studies in individuals with known cochlear hearing loss have yet to be initiated. Developmental studies of the dp-FFR, tracking the response from infancy to early childhood, would also be useful and could be compared with

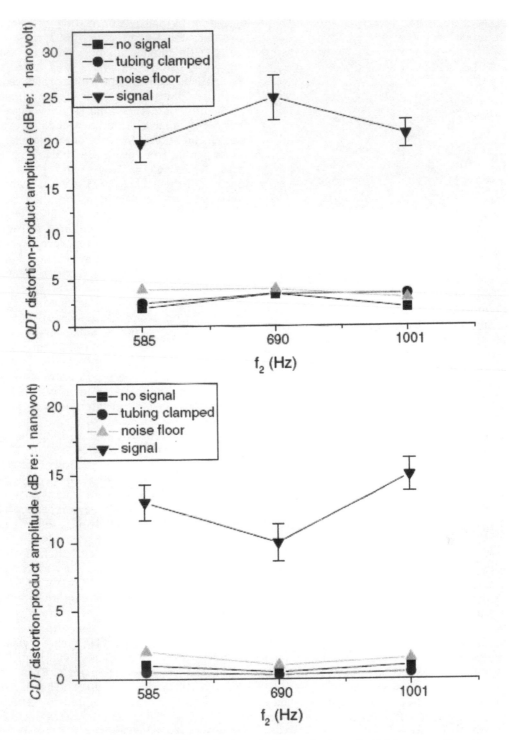

Fig. 7.10 A comparison of averaged dp-FFR amplitudes for control (*circles and squares*) and signal (*inverted triangle*) conditions measured in three individuals. Noise floor estimates (*triangles*) are also shown. Top panel: dp-FFR amplitudes at the QDT frequency. Bottom panel: dp-FFR amplitudes at the CDT frequency. (From Bhagat, S. P., & Champlin, C. A. (2004). Evaluation of distortion products by the human auditory system. *Hearing Research*, *193*(1–2), 51–67, with permission.)

Table 7.2 Typical Parameters for Recording Distortion-Product Frequency-Following Responses

Recording Parameter	Requirements
Signal	Two-tone complex
Number of channels	One to three
Differential amplifier gain	200,000 to 300,000 ×
Bandpass filter	30 to 3000 Hz
Analysis time	Signal duration*
Number of averages	≥ 2000
Artifact ejection	On

*An additional 10 to 20 msec is typically required.

developmental studies of DPOAEs. Possible factors that may confound efforts to fully apply dp-FFRs clinically include their high response thresholds and low-frequency range. Efforts designed to extend the capability of recording dp-FFRs at lower intensity levels and at higher frequencies, including the use of horizontal electrode montages, may assist in the inclusion of the dp-FFR test as a useful tool in the AEP diagnostic test battery.

♦ Frequency-Following Responses as Neuronal Indicators of Brainstem Speech Processing

It is clear that the spectra of English vowels contain formant peaks and that listeners rely on the identification of the formants to distinguish between different vowels. Insight into the neural processing underlying perception has been provided by studies examining FFRs acquired with vowel-like sounds. Krishnan (1999) collected FFR waveforms from listeners with normal hearing that were acquired in response to two-tone signals designed to resemble formant frequencies found in common English vowels. Spectral analysis of these FFR waveforms revealed spectral peaks that corresponded well with the first and second formant frequencies. These findings suggested that brainstem neurons were capable of

encoding frequency information pertaining to different vowels. Krishnan (2002) elaborated upon the previous findings with two-tone signals by using three synthesized vowels to record FFRs in listeners with normal hearing. Harmonics near the first two formant frequencies of each synthesized vowel were easily recognized in the spectral analyses of the FFR waveforms, and the peaks were larger for synthesized vowels presented at higher intensity levels (**Fig. 7.11**). The fact that the spectra of the averaged FFR waveforms preserve important frequency information near the first and second formant frequencies of the synthesized vowels reinforces the idea that neurons at the brainstem level are capable of exhibiting phase-locked discharges to complex signals, such as speech sounds. Although vowel identification and discrimination are probably highly dependent on ensemble neuronal activity in cortical regions of the cortex, accurate representations of the vowels in neuronal output from brainstem neurons may facilitate these perceptual processes. Speech perception studies have shown that under certain conditions, the first formant of vowels can interfere with identification of the second formant. Krishnan and Agrawal (2010) used two-tone analogs of vowel formant frequencies to record FFRs and found that lowering the level of the first formant tone or increasing the spectral distance between the formant tones enhanced the amplitude of the FFR spectral peak corresponding to the second formant tone. These findings may shed light on the neuronal processes at the brainstem level that possibly contribute to formant masking and release from formant masking.

Additional information on the encoding of speechlike sounds has been provided by the speech-evoked brainstem response elicited by a synthesized /da/ speech syllable (Chandrasekaran and Kraus, 2010; Hornickel, Skoe, and Kraus, 2009; Krizman, Skoe, and Kraus 2010; Russo et al 2004). The electrophysiologic waveform acquired in response to the /da/ syllable contains a transient response to the syllable onset and a sustained FFR related to the fundamental frequency of the syllable and its harmonics (**Fig. 7.12**). Interpreting the morphology of the speech-evoked brainstem response is complicated,

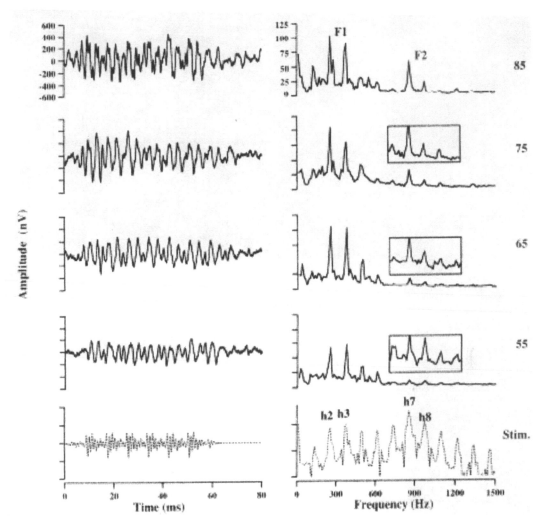

Fig. 7.11 Grand averaged FFR waveforms (*left panels*) and FFR spectra (*right panels*) for the synthesized vowel /u/ at intensities from 55 to 85 dB nHL (normal hearing level). The acoustic signal is displayed at the bottom of the left and right panels. (From Krishnan, A. (2002). Human frequency-following responses: Representation of steady-state synthetic vowels. *Hearing Research*, *166*(1–2), 192–201, with permission.)

but it is believed that the transient component is indicative of neuronal processing of rapid transitions in the/da/syllable, whereas the FFR reflects processing of voicing in the syllable. Under quiet conditions, both the transient and FFR components are evident, but the addition of background noise sharply attenuates the transient component, whereas the FFR remains (Russo et al, 2004). The transient component of the speech-evoked brainstem response also exhibits greater decline with rapid presentation rates of the syllable than the FFR component phase-locked to the fundamental frequency of the syllable. Like the transient response, higher-frequency components in the FFR are vulnerable to higher rates, suggesting that the neural generators of the speech-evoked FFR are diffuse (Krizman et al, 2010). Different neural tracts within the brainstem are the most likely candidates, as several lines of evidence indicate that the speech-evoked FFR does not originate from cochlear or cortical sources (Chandrasekaran and Kraus, 2010). Therefore, the

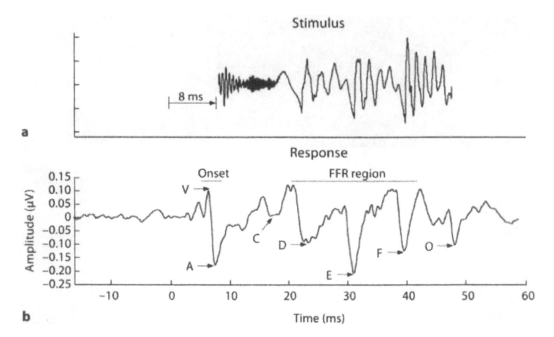

Fig. 7.12 (A) The /da/ signal waveform and **(B)** the speech-evoked brainstem response waveform from one individual. The onset and FFR regions of the speech-evoked brainstem response are indicated. (From Hornickel, J., Skoe, E., & Kraus, N. (2009). Subcortical laterality of speech encoding. *Audiology and Neuro-Otology, 14*(3), 198–207, with permission.)

speech-evoked FFR offers a means to examine speech processing in the brainstem. It is widely accepted that the left cortical hemisphere of the brain in most individuals is specialized to process speech and language. Behavioral dichotic listening studies have indicated that a right ear advantage exists for linguistic stimuli, consistent with the left cortical hemisphere specialization. Using the speech-evoked brainstem response to explore this topic in subcortical neurons, Hornickel et al (2009) found shorter waveform latencies and more robust FFR components were evident when the /da/ syllable was presented to right ears compared with left ears.

✦ Summary

The two best known electrophysiologic responses originating from the brainstem are the ABR and the FFR. The ABR provides information concerning the neural response to transient signals and can be recorded at near-threshold levels. It has numerous applications and is the most commonly used AEP in the clinic. In contrast, the FFR provides information concerning the neural response to longer steady-state signals, can be recorded only at levels considerably above threshold, and has largely been ignored in the clinical arena. Recent innovations in evoking, recording, and analyzing the FFR have rekindled interest in its clinical applications. Preliminary clinical studies have shown that the FFR can document the effects of aging on pitch perception (Clinard, Tremblay, and Krishnan, 2010) and may provide an objective measure to distinguish between language-impaired children and their typically developing peers (Basu, Krishnan, and Weber-Fox, 2010; Wible, Nicol, and Kraus, 2004). Confirmation of this preliminary work is warranted and will enable the FFR to transition from the research laboratory to the clinic.

References

Ballachanda, B. B., & Moushegian, G. (2000). Frequency-following response: Effects of interaural time and intensity differences. *Journal of the American Academy of Audiology, 11*(1), 1–11. PubMed

Ballachanda, B. B., Rupert, A., & Moushegian, G. (1994). Asymmetric frequency-following responses. *Journal of the American Academy of Audiology, 5*(2), 133–137. PubMed

Basu, M., Krishnan, A., & Weber-Fox, C. (2010). Brainstem correlates of temporal auditory processing in children with specific language impairment. *Developmental Science, 13*(1), 77–91. PubMed

Batra, R., Kuwada, S., & Maher, V. L. (1986). The frequency-following response to continuous tones in humans. *Hearing Research, 21*(2), 167–177. PubMed

Bhagat, S. P., & Champlin, C. A. (2004). Evaluation of distortion products produced by the human auditory system. *Hearing Research, 193*(1–2), 51–67. PubMed

Chandrasekaran, B., & Kraus, N. (2010). The scalp-recorded brainstem response to speech: Neural origins and plasticity. *Psychophysiology, 47*(2), 236–246. PubMed

Chimento, T. C., & Schreiner, C. E. (1990). Selectively eliminating cochlear microphonic contamination from the frequency-following response. *Electroencephalography and Clinical Neurophysiology, 75*(2), 88–96. PubMed

Clinard, C. G., Tremblay, K. L., & Krishnan, A. R. (2010). Aging alters the perception and physiological representation of frequency: Evidence from human frequency-following response recordings. *Hearing Research, 264*(1–2), 48–55. PubMed

Davis, H., & Hirsh, S. K. (1976). The audiometric utility of brain stem responses to low-frequency sounds. *Audiology, 15*(3), 181–195. PubMed

De Boer, E., Machiels, M. B., & Kruidenier, C. (1977). Low-level frequency-following response. *Audiology, 16*(3), 229–240. PubMed

Elsisy, H., & Krishnan, A. (2008). Comparison of the acoustic and neural distortion product at 2f1-f2 in normal-hearing adults. *International Journal of Audiology, 47*(7), 431–438. PubMed

Galbraith, G. C., Bagasan, B., & Sulahian, J. (2001). Brainstem frequency-following response recorded from one vertical and three horizontal electrode derivations. *Perceptual and Motor Skills, 92*(1), 99–106. PubMed

Galbraith, G. C., Threadgill, M. R., Hemsley, J., Salour, K., Songdej, N., Ton, J., et al. (2000). Putative measure of peripheral and brainstem frequency-following in humans. *Neuroscience Letters, 292*(2), 123–127. PubMed

Gerken, G. M., Moushegian, G., Stillman, R. D., & Rupert, A. L. (1975). Human frequency-following responses to monaural and binaural stimuli. *Electroencephalography and Clinical Neurophysiology, 38*(4), 379–386. PubMed

Hoormann, J., Falkenstein, M., Hohnsbein, J., & Blanke, L. (1992). The human frequency-following response (FFR): Normal variability and relation to the click-evoked brainstem response. *Hearing Research, 59*(2), 179–188. PubMed

Hornickel, J., Skoe, E., & Kraus, N. (2009). Subcortical laterality of speech encoding. *Audiology and Neuro-Otology, 14*(3), 198–207. PubMed

Krishnan, A. (1999). Human frequency-following responses to two-tone approximations of steady-state vowels. *Audiology and Neuro-Otology, 4*(2), 95–103. PubMed

Krishnan, A. (2002). Human frequency-following responses: representation of steady-state synthetic vowels. *Hearing Research, 166*(1–2), 192–201. PubMed

Krishnan, A., & Agrawal, S. (2010). Human frequency-following response to speech-like sounds: Correlates of off-frequency masking. *Audiology and Neuro-Otology, 15*(4), 221–228. PubMed

Krizman, J. L., Skoe, E., & Kraus, N. (2010). Stimulus rate and subcortical auditory processing of speech. *Audiology and Neuro-Otology, 15*(5), 332–342. PubMed

Moushegian, G., Rupert, A. L., & Stillman, R. D. (1973). Laboratory note: Scalp-recorded early responses in man to frequencies in the speech range. *Electroencephalography and Clinical Neurophysiology, 35*(6), 665–667. PubMed

Pandya, P. K., & Krishnan, A. (2004). Human frequency-following response correlates of the distortion product at 2F1-F2. *Journal of the American Academy of Audiology, 15*(3), 184–197. PubMed

Purcell, D. W., John, M. S., & Picton, T. W. (2003). Concurrent measurement of distortion product otoacoustic emissions and auditory steady state evoked potentials. *Hearing Research, 176*(1–2), 128–141. PubMed

Rickman, M. D., Chertoff, M. E., & Hecox, K. E. (1991). Electrophysiological evidence of nonlinear distortion products to two-tone stimuli. *Journal of the Acoustical Society of America, 89*(6), 2818–2826. PubMed

Russo, N., Nicol, T., Musacchia, G., & Kraus, N. (2004). Brainstem responses to speech syllables. *Clinical Neurophysiology, 115*(9), 2021–2030. PubMed

Sohmer, H., Pratt, H., & Kinarti, R. (1977). Sources of frequency following responses (FFR) in man. *Electroencephalography and Clinical Neurophysiology, 42*(5), 656–664. PubMed

Wible, B., Nicol, T., & Kraus, N. (2004). Atypical brainstem representation of onset and formant structure of speech sounds in children with language-based learning problems. *Biological Psychology, 67*(3), 299–317. PubMed

Worden, F. G., & Marsh, J. T. (1968). Frequency-following (microphonic-like) neural responses evoked by sound. *Electroencephalography and Clinical Neurophysiology, 25*(1), 42–52. PubMed

Yamada, O., Marsh, R. R., & Handler, S. D. (1982). Contributing generator of frequency-following response in man. *Scandinavian Audiology, 11*(1), 53–56. PubMed

Chapter 8

Development of Auditory Steady-State Responses

Elizabeth D. Leigh-Paffenroth

The auditory steady-state response (ASSR) is an auditory evoked potential (AEP) that is phase-locked to the amplitude or frequency modulations in a steady-state signal. The neural response elicited by the steady-state signal reflects the rate of stimulus modulation. The first ASSR was described by Galambos, Makeig, and Talmachoff (1981) as the 40-Hz response composed of the superimposition of the Na-Pa components of the middle latency response (MLR) evoked by clicks and short-duration tone bursts presented every 25 msec (**Fig. 8.1**). Galambos et al (1981) showed that the 40-Hz response could be reliably recorded at stimulus levels near behavioral thresholds for audiometric frequencies. The amplitude of the 40-Hz response decreased as stimulus intensity was reduced, and the amplitude-intensity function was steepest near threshold. These results showed promise for the use of the 40-Hz response as an objective tool for estimating hearing sensitivity (Picton, John, Dimitrijevic, and Purcell, 2003).

The 40-Hz event-related potential (ERP) is an example of a steady-state response (SSR) in the MLR when the carrier frequency is presented at a rate near 40 Hz. The discovery of the ASSR at 40 Hz provided an opportunity for investigators to further explore the clinical usefulness of such responses. To date the ASSR has been used for threshold estimation (Chambers and Meyer, 1993; Lins, Picton, Boucher, Durieux-Smith, Champagne, Moran, et al, 1996; Mauer, Döring, Hamacher, and Bell, 1997; Ménard, Gallego, Truy, Berger-Vachon, Durrant, and Collet, 2004; Picton, Dimitrijevic, Perez-Abalo, and van Roon, 2005; Rance, Roper, Symons, Moody, Poulis, Dourlay, et al, 2005; Stapells, Linden, Suffield, Hamel, and Picton, 1984; Swanepoel and Erasmus, 2007; Vander Werff and Brown, 2005; Yang, Chen, and Hwang, 2008) and supra-threshold measures of complex stimuli (Cone and Garinis, 2009; Dimitrijevic, John, and Picton, 2004; Dimitrijevic, John, van Roon, Purcell, Adamonis, Ostroff, et al, 2002; Grose, Mamo, and Hall, 2009; Leigh-Paffenroth and Fowler, 2006). Other steady-state AEPs are the cochlear microphonic (CM) and the frequency-following response (FFR). What is now generally referred to as the ASSR has also previously been described as the amplitude-modulated following response (AMFR), the envelope-following response (EFR), the steady-state response (SSR), and the auditory steady-state evoked potential (ASSEP).

This chapter covers a review of the literature related to and should assist clinicians in obtaining a basic understanding of ASSRs. Although some information is presented later on clinical applications, readers are directed to Chapter 15 for more practical information on collecting ASSRs in the clinic.

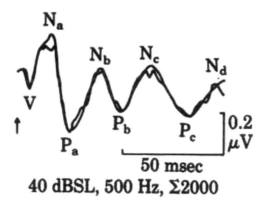

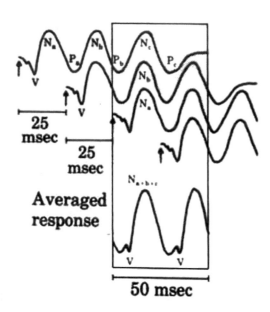

Fig. 8.1 The auditory 40-Hz response as the original steady-state response. The top portion of the figure shows a normal middle latency response (MLR) to a 500-Hz tone burst. The bottom portion of the figure illustrates how overlapping MLR waveforms form the basis of the 40-Hz response when stimuli are presented every 25 msec. The inset box shows how one repeating component of the 40-Hz response is likely composed of summed Na, Nb, and Nc components of consecutive and overlapping MLRs. (From Galambos, R., Makeig, S., & Talmachoff, P. J. (1981). A 40 Hz auditory potential recorded from the human scalp. *Proceedings of the National Academy of Science USA*, *78*(4), 2643–2647, with permission by Scott Makeig, PhD.)

♦ Description

SSRs such as the CM, FFR, and ASSR are different from transient responses, such as the auditory brainstem response (ABR), MLR, and late-evoked cortical potentials (e.g., P1, N1, P2, and P300). Steady-state potentials are sustained responses that maintain amplitude and phase over extended stimulus presentations and recording time. Transient potentials are responses that fluctuate in amplitude and latency with multiple stimulus presentations (Plourde, Stapells, and Picton, 1991). The transient response occurs when the presentation rate of the stimulus allows for the neural generators to recover from one stimulus event before the next stimulus event is presented. The steady-state response occurs when the presentation rate of a stimulus is fast enough to create overlapping responses to the stimulus. The transient responses and the SSRs may have similar neural generators or functionally different neural generators that could provide independent information about auditory processing. It is because the auditory system is not completely linear that the transient responses and the SSRs are unique when compared with one another. In contrast to CM and FFR, ASSRs are analyzed more commonly in the frequency domain using automated detection algorithms rather than in the time domain by reading the evoked potential waveforms. In other words, clinicians will rely more on the results of spectral or phase analysis techniques. These analysis techniques are described later in this chapter, as well as in Chapters 3 and 15.

The ASSR stimulus consists of a pure tone modulated at a specific rate and at a specific depth of modulation. That is, there is a carrier frequency (f_c), a modulation frequency (f_m), and a modulation depth (% modulation) for each steady-state signal. Each of these stimulus characteristics can be manipulated independently and will produce a more or less robust response in any given listener. The result is an electrical response recorded from the scalp that mimics, or follows, the temporal and spectral characteristics of the evoking signal (**Fig. 8.2**).

In general, the best ASSRs occur for low carrier frequencies (i.e., 500 Hz is better than 1000 Hz, which is better than 2000 Hz, etc.)

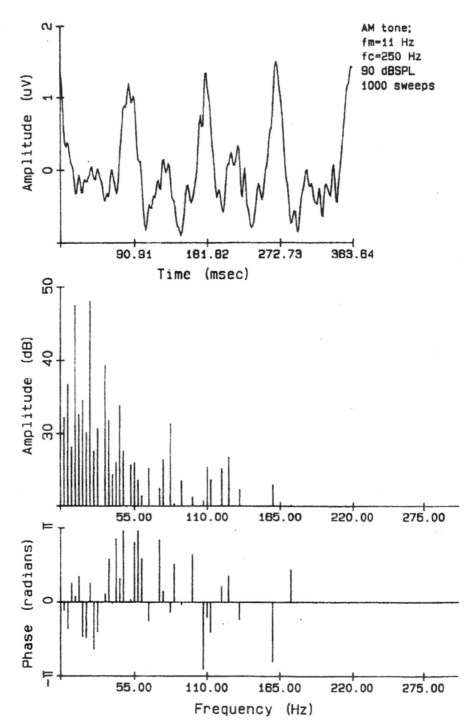

Fig. 8.2 Auditory steady-state response (ASSR) with amplitude and phase spectra from an adult with normal hearing. The stimulus is a 90-dB SPL (sound pressure level), amplitude-modulated 250 Hz carrier tone (f_c) with a modulation frequency of 11 Hz (f_m). In the amplitude spectra, the first four harmonics of the modulation frequency can be seen. (From Rickards, F.W. [1982]. Auditory steady-state evoked potentials in humans to continuous amplitude-modulated tones. Unpublished PhD thesis, University of Melbourne, Melbourne, with permission.)

and higher depths of modulation (e.g., 90% is better than 20%) (Levi, Folsom, and Dobie, 1993; Picton, Skinner, Champagne, Kellett, and Maiste, 1987). The amplitude growth of ASSRs to increasing modulation depth is somewhat linear from 0% up to ~80% modulation, after which further increases in depth do not result in a significantly larger ASSR (Kuwada, Batra, and Maher, 1986). The best modulation frequency is dependent on the listener's arousal state and age. In awake adults, the 40-Hz modulation rate elicits the most robust response (Aoyagi, Kiren, Furuse, Fuse, Suzuki, Yokota, et al, 1994b; Dobie and Wilson, 1998), but in asleep adults, and infants, higher modulation rates (e.g., f_m = 80 Hz) provide the most robust response (Aoyagi et al, 1994b; Cone-Wesson, Dowell, Tomlin, Rance, and Ming, 2002a; Levi et al, 1993). ASSRs have been recorded at modulation rates from ~10 to 180 Hz (Cohen, Rickards, and Clark, 1991).

◆ Neural Generators

The neural generators of the ASSR are complex and vary, depending on the modulation rate of the stimulus. High modulation frequencies (e.g., f_m = 90 Hz) evoke responses primarily from subcortical regions of the auditory system, and low modulation frequencies (e.g., f_m = 40 Hz) evoke responses primarily from cortical regions of the auditory system (Herdman, Lins, van Roon, Stapells, Scherg, and Picton, 2002). Evidence that the ASSR has multiple neural generator sources has been provided by several investigators (Kuwada, Anderson, Batra, Fitzpatrick, Teissier, and D'Angelo, 2002; Pantev, Roberts, Elbert, Ross, and Wienbruch, 1996; Santarelli and Conti, 1999). Kuwada et al (2002) investigated the sources of the neural generators responsible for the ASSR at different modulation rates in unanesthetized rabbits. The surface-recorded ASSR had multiple generators dependent on the modulation rate. At modulation rates lower than ~80 Hz, the cortical regions of the auditory system dominate the response. At modulation rates greater than 80 Hz, the ASSR source has two primary contributors, the midbrain or pontine and the

superior olivary complex or cochlear nucleus. Santarelli and colleagues (Azzena, Conti, Santarelli, Ottaviani, Paludetti, and Maurizi, 1995; Conti, Santarelli, Grassi, Ottaviani, and Azzena, 1999; Santarelli and Conti, 1999) have investigated the source of the ASSR at different modulation rates and compared these data to data obtained from the 40-Hz transient response. Overall, the authors offer clear evidence that the ASSR is not composed of overlapping transient responses, except at the modulation rate of 40 Hz. The conclusions were based on the following evidence reviewed by Santarelli and Conti (1999): (1) the 40-Hz transient response and the 40 Hz ASSR have opposite tonotopic organization; (2) predicted and observed responses of the transient and SSRs matched only at 40 Hz, not at 20, 30, 50, or 60 Hz; and (3) predicted amplitude was larger than recorded amplitude at all rates, except 40 Hz, where the amplitudes matched.

Schoonhoven, Boden, Verbunt, and de Munck (2003) recorded ASSRs by magnetoencephalography (MEG) in response to 40 and 80-Hz modulation rates in subjects with normal hearing. The purpose was to determine the source of the response when the ASSR was modulated at low versus high rates. Data from electrophysiologic studies suggest that the 40-Hz ASSR is primarily from cortical structures, but that the 80-Hz ASSR has strong contributions from the subcortical regions, such as the thalamus. ASSRs recorded by MEG revealed bilateral activation in the auditory cortex (Schoonhoven et al, 2003). Neural generator sources for MEG responses may be different from evoked potential sources based on these findings.

◆ Response Parameters

Response Detection and Amplitude

ASSR measurements include both the presence of a response (detection) and the robustness of the response (amplitude). The presence of a response is determined by an algorithm based on the probability that the response is present at the frequency of modulation. If the probability criterion is met, then an ASSR was detected. The magnitude of the detected response is measured in the frequency domain as absolute amplitude or as signal-to-noise-ratio (SNR) amplitude. Discrete frequency bins at the modulation frequency are used to calculate the ASSR amplitude. Amplitude of the ASSR is an order of magnitude smaller than other AEPs, such as the ABR, ranging from ~30 nV to greater than 100 nV, depending on the stimulus, subject state, and response detection algorithm used to record the response. Several factors (e.g., intensity, f_c, f_m, and subject state) affect the presence of the ASSR and the amplitude of the response; these factors are discussed in detail later in the Stimulus Parameters section.

Phase Latency

The measurement of latency for steady-state responses is complicated and can be estimated only by converting the response phase to latency (John and Picton, 2000). Phase is a circular measure unlike the poststimulus latency typical of other evoked potentials, which is a linear measure. The ASSR response can be recorded in the time domain, then converted into the frequency domain by a fast Fourier transform (FFT). The stimulus frequency components in the FFT of the response then can be transformed into vector units with amplitude and phase. This results in an estimate of apparent latency that might be useful in differentiating normal and impaired ears (John and Picton, 2000).

Stimulus Parameters

The steady-state stimulus requires the combination of several sinusoids (through multiplication or addition) to form a sinusoidally amplitude modulated (AM) signal containing both the carrier frequency and the modulation frequecy. **Figure 8.3** illustrates the simplest method for creating an AM signal, summing the larger f_c frequency (500 Hz) and the smaller side band f_m frequencies (460 and 540 Hz). In a series of experiments, Rickards and colleagues (Rickards and Clark, 1982; Rickards, Tan, Cohen, Wilson, Drew, and Clark, 1994) showed that the steady-state potential in response to an AM continuous tone could be recorded for modulation rates of 4 to 448 Hz, for carrier frequencies from 250 to 4000 Hz, and at presentation levels of 30 to 100 dB SPL (sound pressure level). The

ASSRs were quantified by the magnitude and the phase of the first and second harmonics. Results showed that the response latency and response amplitude were affected by the modulation rate. The response latency was longest for modulation rates lower than 20 Hz and shortest for modulation rates greater than 60 Hz. The response amplitude decreased with increasing modulation rate, with a peak in the amplitude-rate function at ~40 Hz.

The effects of modulation depth, modulation rate, carrier frequency, and stimulus intensity on ASSRs were studied later in subjects with normal hearing (Kuwada et al, 1986; Picton, Skinner, Champagne, Kellett, and Maiste, 1987) and in subjects with hearing loss (Kuwada, Batra, and Maher, 1986; Milford and Birchall, 1989). Results showed that as AM modulation depth increased the ASSR amplitude and detection rate increased. ASSR amplitude was largest between the modulation rates of 25 and 55 Hz with an averaged best rate at 39.1 Hz. The most robust responses were recorded for the lower carrier frequencies (≤1000 Hz) (Kuwada, Batra, and Maher, 1986; Picton et al, 1987) compared with carrier frequencies greater than 2000 Hz. ASSR amplitude increased with increasing stimulus intensity, but in subjects with hearing loss, there were unexplained interactions between higher stimulus levels (>60 dB HL [hearing level]) and carrier frequency. The differences in amplitude-intensity functions between subjects with and without hearing loss suggest that abnormal cochlear mechanics may play a role in suprathreshold responses for subjects with hearing loss.

Intensity

As stimulus intensity increases, ASSR amplitude increases, however, this effect also interacts with carrier frequency. Kuwada and colleagues (1986) plotted amplitude-intensity functions in subjects with normal hearing for carrier frequencies of 250, 1000, 4000, and 8000 Hz. ASSR amplitude increased with increasing intensity, but the slopes for the 250- and 1000-Hz functions were steeper than the 4000- and 8000-Hz functions. Rodriguez, Picton, Linden, Hamel, and Laframboise (1986) and Rodriguez and colleagues (1986) measured the effects of intensity and frequency on

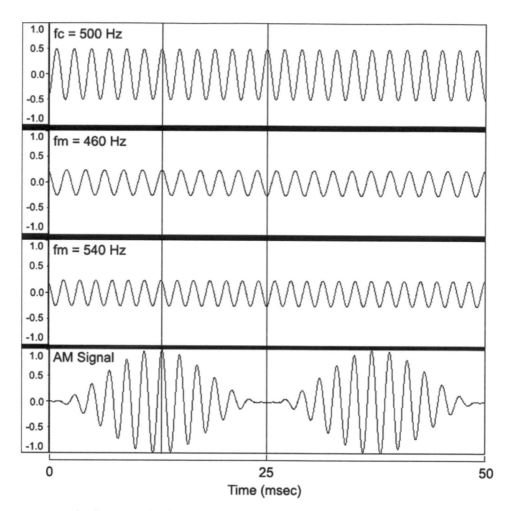

Fig. 8.3 Example of 40-Hz amplitude-modulated (AM) stimulus construction by the addition of three pure tones. The 500-Hz tone (*top*) is the carrier frequency (f_c); the 460- and 540-Hz tones (*middle two*) are the sideband tones at the 40-Hz modulation frequency (f_m). The resultant AM stimulus (*bottom*) is the sum of the three tones. The two vertical lines across the figure indicate areas of construction ($\sim$12.5 msec) and destruction ($\sim$25 msec) in the resultant AM stimulus.

the ASSR in subjects with normal hearing and in subjects with hearing loss. In subjects with normal hearing, the ASSR amplitude increased with increasing intensity above threshold. Similar findings were noted for amplitude intensity functions. The amplitude intensity slopes were steeper for the 500- and 1000-Hz ASSRs compared with the 2000- and 4000-Hz ASSRs. ASSRs recorded from subjects with hearing loss have a steeer amplitude intensity slope than ASSRs recorded in subjects with normal hearing. The amplitudes were larger for the 500-Hz ASSR than for the 2000-Hz

ASSR. An interesting and as yet unexplained result was that the subjects with hearing loss had larger 2000-Hz ASSR amplitudes than the subjects with normal hearing (Rodriguez, Picton, Linden, Hamel, and Laframboise, 1986). One possible explanation is cochlear recruitment at higher sound pressure levels for specific places along the basilar membrane.

Picton, van Roon, and John (2007) measured ASSRs to sweeps of ascending and descending intensity and found that thresholds could be estimated by this method as accurately as thresholds estimated by discrete intensity steps. The 1000- and 2000-Hz ASSRs saturated at intensities > ~60 dB SPL, but the 500- and 4000-Hz ASSRs continued to increase in amplitude greater than 60 dB SPL. Thresholds obtained in a sweep intensity method offer advantages over thresholds obtained in a discrete intensity step method. The sweep recording can provide more data points in less time than the discrete recording method. The discrete recording method, however, can be used to increase the number of data points near threshold. Another factor to consider is the difference in the amplitude intensity functions between ASSRs recorded in normal and simulated hearing loss. The linear functions in the normal hearing subjects led to more accurate extrapolation to threshold, which is not possible in the nonlinear functions found in the simulated hearing loss condition. The authors offer three considerations when using the sweep intensity method to estimate behavioral thresholds: (1) test time should increase at intensities near threshold due to the lower SNRs in the ASSRs, (2) multiple frequency ASSRs show interactions of frequencies for 1000 and 2000 Hz at higher intensities, and (3) amplitude intensity functions are linear in normal ears but nonlinear in ears with hearing loss.

Carrier Frequency

In general, investigations of the effects of carrier frequency have been for the audiometric frequencies between 500 and 4000 Hz. The limited frequency range is due to the focus of ASSR research on estimating behavioral hearing sensitivity. Additional applications will be discussed later in the chapter.

The most robust ASSRs are measured from stimuli with low carrier frequencies. Levi and colleagues (1993) measured responses to stimuli presented at the frequencies of 500 and 2000 Hz amplitude modulated at 95% and at rates varying from 10 to 80 Hz in infants and young adults. Responses occurred more often at 500 Hz compared with 2000 Hz for both infants and adults. Similar results for carrier frequency and modulation rate were reported by Aoyagi and colleagues (1994a), who investigated ASSRs in adults with normal hearing. Responses were recorded to stimuli presented at the frequencies of 500, 1000, 2000, and

4000 Hz, amplitude modulated at 95% for modulation rates from 20 to 120 Hz. The most robust responses occurred for the frequencies of 500 and 1000 Hz.

John and Picton (2000) converted phase into latency measures to determine whether the ASSR phase changed in a systematic manner with regard to stimulus carrier frequency. As carrier frequency increased, latency decreased. This latency trend was also seen with an increase in presentation level. The authors suggest that these changes are due to (1) the time it takes for the acoustic energy to reach the responding hair cells on the basilar membrane and (2) the time it takes for the hair cell to begin and complete the transduction process. The effects of carrier frequency on the ASSR appear to be related to cochlear mechanics.

> **Pearl**
>
> Similar to the effect that tone burst frequency has on the latency of the ABR, carrier frequencies affect latency measures within the ASSR response such that higher carrier frequencies result in decreased latencies. These effects appear to be related to cochlear mechanics (e.g., traveling waves).

Modulation Rate

The best rate of modulation depends primarily on the age of the individual and his or her sleep state (Levi et al, 1993). Responses are larger and occur more often at a modulation rate of 40 Hz for adults compared with infants who had more responses at a modulation rate of 80 Hz. Lins and Picton (1995) measured 1000-Hz ASSRs modulated at 39, 49, 81, and 93 Hz presented at 60 dB SPL. The results showed that the 40-Hz ASSRs were 3 to 4 times larger than the 80-Hz ASSRs. In addition, the 40 Hz ASSR amplitude was significantly reduced during sleep, but the 80 Hz ASSR amplitude was maintained. Aoyagi and colleagues (1994a,b) investigated ASSRs in adults with normal hearing. Responses were recorded to stimuli presented at rates from 20 to 120 Hz in 20-Hz steps. The most robust responses were found at rates of 40 and 80 Hz.

Modulation Depth

Amplitude-modulated ASSRs change as a function of modulation depth (i.e., from unmodulated to 100% AM) (Milford and Birchall, 1989; Picton et al, 1987; Rees, Green, and Kay, 1986). Milford and Birchall (1989) recorded AM ASSRs at the frequencies of 1000, 2000, 4000, and 8000 Hz modulated at 40 Hz at a range of modulation depths (e.g., 25–100%) in subjects with and without hearing loss. Maximal response at modulation depths of 75 to 95% were noted. Similarly, Rees et al (1986) measured AM ASSRs in adults with normal hearing for a 1000-Hz tone at the modulation rates of 4, 10, and 80 Hz. The response magnitude increased linearly from 0 to 100% modulation. In contrast, Kuwada et al (1986) reported that in subjects with varying degrees of hearing loss, the response to increasing modulation depth was somewhat linear from 0% up to ~50% modulation, after which further increases in depth did not result in significantly larger ASSRs. All of these studies confirmed that ASSRs improve as modulation depth increases from unmodulated signals to highly modulated signals.

Single versus Multiple ASSRs

One advantage of ASSRs is that multiple frequencies can be presented simultaneously, each at a different rate of modulation. Different modulation rates are used for each carrier frequency, so the responses can be analyzed separately. The multiple-frequency ASSR has been used to estimate hearing sensitivity and to assess the auditory system's response to complex stimuli. ASSRs show distinct place specificity along the basilar membrane for audiometric frequencies (500, 1000, 2000, and 4000 Hz) presented at 60 dB SPL or lower (Herdman et al, 2002), similar to the place specificity for the ABR and MLR.

ASSR amplitude is not significantly changed by the presence of more than one carrier frequency under certain conditions. Lins and Picton (1995) showed that amplitudes were not significantly different when ASSRs were presented alone, in a combination of four frequencies in one ear, or in a combination of eight frequencies in both ears. Luts and Wouters (2005) examined multiple- and single-frequency ASSR in normal and hearing-impaired listeners and found that the multiple-frequency ASSR technique was the better technique overall, but both techniques worked equally well for the hearing-impaired subjects. Standard error for threshold was between 7 and 12 dB across all frequencies. Approximately 55% of ASSR thresholds were within 5 dB of the behavioral threshold, and 94% were within 15 dB. An increase in test time improved the accuracy of threshold estimation.

The presentation of multiple-frequency ASSRs is a potential problem when stimuli are given at intensities greater than 60 dB SPL. For example, Picton, van Roon, and John (2009) reported significant decreases in ASSR amplitude when multiple-frequency ASSRs were modulated from 80 and 101 Hz and presented at 73 dB SPL. Results showed that the 500-Hz ASSRs masked the 1000- and 2000-Hz ASSRs and that the 4000 Hz ASSR reduced the 2000-Hz ASSR. To illustrate this problem on a more basic level, Lins and Picton (1995) demonstrated a masking effect (i.e., reduced ASSR amplitude) when presenting to the same ear a carrier frequency tone (e.g., f_c = 1000 Hz) modulated with two different frequencies (e.g., f_m = 81 Hz and 97 Hz); the lower f_m signal presented at 60 dB SPL, and the higher f_m signal presented at 66 dB SPL. In addition to the masking effect, distortion products were produced that were combinations of the two modulating frequencies. These findings suggest that the interactions of multiple carrier frequencies at higher presentation levels greater than 60 dB SPL require further investigation.

Luts, Desloovere, and Wouters (2006) found that the multiple-frequency ASSR was smaller for the younger infants (< 41 weeks) compared with the older infants (> 41 weeks) and adults. Adults had larger ASSRs than the older infants. This was due to the increase in the noise in the younger infant recordings, especially near threshold. For threshold comparisons, 35% of the ASSR thresholds were within 5 dB of the behavioral threshold, and 61% were within 10 dB. Dichotic multiple-frequency ASSRs are measureable in infants, but they should be recorded in sleep and for ~10 minutes for each per trial to optimize the response.

Van Maanen and Stapells (2009) recorded ASSR thresholds in 54 subjects aged 0.7 to 66.2 months. ASSR thresholds were measured at 500, 1000, 2000, and 4000 Hz as single frequencies and as a multiple frequency stimulus that included all four frequencies. Average thresholds for the single-stimulus frequencies ranged from 15 to 36 dB HL, whereas multiple-frequency ASSR average thresholds were much higher (32–49 dB HL). ASSR screening protocols should take these data into consideration when establishing screening levels for normal hearing.

In conclusion, multiple-frequency ASSRs can be recorded when carrier frequencies are separated by one octave, are presented in different ears, and presentation levels are lower than 60 dB SPL. Multiple-frequency behavioral should be useful in reducing test time for estimation of behavioral threshold (Lins and Picton, 1995). The ASSR offers a complementary technique to the ABR, particularly for low-frequency hearing assessment.

◆ Measurement Parameters

Electrode Montage

Van der Reijden, Mens, and Snik (2005) reported on optimized electrode montage for ASSRs in infants 0 to 5 months of age. Various electrode positions were assessed, including inion, Pz, nape of neck, Fpz, M2, M1, F4, F3, A2, A1, and Cz. The fewest responses were recorded from inion to Cz in infants, and the most ASSRs were recorded from ipsilateral mastoid to Cz. This is in contrast to adult data, which showed that the best electrode montage was inion referenced to Cz (van der Reijden et al,

2004). Electrode montage for infants should be ipsilateral mastoid to Cz and for adults, inion to Cz. For children older than 6 months, both ipsilateral mastoid to Cz and inion to Cz should be recorded because the closure of the posterolateral fontanelles is likely the cause for the discrepancy between infants and adults, and the time of close is not known exactly.

The electrode placement for single- versus multiple-frequency ASSRs has been recently investigated. Van Dun, Wouters, and Moonen (2009) reported that optimal electrode placement was dependent on the modulation rate of the ASSR and the number of carrier frequencies used. The optimal electrode placement for single-frequency ASSRs at 80 to 100 Hz was the back of the head and the mastoids. The optimal electrode placement for multiple-frequency ASSRs at 80 to 100 Hz was for electrodes placed at Oz, P3, and mastoid, with Cz as reference and ground electrode on the clavicle. At 10 Hz, the optimal electrode placement for single-frequency ASSRs was the back of the head (Oz, P4, and P3) and the mastoids, but for multiple-frequency ASSRs, the best electrode placement was F4, F3, with Cz as reference and ground electrode on the clavicle.

Bone-Conducted ASSRs

Bone-conducted ASSRs have the potential for high artifact and false-positive response detection even at low to moderate stimulus presentation levels. The likelihood of recording a response that is actually an electromagnetic stimulus artifact is much higher for bone-conducted ASSRs than for air-conducted ASSRs. The artifact is produced by the bone oscillator and cable, which must be shielded to prevent electrical artifact from being picked up by the electrodes or electrode leads. Stimulus artifact in the bone-conducted response can be reduced by the following: (1) increasing the sampling rate from 1000 Hz to 1250 or 1600 Hz; (2) screening the transducer and the transducer cable with braided mu-metal shielding, then connecting the transducer and cable to ground; and (3) placing the transducer and cable away from the electrode leads (Brooke, Brennan, and Stevens, 2009). These factors significantly reduce the electromagnetic stimulus artifact in the ASSR, especially above moderate stimulus levels (e.g., ≥60 dB HL).

Bone-conducted thresholds are important when the possibility of a conductive hearing loss exists, especially in infants and children who cannot provide accurate behavioral responses. Several factors can influence bone-conducted ASSR thresholds, such as placement and coupling of the oscillator to the skull and the presence or absence of an occlusion effect. Infants present several problems in testing because of smaller head size, prohibiting the use of adult- and child-size steel headbands and the need to keep the infant asleep. Careful placement of the bone oscillator with maximum comfort is required to prevent waking the infant during testing.

Small, Hatton, and Stapells (2007) investigated the effects of bone oscillator placement (e.g., forehead, temporal bone, and mastoid sites), the occlusion effect, and bone oscillator coupling (steel headband, handheld placement, or elastic band) on ASSR thresholds in infants. No significant differences in threshold or amplitude were found between temporal bone and mastoid sites, between occluded and non-occluded ears, or among the coupling methods. It is possible to record bone-conducted ASSRs in infants younger than 6 months using an elastic band or handheld method (with proper training), a mastoid or temporal bone placement, and with ears occluded or not. The forehead placement should be avoided because of significantly poorer thresholds than those seen with mastoid or temporal bone placement.

Small and Stapells (2008) reported that infants 2 to 11 months of age had ~10 to 20 dB of interaural attenuation for bone-conducted ASSRs for the octave frequencies between 500 and 4000 Hz. Adults 18 to 40 years of age showed no interaural attenuation for bone-conducted ASSRs. These results should be considered when using bone-conducted ASSRs to isolate the cochlear contributions in infants younger than 12 months. Bone-conducted ASSR thresholds are 9 to 15 dB poorer than bone-conducted behavioral thresholds for the octave frequencies between 500 and 4000 Hz (Lins et al, 1996; Small and Stapells, 2008). The clinical use of ASSR bone-conducted asymmetries will depend on the publication of normative data from infants with sensorineural, conductive, and mixed hearing losses.

When recording ASSRs at near-threshold levels, it is often important to present contralateral masking to isolate the test ear. Maki, Kawase, and Kobayashi (2009) measured the effects of contralateral noise on ASSRs recorded at 40 and 80 Hz modulation rates in 11 subjects with normal hearing. Large effects were found at 40 Hz (reduction in amplitude and fewer responses detected), but minimal effects were found at 80 Hz. These results suggest that the use of contralateral masking to isolate the test ear for high modulation rates (e.g., 80 Hz) is feasible.

Response Detection

Traditionally, phase-locked responses have been identified in the time domain by plotting the voltage of the recording electrode as a function of post-stimulus time. The presence or absence of a response is then identified by visual inspection of the time waveform as the observer attempts to determine whether the peaks in the response correspond to the frequency of the stimulus. The subjective nature of time waveform analyses reduces the reliability of the measurement and may lead to an underestimation of auditory sensitivity (Aoyagi, Fuse, Suzuki, Kim, and Koike, 1993). Objective analysis techniques, which are used to determine whether or not a phase-locked response has occurred are a methodologic advantage over subjective time waveform analysis. Because the ASSR follows the temporal and spectral characteristics of the eliciting signal, a comparison between the stimulus and the response can be made. Automated detection algorithms based on known statistical properties of background electroencephalographic (EEG) noise and on the statistical properties of the ASSR have been used to analyze these potentials (Aoyagi, Suzuki, Yokota, Furuse, Watanabe, and Ito, 1999; Dobie and Wilson, 1994). One automated detection algorithm is phase coherence squared (PC^2), which is used to determine whether or not the phase of the response is randomly distributed (i.e., in phase with the stimulus). If the phase is randomly distributed, then a response that can be detected above the noise has not occurred. If the phase of the response is not randomly distributed, then a response has occurred within a certain probability (e.g., $p \leq .001$) (Champlin, 1992; Stapells, Makeig, and Galambos, 1987).

An ASSR threshold is defined as the lowest level at which a response is detected at the specific modulation frequency. To avoid erroneous measures, it is often necessary to establish strict criteria for ASSR thresholds. This is based on how often an ASSR at that frequency was detected at intensities above the threshold. For example, one criterion would be to require a response be present at the two levels immediately above the threshold or that a response to be present 50% of the time at all levels above the threshold.

◆ Subject Effects

Awake and Sleep States

Cohen and colleagues (1991) measured ASSR thresholds in sleeping and sedated subjects with normal hearing compared with awake adults. In awake subjects, the 500-Hz ASSR was the largest and the ASSR amplitude decreased with increasing frequency from 500 to 4000 Hz. The largest ASSR amplitudes occurred for modulation frequencies from 30 to 60 Hz, with the next best modulation frequency range from 80 to 120 Hz. With sleep, however, ASSR amplitudes were reduced. Similarly, Plourde et al (1991) found that the 40-Hz ASSR was reduced in amplitude during sleep compared with the awake state and that ASSR amplitude was further reduced by anesthesia.

Actively attending to the ASSR stimulus has shown no effect on the amplitude or the phase of the response at 40 Hz (Lazzouni, Ross, Voss, and Lepore, 2010; Linden, Picton, Hamel, and Campbell, 1987). However, if a hemispheric study is conducted, ASSRs have been found to be more robust over the left hemisphere when subjects attended to a change in the temporal envelop (rhythm) of stimuli presented to the right ear when compared with the left stimulation/right hemisphere condition (Ross, Picton, Herdman, and Pantev, 2004). The effect of attention on the ASSR has yet to be understood clearly.

Maturation Effects

Maurizi and colleagues (Maurizi, Amladori, Paludetti, Ottaviani, Rosignoli, and Luciano, 1990) recorded 40-Hz ASSRs to a 500-Hz stimulus in newborns and children aged 5 to 8. Results showed that the ASSR threshold in newborns was ~40 dB nHL (normal hearing level) and ~20 dB nHL in the children. The 40-Hz ASSR was more stable and repeatable from test to test in children compared with newborns. The authors concluded that the 40-Hz ASSR was not reliable for estimating low-frequency thresholds in newborns. As mentioned, ASSR is more robust in children for 80-Hz modulation frequency and more robust at 40 Hz in adults. Pethe, Mühler, Siewert, and von Specht (2004) studied ASSR in subjects aged 2 months to 14 years. They found that the age at which the 40-Hz ASSR became larger than the 80-Hz ASSR was 13 years of age, and by 14 years of age, the 40-Hz ASSR was similar to the adult 40-Hz ASSR.

Savio, Cárdenas, Pérez Abalo, González, and Valdés (2001) found significant changes in ASSR maturation in infants (up to 12 months of age). Their research showed that ASSR detectability increased with increasing age and that the rate of increase was steeper for the higher frequencies. The ASSR thresholds also decreased with increasing age, and this effect was also more rapid for the higher carrier frequencies. Amplitude increased with increasing age, especially for the 0- to 6-month age group, although this change was not as pronounced for 500 Hz as it was for higher-frequency ASSRs.

ASSR detection rate and amplitude increase with increasing age from infancy to early adulthood (Aoyagi et al, 1994a; Rojas, Maharajh, Teale, Kleman, Benkers, Carlson, et al, 2006). Purcell, John, Schneider, and Picton (2004) found significant differences in the best modulation rate between young and older subject groups. The young group had a peak at 41 Hz, and the older group had a peak at 37 Hz. Poulsen, Picton, and Paus (2007) recorded ASSRs in 19- to 45-year-olds to determine the effect of middle age on ASSR amplitude and latency. The steady-state responses were measured with fixed and varied modulation rates. The 40-Hz ASSRs increased in amplitude and decreased in variability with an increase in age. Additionally, the modulation frequency eliciting the largest amplitude increased with increasing age.

◆ Clinical Applications

Threshold Estimation

The primary clinical application for the ASSR is behavioral threshold estimation. The ASSR has been used for neonatal hearing screenings (Cone-Wesson, Parker, Swiderski, and Rickards, 2002b; Savio et al, 2001) and to estimate hearing thresholds in children (Lins et al, 1996; Mauer et al, 1997; Rance et al, 2005; Swanepoel and Erasmus, 2007; Yang et al, 2008), adults (Chambers and Meyer, 1993; Griffiths and Chambers, 1991; Lins et al, 1996; Mauer et al, 1997; Picton, Dimitrijevic, Perez-Abalo, and van Roon, 2005; Vander Werff and Brown, 2005), and cochlear implant patients (Mauer et al, 1997; Ménard et al, 2004). A brief summary of hearing threshold estimation will be presented.

The accuracy of threshold estimation by ASSRs depends primarily on the age of the subject and the underlying behavioral threshold. In young children, the ASSR threshold is, on average, ~23 to 31 dB higher than behavioral thresholds (Rance et al, 2005). In adults with normal hearing, threshold differences between ASSRs and behavioral responses were 11 to 14 dB for 500, 1000, 2000, and 4000 Hz (Lins et al, 1996). In well babies, the threshold differences were larger, 29 to 45 dB (Lins et al, 1996). The ASSR is a better predictor of behavioral threshold at 2000 and 4000 Hz than at 500 and 1000 Hz, with the best threshold prediction at 2000 Hz. The ASSR frequencies from 1000 to 4000 Hz are significantly closer to behavioral thresholds than the 500-Hz ASSR in adults with normal hearing and well babies (Lins et al, 1996; Swanepoel and Erasmus, 2007).

Strong correlations between behavioral threshold and ASSR threshold ($r = 0.96-0.98$) have been found for infants (Rance et al, 2005). In adolescents with known hearing loss, the correlations between ASSR thresholds and behavioral thresholds are from $r = 0.7$ to 0.9 (Lins et al, 1996; Swanepoel and Erasmus, 2007). The ASSR was a better predictor of behavioral thresholds for subjects with moderate to profound hearing loss than for subjects with mild hearing loss or normal hearing (Ozdek, Karacay, Saylam, Tatar, Aygener, and Korkmaz, 2010; Swanepoel and Erasmus, 2007). This is important for cochlear implant users where stimulus artifact is a problem for other AEP measures. In cochlear implant patients, ASSRs have been recorded at greater than 60 dB HL with no stimulus artifact (Mauer et al, 1997).

Special Consideration

ASSRs appear to be better predictors of hearing sensitivity for patients with moderate to profound hearing losses compared with those with mild hearing loss or normal hearing.

Special Consideration

Because of the continuous nature of ASSR stimuli, they may hold greater promise for threshold estimation in cochlear implant users compared with other AEPs, which may be susceptible to stimulus-related cochlear implant artifact.

Finally, there is a trade-off between recording time and accuracy of threshold prediction. Shorter test time results in larger differences between physiologic and behavioral thresholds, such as 19 ± 10 dB for 6-minute recordings (Luts and Wouters, 2005), 13 ± 8 for 8-minute recordings (Kaf, Sabo, Durrant, and Rubinstein, 2006), and 38 ± 20 for 1.5-minute recordings (Luts and Wouters, 2005). In hearing-impaired ears, the abrupt rise in amplitude just above threshold permits physiologic threshold estimates to be closer to behavioral thresholds. Collapsed across frequencies, the difference between the ASSR estimated threshold and the behavioral threshold has been reported to be 13 ± 10 dB (Lins and Picton, 1995), 9 ± 11 dB (Herdman and Stapells, 2003), 8 ± 10 (Dimitrijevic et al, 2002), and 9 ± 7 dB (Vander Werff and Brown, 2005).

Suprathreshold Applications

ASSRs can be used to identify poor neural temporal coding that may underlie poor speech perception or neural synchrony disorders such as auditory neuropathy spectrum disorder (ANSD). Temporal cues in a signal are coded by certain neurons, which lock on to the dynamic timing patterns present in the harmonics and in the envelope of the signal. In other words, one neural code for temporal processing is based on the phase-locking ability of neurons. Neurons in the auditory system phase lock to low-frequency stimuli (Rose, Brugge, Anderson, and Hind, 1967) and to the low-frequency envelope of high-frequency stimuli (Møller, 1974; Rees and Møller, 1983; Yin, Kuwada, and Sujaku, 1984). The electrical potentials produced in response to temporal features of a signal can be recorded from the scalp to show phase-locking ability in individual listeners. Only recently have investigators begun to use suprathreshold ASSRs to improve our understanding of how the auditory system responds to speechlike stimuli. Speech is characterized, in part, by dynamic changes in amplitude and frequency, which the auditory system must resolve for accurate speech perception to occur. Several important speech features (e.g., voice onset time and fundamental frequency) occur at high rates of amplitude and frequency modulation.

The relationship between ASSRs and word recognition performance has been examined in young normal-hearing subjects (Dimitrijevic, John, van Roon, and Picton, 2001), older adult subjects with and without hearing loss (Dimitrijevic et al, 2004), and younger and older adult subjects with minimal hearing loss (Leigh-Paffenroth and Fowler, 2006). Additionally, significant relationships between phoneme feature detection and ASSRs have been found for infants (Cone and Garinis, 2009). Finally, Santarelli and Conti (1999) showed a significant correlation between phoneme identification score and ASSR amplitude.

Dimitrijevic et al (2001) showed that ASSR amplitude and detection increased with increasing presentation level and that word recognition performance improved as presentation level increased in young subjects with normal hearing. A significant correlation was found between the number of ASSRs detected and ASSR amplitude with percent correct-word recognition performance.

Suprathreshold ASSRs have been used to investigate temporal processing in subjects with dyslexia. McAnally and Stein (1997) found significantly smaller ASSRs in a group of dyslexic subjects compared with a group of nondyslexic subjects. A significant relationship between a behavioral measure of temporal processing (temporal modulation transfer functions) and ASSR amplitude was also seen in dyslexic individuals (Menell, McAnally, and Stein, 1999). These results show that listeners with poor temporal processing have less phase locking to AM stimuli, suggesting a role for ASSRs in the measurement of temporal processing.

The ASSR also has been used to show age-related changes in the coding of time-altered signals (Grose et al, 2009; Leigh-Paffenroth and Fowler, 2006). Younger listeners, as opposed to older listeners, showed an advantage in phase locking for low-frequency ASSRs (e.g., 500 Hz) compared with high-frequency ASSRs (e.g., 2000 Hz). Fewer 500-Hz ASSRs were detected for the older subjects at the 90-Hz modulation rate compared with younger subjects, and this decreased detection was significantly correlated to word-recognition performance (Leigh-Paffenroth and Fowler, 2006). This work suggests that age effects exist for measures of temporal processing and indicates the need for further assessment of the relation between SSRs from a range of ASSR parameters and speech-understanding performance in a competing message, including data from listeners with poor word recognition performance.

◆ Summary

The ASSR is elicited by pure tones, which are modulated in amplitude and/or frequency and have been used typically as an objective estimate of behavioral pure-tone thresholds. Single- and multiple-frequency ASSRs can be presented either monotically or dichotically to elicit the ASSR. ASSRs have been used as a hearing screening tool, to estimate pure-tone thresholds, to assess temporal processing ability, and to investigate auditory processing of speechlike stimuli. Recently, ASSRs to complex tonal stimuli have shown significant correlations with measures of word recognition in adults. New applications offer the possibility to improve our understanding of auditory processing at subcortical and cortical levels.

References

Aoyagi, M., Fuse, T., Suzuki, T., Kim, Y., & Koike, Y. (1993). An application of phase spectral analysis to amplitude-modulation following response. *Acta Oto-Laryngologica, 504*(Suppl), 82–88. PubMed

Aoyagi, M., Kiren, T., Furuse, H., Fuse, T., Suzuki, Y., Yokota, M., et al. (1994a). Effects of aging on amplitude-modulation following response. *Acta Oto-Laryngologica, 511*(Suppl), 15–22. PubMed

Aoyagi, M., Kiren, T., Furuse, H., Fuse, T., Suzuki, Y., Yokota, M., et al. (1994b). Pure-tone threshold prediction by 80-Hz amplitude-modulation following response. *Acta Oto-Laryngologica, 511*(Suppl), 7–14. PubMed

Aoyagi, M., Suzuki, Y., Yokota, M., Furuse, H., Watanabe, T., & Ito, T. (1999). Reliability of 80-Hz amplitude-modulation-following response detected by phase coherence. *Audiology and Neuro-Otology, 4*(1), 28–37. PubMed

Azzena, G. B., Conti, G., Santarelli, R., Ottaviani, F., Paludetti, G., & Maurizi, M. (1995). Generation of human auditory steady-state responses (SSRs): 1. Stimulus rate effects. *Hearing Research, 83*(1–2), 1–8. PubMed

Brooke, R. E., Brennan, S. K., & Stevens, J. C. (2009). Bone conduction auditory steady state response: Investigations into reducing artifact. *Ear and Hearing, 30*(1), 23–30. PubMed

Chambers, R. D., & Meyer, T. A. (1993). Reliability of threshold estimation in hearing-impaired adults using the AMFR. *Journal of the American Academy of Audiology, 4*(1), 22–32. PubMed

Champlin, C. A. (1992). Method for detecting auditory steady-state potentials recorded from humans. *Hearing Research, 58*(1), 63–69. PubMed

Cohen, L. T., Rickards, F. W., & Clark, G. M. (1991). A comparison of steady-state evoked potentials to modulated tones in awake and sleeping humans. *Journal of the Acoustical Society of America, 90*(5), 2467–2479. PubMed

Cone, B., & Garinis, A. (2009). Auditory steady-state responses and speech feature discrimination in infants. *Journal of the American Academy of Audiology, 20*(10), 629–643. PubMed

Cone-Wesson, B., Dowell, R. C., Tomlin, D., Rance, G., & Ming, W. J. (2002). The auditory steady-state response: comparisons with the auditory brainstem response. *Journal of the American Academy of Audiology, 13*(4), 173–187.

Cone-Wesson, B., Parker, J., Swiderski, N., & Rickards, F. (2002). The auditory steady-state response: Full-term and premature neonates. *Journal of the American Academy of Audiology, 13*(5), 260–269. PubMed

Conti, G., Santarelli, R., Grassi, C., Ottaviani, F., & Azzena, G. B. (1999). Auditory steady-state responses to click trains from the rat temporal cortex. *Clinical Neurophysiology, 110*(1), 62–70. PubMed

Dimitrijevic, A., John, M. S., & Picton, T. W. (2004). Auditory steady-state responses and word recognition scores in normal-hearing and hearing-impaired adults. *Ear and Hearing, 25*(1), 68–84. PubMed

Dimitrijevic, A., John, M. S., van Roon, P., & Picton, T. W. (2001). Human auditory steady-state responses to tones independently modulated in both frequency and amplitude. *Ear and Hearing, 22*(2), 100–111. PubMed

Dimitrijevic, A., John, M. S., van Roon, P., Purcell, D. W., Adamonis, J., Ostroff, J., et al. (2002). Estimating the audiogram using multiple auditory steady-state responses. *Journal of the American Academy of Audiology, 13*(4), 205–224. PubMed

Dobie, R. A., & Wilson, M. J. (1994). Objective detection of 40 Hz auditory evoked potentials: Phase coherence vs. magnitude-squared coherence. *Electroencephalography and Clinical Neurophysiology, 92*(5), 405–413. PubMed

Dobie, R. A., & Wilson, M. J. (1998). Low-level steady-state auditory evoked potentials: Effects of rate and sedation on detectability. *Journal of the Acoustical Society of America, 104*(6), 3482–3488. PubMed

Galambos, R., Makeig, S., & Talmachoff, P. J. (1981). A 40-Hz auditory potential recorded from the human scalp. *Proceedings of the National Academy of Sciences USA, 78*(4), 2643–2647. PubMed

Griffiths, S. K., & Chambers, R. D. (1991). The amplitude modulation-following response as an audiometric tool. *Ear and Hearing, 12*(4), 235–241. PubMed

Grose, J. H., Mamo, S. K., & Hall, J. W. III (2009). Age effects in temporal envelope processing: Speech unmasking and auditory steady state responses. *Ear and Hearing, 30*(5), 568–575. PubMed

Herdman, A. T., Lins, O., van Roon, P., Stapells, D. R., Scherg, M., & Picton, T. W. (2002). Intracerebral sources of human auditory steady-state responses. *Brain Topography, 15*(2), 69–86. PubMed

Herdman, A. T., & Stapells, D. K. (2003). Auditory steady-state response thresholds of adults with sensorineural hearing impairments. *International Journal of Audiology, 42*(5), 237–248. PubMed

John, M. S., & Picton, T. W. (2000). Human auditory steady-state responses to amplitude-modulated tones: Phase and latency measurements. *Hearing Research, 141*(1–2), 57–79. PubMed

Kaf, W. A., Sabo, D. L., Durrant, J. D., & Rubinstein, E. (2006). Reliability of electric response audiometry using 80 Hz auditory steady-state responses. *International Journal of Audiology, 45*(8), 477–486. PubMed

Kuwada, S., Anderson, J. S., Batra, R., Fitzpatrick, D. C., Teissier, N., & D'Angelo, W. R. (2002). Sources of the scalp-recorded amplitude-modulation following response. *Journal of the American Academy of Audiology, 13*(4), 188–204. PubMed

Kuwada, S., Batra, R., & Maher, V. L. (1986). Scalp potentials of normal and hearing-impaired subjects in response to sinusoidally amplitude-modulated tones. *Hearing Research, 21*(2), 179–192. PubMed

Lazzouni, L., Ross, B., Voss, P., & Lepore, F. (2010). Neuromagnetic auditory steady-state responses to amplitude modulated sounds following dichotic or monaural presentation. *Clinical Neurophysiology, 121*(2), 200–207. PubMed

Leigh-Paffenroth, E. D., & Fowler, C. G. (2006). Amplitude-modulated auditory steady-state responses in younger and older listeners. *Journal of the American Academy of Audiology, 17*(8), 582–597. PubMed

Levi, E. C., Folsom, R. C., & Dobie, R. A. (1993). Amplitude-modulation following response (AMFR): Effects of modulation rate, carrier frequency, age, and state. *Hearing Research, 68*(1), 42–52. PubMed

Linden, R. D., Picton, T. W., Hamel, G., & Campbell, K. B. (1987). Human auditory steady-state evoked potentials during selective attention. *Electroencephalography and Clinical Neurophysiology, 66*(2), 145–159. PubMed

Lins, O. G., & Picton, T. W. (1995). Auditory steady-state responses to multiple simultaneous stimuli. *Electroencephalography and Clinical Neurophysiology, 96*(5), 420–432. PubMed

Lins, O. G., Picton, T. W., Boucher, B. L., Durieux-Smith, A., Champagne, S. C., Moran, L. M., et al. (1996). Frequency-specific audiometry using steady-state responses. *Ear and Hearing, 17*(2), 81–96. PubMed

Luts, H., Desloovere, C., & Wouters, J. (2006). Clinical application of dichotic multiple-stimulus auditory steady-state responses in high-risk newborns and young children. *Audiology and Neuro-Otology, 11*(1), 24–37. PubMed

Luts, H., & Wouters, J. (2005). Comparison of MASTER and AUDERA for measurement of auditory steady-state responses. *International Journal of Audiology, 44*(4), 244–253. PubMed

Maki, A., Kawase, T., & Kobayashi, T. (2009). Effects of contralateral noise on 40-Hz and 80-Hz auditory steady-state responses. *Ear and Hearing, 30*(5), 584–589. PubMed

Mauer, G., Döring, W. H., Hamacher, V., & Bell, C. (1997). Amplitude modulation following response in children as a clinical audiometric tool. *American Journal of Otology, 18*(6, Suppl), S111–S112. PubMed

Maurizi, M., Almadori, G., Paludetti, G., Ottaviani, F., Rosignoli, M., & Luciano, R. (1990). 40-Hz steady-state responses in newborns and in children. *Audiology, 29*(6), 322–328.

McAnally, K. I., & Stein, J. F. (1997). Scalp potentials evoked by amplitude-modulated tones in dyslexia. *Journal of Speech, Language, and Hearing Research, 40*(4), 939–945. PubMed

Ménard, M., Gallego, S., Truy, E., Berger-Vachon, C., Durrant, J. D., & Collet, L. (2004). Auditory steady-state response evaluation of auditory thresholds in cochlear implant patients. *International Journal of Audiology, 43*(Suppl 1), S39–S43. PubMed

Menell, P., McAnally, K. I., & Stein, J. F. (1999). Psychophysical sensitivity and physiological response to amplitude modulation in adult dyslexic listeners. *Journal of Speech, Language, and Hearing Research, 42*(4), 797–803. PubMed

Milford, C. A., & Birchall, J. P. (1989). Steady-state auditory evoked potentials to amplitude-modulated tones in hearing-impaired subjects. *British Journal of Audiology, 23*(2), 137–142. PubMed

Møller, A. R. (1974). Coding of sounds with rapidly varying spectrum in the cochlear nucleus. *Journal of the Acoustical Society of America, 55*(3), 631–640. PubMed

Ozdek, A., Karacay, M., Saylam, G., Tatar, E., Aygener, N., & Korkmaz, M. H. (2010, Jan). Comparison of pure tone audiometry and auditory steady-state responses in subjects with normal hearing and hearing loss. *European Archives of Oto-Rhino-Laryngology, 267*(1), 43–49. PubMed

Pantev, C., Roberts, L. E., Elbert, T., Ross, B., & Wienbruch, C. (1996). Tonotopic organization of the sources of human auditory steady-state responses. *Hearing Research, 101*(1–2), 62–74. PubMed

Pethe, J., Mühler, R., Siewert, K., & von Specht, H. (2004). Near-threshold recordings of amplitude modulation following responses (AMFR) in children of different ages. *International Journal of Audiology, 43*(6), 339–345. PubMed

Picton, T. W., Dimitrijevic, A., Perez-Abalo, M. C., & van Roon, P. (2005). Estimating audiometric thresholds using auditory steady-state responses. *Journal of the American Academy of Audiology, 16*(3), 140–156. PubMed

Picton, T. W., John, M. S., Dimitrijevic, A., & Purcell, D. (2003). Human auditory steady-state responses. *International Journal of Audiology, 42*(4), 177–219. PubMed

Picton, T. W., Skinner, C. R., Champagne, S. C., Kellett, A. J., & Maiste, A. C. (1987). Potentials evoked by the sinusoidal modulation of the amplitude or frequency of a tone. *Journal of the Acoustical Society of America, 82*(1), 165–178. PubMed

Picton, T. W., van Roon, P., & John, M. S. (2007). Human auditory steady-state responses during sweeps of intensity. *Ear and Hearing, 28*(4), 542–557. PubMed

Picton, T. W., van Roon, P., & John, M. S. (2009). Multiple auditory steady state responses (80–101 Hz): Effects of ear, gender, handedness, intensity and modulation rate. *Ear and Hearing, 30*(1), 100–109. PubMed

Plourde, G., Stapells, D. R., & Picton, T. W. (1991). The human auditory steady-state evoked potentials. *Acta Oto-Laryngologica, 491*(Suppl), 153–159, discussion 160. PubMed

Poulsen, C., Picton, T. W., & Paus, T. (2007). Age-related changes in transient and oscillatory brain responses to auditory stimulation in healthy adults 19–45 years old. *Cerebral Cortex, 17*(6), 1454–1467. PubMed

Purcell, D. W., John, S. M., Schneider, B. A., & Picton, T. W. (2004). Human temporal auditory acuity as assessed by envelope following responses. *Journal of the Acoustical Society of America, 116*(6), 3581–3593. PubMed

Rance, G., Roper, R., Symons, L., Moody, L. J., Poulis, C., Dourlay, M., et al. (2005). Hearing threshold estimation in infants using auditory steady-state responses. *Journal of the American Academy of Audiology, 16*(5), 291–300. PubMed

Rees, A., Green, G. G., & Kay, R. H. (1986). Steady-state evoked responses to sinusoidally amplitude-modulated sounds recorded in man. *Hearing Research, 23*(2), 123–133. PubMed

Rees, A., & Møller, A. R. (1983). Responses of neurons in the inferior colliculus of the rat to AM and FM tones. *Hearing Research, 10*(3), 301–330. PubMed

Rickards, F., & Clark, G. M. (1982). Steady-state evoked potentials in humans to amplitude modulated tones. *Journal of the Acoustical Society of America, 72*(1, Suppl), S54.

Rickards, F. W., Tan, L. E., Cohen, L. T., Wilson, O. J., Drew, J. H., & Clark, G. M. (1994). Auditory steady-state evoked potential in newborns. *British Journal of Audiology, 28*(6), 327–337. PubMed

Rodriguez, R., Picton, T., Linden, D., Hamel, G., & Laframboise, G. (1986). Human auditory steady state responses: Effects of intensity and frequency. *Ear and Hearing, 7*(5), 300–313. PubMed

Rojas, D. C., Maharajh, K., Teale, P. D., Kleman, M. R., Benkers, T. L., Carlson, J. P., et al. (2006). Development of the 40 Hz steady state auditory evoked magnetic field from ages 5 to 52. *Clinical Neurophysiology, 117*(1), 110–117. PubMed

Rose, J. E., Brugge, J. F., Anderson, D. J., & Hind, J. E. (1967). Phase-locked response to low-frequency tones in single auditory nerve fibers of the squirrel monkey. *Journal of Neurophysiology, 30*(4), 769–793. PubMed

Ross, B., Picton, T. W., Herdman, A. T., & Pantev, C. (2004). The effect of attention on the auditory steady-state response. *Neurology and Clinical Neurophysiology, 2004,* 22. PubMed

Santarelli, R., & Conti, G. (1999). Generation of auditory steady-state responses: Linearity assessment. *Scandinavian Audiology, 51*(Suppl), 23–32. PubMed

Savio, G., Cárdenas, J., Pérez Abalo, M., González, A., & Valdés, J. (2001). The low and high frequency auditory steady state responses mature at different rates. *Audiology and Neuro-Otology, 6*(5), 279–287. PubMed

Schoonhoven, R., Boden, C. J., Verbunt, J. P., & de Munck, J. C. (2003). A whole head MEG study of the amplitude-modulation-following response: Phase coherence, group delay and dipole source analysis. *Clinical Neurophysiology, 114*(11), 2096–2106. PubMed

Small, S. A., Hatton, J. L., & Stapells, D. R. (2007). Effects of bone oscillator coupling method, placement location, and occlusion on bone-conduction auditory steady-state responses in infants. *Ear and Hearing, 28*(1), 83–98. PubMed

Small, S. A., & Stapells, D. R. (2008). Normal ipsilateral/contralateral asymmetries in infant multiple auditory steady-state responses to air- and bone-conduction stimuli. *Ear and Hearing, 29*(2), 185–198. PubMed

Stapells, D. R., Linden, D., Suffield, J. B., Hamel, G., & Picton, T. W. (1984). Human auditory steady state potentials. *Ear and Hearing, 5*(2), 105–113. PubMed

Stapells, D. R., Makeig, S., & Galambos, R. (1987). Auditory steady-state responses: threshold prediction using phase coherence. *Electroencephalography and Clinical Neurophysiology, 67*(3), 260–270. PubMed

Swanepoel, D., & Erasmus, H. (2007). Auditory steady-state responses for estimating moderate hearing loss. *European Archives of Oto-Rhino-Laryngology, 264*(7), 755–759. PubMed

Swanepoel, D., Hugo, R., & Roode, R. (2004). Auditory steady-state responses for children with severe to profound hearing loss. *Archives of Otolaryngology—Head and Neck Surgery, 130*(5), 531–535. PubMed

van der Reijden, C. S., Mens, L. H., & Snik, A. F. (2004). Signal-to-noise ratios of the auditory steady-state response from fifty-five EEG derivations in adults. *Journal of the American Academy of Audiology, 15*(10), 692–701. PubMed

van der Reijden, C. S., Mens, L. H., & Snik, A. F. (2005). EEG derivations providing auditory steady-state responses with high signal-to-noise ratios in infants. *Ear and Hearing, 26*(3), 299–309. PubMed

Van Dun, B., Wouters, J., & Moonen, M. (2009). Optimal electrode selection for multi-channel electroencephalogram based detection of auditory steady-state responses. *Journal of the Acoustical Society of America, 126*(1), 254–268. PubMed

Van Maanen, A., & Stapells, D. R. (2009). Normal multiple auditory steady-state response thresholds to air-conducted stimuli in infants. *Journal of the American Academy of Audiology, 20*(3), 196–207. PubMed

Vander Werff, K. R., & Brown, C. J. (2005). Effect of audiometric configuration on threshold and suprathreshold auditory steady-state responses. *Ear and Hearing, 26*(3), 310–326. PubMed

Yang, C. H., Chen, H. C., & Hwang, C. F. (2008). The prediction of hearing thresholds with auditory steady-state responses for cochlear implanted children. *International Journal of Pediatric Otorhinolaryngology, 72*(5), 609–617. PubMed

Yin, T. C., Kuwada, S., & Sujaku, Y. (1984). Interaural time sensitivity of high-frequency neurons in the inferior colliculus. *Journal of the Acoustical Society of America, 76*(5), 1401–1410. PubMed

Chapter 9

Middle Latency Responses

Ashley W. Harkrider

The middle latency response (MLR), also known as the auditory middle latency response (AMLR), was first reported by Geisler, Frishkoph, and Rosenblith (1958). It is a transient auditory evoked potential (AEP) composed of three or four positive and negative peaks that appear ~10 to 80 msec relative to stimulus onset. The MLR follows the auditory brainstem response (ABR) and precedes the obligatory slow cortical potential (SCP) in latency (**Fig. 9.1**). The MLR is larger in amplitude than the ABR and smaller than the SCP. It is believed that the MLR is generated primarily by neurons at the level of the thalamus and the cortex (Borgmann, Ross, Draganova, and Pantev, 2001) in response to acoustic and electrical stimuli, such as clicks, tone bursts, and short-duration speech sounds. The MLR is a far-field response that can be measured non-invasively using surface-recorded electrodes. It is considered to be a mesogenous response, meaning the characteristics are dependent on factors both extrinsic to the subject (e.g., stimulus or recording parameters) and intrinsic to the subject (e.g., arousal level and attention to stimuli). Despite its dependence on intrinsic characteristics, the MLR has been recorded in neonates and in sleeping or sedated animals and humans. However, it is most reliably obtained in awake, cooperative children (10 years and older) and adults who are relaxed and quiet (Kraus, Smith, Reed, Stein, and Cartee, 1985; Tucker and Ruth, 1996). Because of the latency of the MLR, it can be confounded

by postauricular muscle (PAM) artifact (Matas, Neves, Carvalho, and Leite, 2009). For this reason, it is important to support the head and neck of the subject to minimize PAM while recording the MLR. Additionally, most of the energy of the MLR is in the 10- to 100-Hz frequency range. Therefore, it can be confounded by electrical artifact, which has its greatest energy at ~50 to 60 Hz. Unlike with the ABR, a notch-rejection filter centered at 50 or 60 Hz cannot be used to minimize electrical artifact when recording MLRs because it also would reject much of the MLR energy. Despite these potential challenges, the MLR is a robust and clinician-friendly AEP that provides valuable information about the integrity of the auditory system in normal and impaired listeners when measured and interpreted appropriately.

◆ Components of the Middle Latency Response

The components of the MLR are defined as Na, Pa, and Nb, with Pb sometimes included. Nomenclature is based on both polarity and latency. If the component is labeled with an *N*, it is a negative peak; a *P* indicates a positive peak. Peaks with *a* designations precede peaks with *b* designations in latency. The earlier components of the MLR (Na, Pa) appear to be generated from both subcortical and cortical

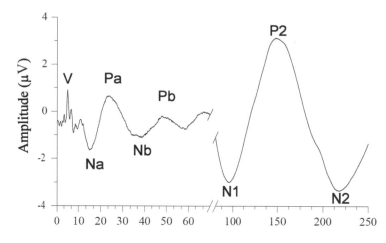

Fig. 9.1 Grand average waveforms depicting the auditory brainstem response (ABR), middle latency response (MLR), and slow cortical potential (SCP) in aggregate, obtained from a group of young adults with normal hearing. (SCPs were recorded separately and appended to the simultaneously recorded ABRs and MLRs, which explains the break in the horizontal axis.)

structures around the level of the thalamocortical radiations, whereas the later components (Nb, Pb) originate primarily from the cortex.

Na

Na typically falls ~18 to 20 msec relative to stimulus onset, depending on the type of stimulus used. Both subcortical and cortical structures appear to contribute to wave Na (Hashimoto, 1982; Jacobson, Privitera, Neils, Grayson, and Yeh, 1990; Kileny, Paccioretti, and Wilson, 1987; Scherg, Vasajar, anf Picton, 1989). The Na component is recorded reliably in individuals with normal auditory systems and serves as a robust visual marker for the onset of the MLR. It is an obligatory response that is dictated by stimulus and recording parameters and generally is unaffected by subject state with the exception of muscular artifact (see section on PAM below). This may be due to the fact that the mesencephalic reticular formation does not appear to contribute to Na (Kraus, McGee, Littman, and Nicol 1992). More recent source localization data attribute the posterior-medial portion of Heschl gyrus and sulcus to the generation of Na (Yvert, Fischer, Bertrand, and Pernier, 2005). Although not quite as systematically as the waves of the ABR, Na is influenced by changes in stimulus intensity, frequency, and rate. Specifically, Na will increase in latency and decrease in amplitude with reductions in intensity and frequency and decrease in latency and amplitude with increases in repetition rate (Bell,

Allen, and Lutman, 2001; Nagle and Musiek, 2009; Nousak and Stapells, 2005; Ozdamar, Bohórquez, and Ray, 2007).

Pa

Wave Pa occurs at ~28 to 33 msec relative to stimulus onset and generally is believed to arise from the temporal lobe and/or thalamocortical pathway (Buchwald, Erwin, Van Lancker, Guthrie, Schwafel, and Tanguay, 1992; Erwin and Buchwald, 1986; Woods, Clayworth, Knight, Simpson, and Naeser, 1987). Recently, more detailed source localization data suggest that Heschl gyrus and sulcus, the planum temporale, and the superior temporal gyrus are simultaneously activated to generate the Pa component (Yvert, Crouzeix, Bertrand, Seither-Preisler, and Pantev, 2001; Yvert et al, 2005). Additionally, Pa amplitude decreases slightly with reductions in arousal, implying a minor contribution of the reticular formation to its presence (Collet, Duclaux, Challamel, and Revol, 1988; Osterhammel, Shallop, and Terkildsen, 1985). It also is affected by stimulus intensity, frequency, and rate. Generally, Pa will decrease in amplitude and increase in latency with decreases in stimulus intensity (Nousak and Stapells, 2005) or frequency. It is less clear how Pa is influenced by stimulus rate, with some studies indicating a decrease in amplitude and latency with an increase in stimulus rate (Nagle and Musiek, 2009; Ozdamar et al, 2007) and others showing no effect (Tucker and Ruth, 1996). Like Na, Pa is reliably recorded in individuals with normal auditory systems. Because of this, Na and Pa are the MLR components that are the most useful for clinical assessments. It is not unusual to see clinical interpretations of MLRs based on the absolute latencies of Na and Pa and the peak-to-peak amplitude of Na-Pa. Mean amplitude for Na-Pa is ~600 nV, although the range of peak-to-peak amplitude within the normal-hearing population is quite large.

Nb

The latency of Nb generally falls ~35 to 45 msec relative to the onset of the stimulus. It is slightly less reliable than the Na and Pa components, perhaps because it is influenced more by arousal and attention. For this reason, it is not surprising that the reticular formation reportedly plays a primary role in generating Nb, as do the supratemporal gyrus (Yvert et al, 2001) and the primary auditory cortex. Because Nb is so variable even among normal individuals, it is not as well studied as Na and Pa. Thus, less is known about the influence of stimulus characteristics (e.g., frequency, intensity, and rate) on the amplitude or latency of the response.

Pb

Often Pb is not included in MLR studies because it is highly variable and inconsistently present in individuals with normal auditory systems (Nelson, Hall, and Jacobson, 1997). Similar to Nb, this variability is likely due to the influence of the reticular formation in its generation. When present, Pb occurs at ~50 to 75 msec relative to stimulus onset and is attributed to activation of the anterolateral portion of Heschl gyrus, the planum temporale, the superior temporal gyrus, secondary auditory cortical areas, and the reticular formation (Yvert et al, 2001, 2005). It has been suggested that Pb may be best visualized using high-level stimuli presented at a slow repetition rate lower than 1/s (Dietrich, Barry, and Parker, 1995; Tucker, Dietrich, Harris, and Pelletier, 2002). However, recent studies demonstrate that both Nb and Pb were present more frequently when maximum-length sequence stimuli at high repetition rates were used versus traditional, slower repetition rate stimuli (Bell, Allen, and Lutman,

2001, 2002; Nagle and Musiek, 2009; Notley, Bell, and Smith, 2010). Pb is also known as P1, P50, or P60 (Tucker, Dietrich, McPherson, and Salamat, 2001) and is sometimes included as the first peak in the series of components that make up the SCP.

◆ Clinical Applications

Behavioral Threshold Estimation

There are several purported advantages to using the MLR for behavioral threshold estimation. First, thalamic and cortical generators of the MLR are not as dependent on neural synchrony as those of the ABR. Therefore, unlike the ABR, MLRs can be recorded despite neural Asynchrony caused by damage at the level of the eighth cranial nerve (CN VIII) or brainstem, allowing for use of the MLR for objective assessment of the peripheral hearing mechanism in these cases. Second, stimuli of longer durations (e.g., tone bursts ≤10 msec) can be used to obtain the MLR, and the response will be almost as robust as if it were evoked by a transient stimulus (e.g., 100-μsec click). This may be an advantage when estimating thresholds because the longer the duration of the stimulus, the more frequency specific it is. Third, MLR testing requires the transduction of auditory information from the periphery to the cortex consistent with the pathway tested during behavioral audiometric examinations. Also, the amplitude of the MLR is larger and the signal-to-noise ratio (SNR) better than that of the ABR (Musiek and Geurkink, 1981; Nousak and Stapells, 2005; Scherg and Volk, 1983). This may be an advantage for detection of an AEP, especially at stimulus levels approaching threshold, although recent data suggest this aspect does not yield more accurate threshold estimates than ABR (Nousak and Stapells, 2005). Lastly, in contrast to wave V of the ABR, which is reduced considerably near threshold in the hearing-impaired versus normal-hearing ear, Na-Pa amplitudes recorded at or near threshold from hearing-impaired ears are only slightly smaller than those recorded from normal-hearing ears at threshold. This suggests that cochlear damage has a greater detrimental effect on the function of the CN VIII and brainstem generators compared with subcortical and cortical generators, where neural redundancy in the central pathways and/or plasticity may allow for more normal responses (Nousak and Stapells, 2005).

When using the MLR for threshold estimation, most often the presence and replicability of the Na-Pa complex are assessed at varying frequencies and intensity levels because Na and Pa have been shown to be recorded reliably to tonal stimuli in normal and hearing-impaired listeners (e.g., Barajas, Exposito, Fernandez, and Martin, 1988; Borgmann et al, 2001; Fukushima and Penteado de Castro, 2007; Kavanagh, Domico, Crews, and McCormick, 1988; Kraus et al, 1985; Maurizi, Ottaviani, Paludetti, Rosignoli, Almadori, and Tassoni, 1984; Nousak and Stapells, 2005; Scherg and Volk, 1983). Minimally, Na and Pa recorded from the ipsilateral side (Cz-Ai) are analyzed,

although contralateral recordings (Cz-Ac) can be beneficial for identification purposes. Generally, thresholds estimated using tone-evoked MLRs in isolation (e.g., Barajas et al, 1988; Kavanagh et al, 1988) or simultaneous with ABR measurement (e.g., Nousak and Stapells, 2005; Scherg and Volk, 1983) are within 10 dB of behavioral thresholds in normal-hearing and hearing-impaired adults if testing conditions are good (**Fig. 9.2**).

Adults typically are capable of remaining awake and quiet during the testing, which would be the preferred patient state when measuring MLRs. However, MLRs can be recorded reliably in the most sleeping adults, even near threshold. Using MLRs to estimate thresholds in infants and young children proves to be more of a challenge for several reasons. First, it is difficult for them to remain quiet when awake, and movement artifact may preclude valid MLR recordings.

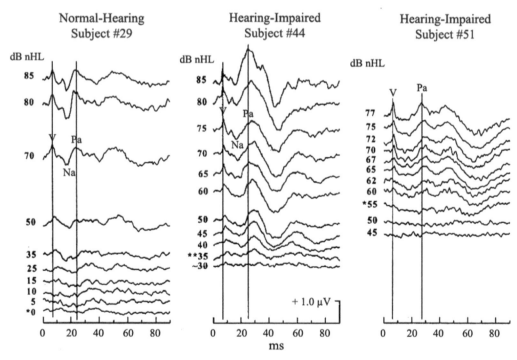

Fig. 9.2 Middle latency responses (MLRs) during auditory threshold estimation in a normal-hearing and two hearing-impaired listeners. Thresholds estimated using the MLR only are marked with a ~, thresholds estimated using auditory brainstem responses (ABRs) only are marked with a **, and thresholds estimated using both ABR and MLR are marked with a *. (From Nousak, J. K.,

& Stapells, D. R. (2005). Auditory brainstem and middle latency responses to 1 kHz tones in noise-masked normally-hearing and sensorineural hearing-impaired adults. *International Journal of Audiology, 44*(6), 336. Copyright 2005 by Informa Plc. Reprinted with permission.)

Second, MLRs in sleeping or sedated infants and young children have been reported to be less reliable and more volatile than in adolescents and adults, possibly because, whereas the subcortical contributors to the earlier MLR components are developed in infants and young children, the cortical generators are not (Kraus et al, 1985; Kraus and McGee, 1990; Stapells, Galambos, Costello, anfd Makieg, 1988). However, although some studies suggest that only 20% of infants have recordable Na and Pa waveforms (e.g., Kraus and McGee, 1990), other data demonstrate that ipsilateral MLRs can be obtained from 90 to 100% of sleeping newborns and young children to both moderate-and low-intensity click stimuli at slow and moderate stimulus rates (Collet et al, 1988; Suzuki and Hirabayashi, 1987; Tucker and Ruth, 1996). Thus, it appears MLRs can be used to estimate behavioral thresholds in infants and young children as long as it is recognized that the morphology of the MLR waveform differs from that of adults. Specifically, whereas Na appears unaffected by age (McPherson, Tures, and Starr, 1989; Schochat and Musiek, 2006; Suzuki and Hirabayashi, 1987), Pa is broader, smaller in amplitude, and its peak latency is closer to 40 msec with no evidence of Nb or Pb in infants relative to adults. Additionally, when stimulating a given ear, neonates and young infants have ipsilateral-only responses, whereas healthy children and adults will have ipsilateral and contralateral responses indistinct from each other (McGee and Kraus, 1996; Schochat and Musiek, 2006; Tucker et al, 2001). In children approximately 5 to 7 years of age, Pa latency decreases to adult values, whereas amplitudes continue to increase, Nb becomes better defined, and response variability decreases into adulthood (Schochat and Musiek, 2006; Suzuki and Hirabayashi, 1987; Tucker and Ruth, 1996). While discussing the influence of maturation on the MLR, it should be noted that some researchers (e.g., Amenedo and Díaz, 1998; Woods and Clayworth, 1986) have demonstrated poorer morphology, larger amplitudes, and longer latencies in older adults (i.e., older than 60 years) compared with younger adults even when hearing thresholds are normal or near normal.

Neurodiagnostic Middle Latency Responses

MLRs may be used to assess central auditory nervous system function. Data suggest that the MLR is a valuable part of the test battery for identifying deficits related to pathologies of the thalamocortical pathways, including but not limited to central/cortical deafness (Musiek, Charette, Morse, and Baran, 2004; Praamstra, Hagoort, Maassen, and Crul, 1991; Setzen et al, 1999; Tanaka, Kamo, Yoshida, and Yamadori, 1991), multiple sclerosis (Musiek et al, 1999; Stach and Hudson, 1990; Versino et al, 1992), auditory processing deficits (Chermak and Musiek, 1997; Fifer and Sierra-Irizarry, 1988; Musiek et al, 1999; Purdy, Kelly, and Davies, 2002), learning disabilities (Arehole, Augustine, and Simhadri, 1995; Purdy, Kelly, and Davies, 2002), traumatic brain injury (Munjal, Panda, and Pathak, 2010; Musiek, Baran, and Shinn, 2004), stroke (Rojas Sosa, Fraire Martínez, Olvera Gómez, and Jáuregui-Renaud, 2009), and dementia (Jessen et al., 2001). MLRs also have been shown to be influenced by commonly used stimulants and depressants affecting neural function, such as acute and chronic nicotine use (Harkrider and Champlin, 2001; Ramkissoon and Chambers, 2008), chronic alcohol use (Ahveninen et al, 1999), and use of anesthetic agents (e.g., Bell, Smith, Allen, and Lutman, 2004; Notley et al, 2010; Sloan, 2002).

Generally, components of the MLR are believed to reflect responses from the primary auditory pathways central to, and possibly including, the inferior colliculus, secondary multisensory divisions of the thalamus and thalamocortical pathways, and the reticular formation. As mentioned, the MLR is not as vulnerable as the ABR to Asynchrony at the level of CN VIII or brainstem, so subcortical and cortical auditory pathways can be assessed even in the presence of CN VIII or lower brainstem abnormalities and an absent or distorted ABR. Moreover, because the MLR is as robust to tone-burst stimuli as it is to click stimuli, neural testing in a patient with peripheral hearing loss can still be performed reliably by choosing a tone-burst frequency in the patient's range of best hearing to evoke the diagnostic MLR.

When using the MLR for neurodiagnostic purposes, most often the morphology, amplitude, and latency of Na and Pa evoked by moderately high-intensity click stimuli presented to each ear separately are assessed at multiple electrode sites. Electrode sites typically include central (i.e., Cz and/or Pz) and left and right hemispheric placements (i.e., C3 and C4, or C5 and C6, or T3 and T4). Response symmetry for ear and hemisphere is expected in the normal individual, making ear or hemispheric differences a good clinical measure (Musiek et al, 1999; Schochat and Musiek, 2006; Tucker et al, 2001). For this reason, possible ear and/or electrode differences in amplitude should be examined. For example, Na-Pa amplitude differences greater than 20 to 50% when comparing contralateral recordings (left ear, right hemisphere vs right ear, left hemisphere) are a sensitive indicator of central auditory nervous system involvement in adults (e.g., Musiek et al, 1999) and children (Purdy et al, 2002). Typically, MLR abnormalities (i.e., waveform absence, decreased amplitudes, and increased latencies) are present at the electrode closest to the lesion, whereas MLRs recorded from electrodes on the opposite side of the lesion are normal (**Fig. 9.3**).

Pearl

During hemispheric studies, ear and/or electrode differences in amplitude may appear in patients. If Na-Pa amplitude at a given electrode is reduced in one ear, this is called an ear effect. An electrode effect occurs when an electrode on one side of the head exhibits consistently smaller Na-Pa amplitudes compared with the contralateral side regardless of ear of stimulation.

When using a test-battery approach, including physiologic tests, such as otoacoustic emissions (OAEs), acoustic reflect thresholds (ARTs), ABRs, MLRs, and SCPs, one can better locate the site of injury or lesion. For example, absent MLRs and SCPs in the presence of normal OAEs, ARTs, and ABRs suggest subcortical/cortical involvement. Present OAEs, absent ARTs and

absent or distorted ABRs, and present MLRs and SCPs suggest involvement of the auditory nerve and/or lower brainstem. Absent OAEs, elevated or absent ARTs, and abnormal ABRs, MLRs, and SCPs may be consistent with moderate to severe cochlear hearing loss. Absent OAEs, elevated ARTs, and normal or near-normal ABRs, MLRs, and SCPs may suggest mild cochlear hearing loss. As always, there are exceptions to these patterns. Nonetheless, MLRs can and should be considered a valuable part of the test battery when assessing potential pathologies of the auditory system or when monitoring recovery from neural damage (**Fig. 9.4**).

Assessing Cochlear Implant Candidacy and Function

Electrically evoked MLRs (EMLRs) are comparable in morphology and threshold to the acoustically evoked MLR (Kelly, Purdy, and Thorne, 2005; Kileny, Kemink, and Miller, 1989; Shallop, Beiter, Goin, and Mischke, 1990), and the absolute latencies are shorter (Miyamoto, 1986). For comparison, Pa falls ~26 msec and Pb ~56 msec to moderate-level electrical stimuli (**Fig. 9.5**). The EMLRs have been used to determine extent of neural survival in animals (e.g., Kileny et al, 1989) and humans (e.g., Black, Lilly, Fowler, and Stypulkowski, 1987; Game, Gibson, and Pauka, 1987; Kileny and Kemink, 1987), which is important information when establishing implant candidacy and/or best ear for implantation. It also has been used to assess activation patterns and performance with cochlear implants in adults (e.g., Firszt, Chambers, and Kraus, 2002; Makhdoum, Groenen, Snik, and van den Broek, 1998; Shallop et al, 1990) and children (Davids, Valero, Papsin, Harrison, and Gordon, 2008a; Davids, Valero, Papsin, Harrison, and Gordon, 2008b; Gordon, Papsin, and Harrison, 2005; Shallop et al, 1990).

One of the limitations to using electrical stimuli to obtain AEPs is that earlier latency neural responses (e.g., EABR) are obscured by stimulus artifact. The EMLR has longer latencies than the electrically evoked ABR (EABR) and is visible beyond the stimulus artifact even when electrical pulses of up to 10 msec in duration are used (Davids et al, 2008a). Further, the amplitude, latency, and morphology of the EMLR appear unaffected by longer durations of elec-

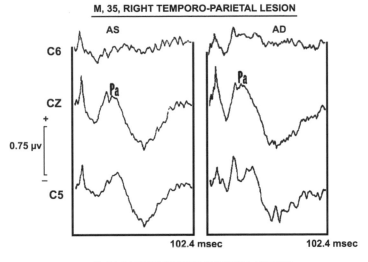

M, 35, RIGHT TEMPORO-PARIETAL LESION

AS   AD

C6

CZ   Pa   Pa

+
0.75 µv
−

C5

102.4 msec   102.4 msec

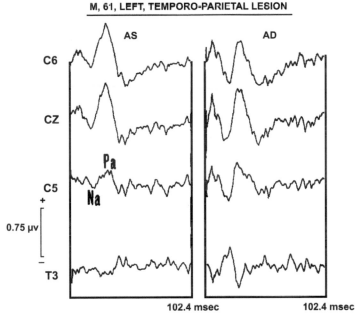

M, 61, LEFT, TEMPORO-PARIETAL LESION

AS   AD

C6

CZ

Pa

C5   Na

+
0.75 µv
−

T3

102.4 msec   102.4 msec

Fig. 9.3 Middle latency response (MLR) waveforms obtained from two individuals, one with damage to the cerebral cortex on the right side (*top panels*) and one with damage to the cerebral cortex on the left side (*bottom panels*). In the top panels, note the common pattern of absent MLRs recorded from electrodes over the damaged right hemisphere and the normal MLRs recorded from the vertex and left hemisphere regardless of ear of stimulation. In the bottom panels, note the other common pattern of reduced MLRs recorded from electrodes over the damaged left hemisphere and the normal MLRs recorded from the vertex and right hemisphere regardless of ear of stimulation. (From Kileny, P., Paccioretti, D., & Wilson, A. F. (1987). Effects of cortical lesions on middle-latency auditory evoked responses (MLR). *Electroencephalography and Clinical Neurophysiology, 66*(2), 114–115. Copyright 1987 by Elsevier. Reprinted with permission.)

trical pulse stimuli (e.g., 10 msec), suggesting that EMLRs may be evoked by stimulus onset rather than duration (Davids et al, 2008a). The ability for robust, unaltered EMLRs to be obtained with longer versus short-duration stimuli is an advantage of the EMLR when testing threshold levels of electrical stimulation. This is in large part because longer stimuli have better frequency specificity, one reason why behavioral thresholds are measured using pure-tone stimuli 500 msec or longer in duration. It may also be due to differences in temporal integration of short, repetitive versus long, continuous stimuli (Davids, Valero, Papsin, Harrison, and Gordon, 2008b). Whatever the explanation, the longer the duration of the electrical stimuli, the more accurately physiologic responses will predict behavioral thresholds.

The EMLR has been effective in assessing cochlear implants and their influence on the

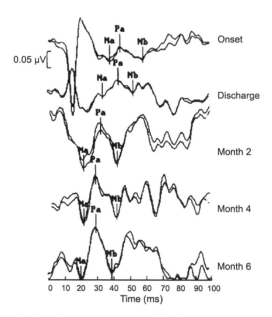

Fig. 9.4 Improvement in middle latency response (MLR) waveforms mirror recovery from stroke. (From Rojas Sosa, M. C., Fraire Martínez, M. I., Olvera Gómez, J. L., & Jáuregui-Renaud, G. (2009). Early auditory middle latency evoked potentials correlates with recovery from aphasia after stroke. *Clinical Neurophysiology*, *120*(1), 138. Copyright 2008 by Elsevier. Reprinted with permission.)

implants. The results of this study demonstrated that EMLR detectability increased, amplitudes increased, and latencies decreased with cochlear implant use. The authors suggested that this reflects plasticity in the midbrain and cortical pathways, following a period of deprivation, in response to an increase in auditory activity via the implant. Unlike the EABR, the percentage of EMLRs obtained at the time of implantation was low, even in awake patients, suggesting it may not be optimal for assessing stimulation levels or function of the device immediately following surgery. This may be especially true in children whose MLRs are affected both by auditory deprivation and by neural pathway immaturity.

Although some studies report that EMLRs are not consistent with behavioral performance in adult cochlear implant users (e.g., Kelly et al, 2005; Makhdoum et al, 1998), others have found significant correlations between EMLR characteristics and speech perception abilities (Firszt et al, 2002; Groenen, Snik, and van den Broek, 1997). Specifically, it appears that similar morphology across electrodes, larger Na-Pa amplitudes, and lower Na-Pa thresholds are associated with better performers during speech perception testing in quiet. Interestingly, the EMLR is more likely to relate to behavioral performance than the EABR or electrically evoked SCPs. To date, no studies reporting EMLR correlations with behavioral performance in children with cochlear implants have been reported.

auditory system of the individual implanted. Gordon and colleagues (2005) examined the plasticity of the auditory system in individuals with varying periods of auditory deprivation (deafness) before and after receiving cochlear

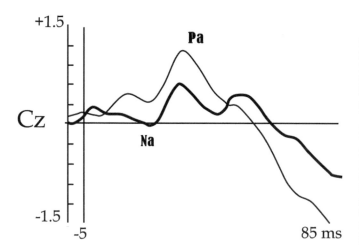

Fig. 9.5 Electrically evoked middle latency response (EMLR) waveforms from cochlear implant users compared with MLR waveforms from normal-hearing listeners. Bold lines represent grand average data from 12 cochlear implant users. Thin lines represent grand average data from 12 normal-hearing listeners. (From Kelly, A.S., Purdy, S.C., & Thorne, P. R. (2005), Electrophysiological and speech perception measures of auditory processing in experienced adult cochlear implant users. *Clinical Neurophysiology*, *116*(6), 1239. Copyright 2005 by Elsevier. Reprinted with permission.)

◆ Recording Considerations for Middle Latency Responses

Table 9.1 includes recommended stimulus, recording, and analysis protocols for MLR testing. The exact parameters chosen will depend on the clinical purpose for measuring the MLR (e.g., audiometric threshold estimation vs neural examination), the patient (e.g., infant vs adult), the capabilities of the AEP equipment, and the testing environment. The ABR and MLR can be measured simultaneously as long as bandpass filter settings, stimulus rates and durations, and number of stimulus averages are adjusted to maximize recording of both AEPs (e.g., Musiek et al, 1999; Tampas and Harkrider, 2006). Simultaneous measurement of the two responses can be a time-saving advantage when recording both responses is recommended for a clinical case.

Number of Electrode Channels Available for Recording

Whenever possible, a four-channel vertical electrode configuration should be used. Noninverting electrodes commonly will include Cz, C3, and C4, with the earlobe of the test ear (Ai), the tip of the nose, or the nape of the neck as the inverting electrode. The ground electrode can be placed on the forehead (Fz or Fpz) or the earlobe contralateral (Ac) to the stimulated ear. The electrodes associated with the fourth channel should be placed above and below one of the eyes so that the electro-oculogram can be used to develop an eyeblink rejection rule during data collection. Similar to PAM, eyeblink artifact resembles the MLR in amplitude, latency, and morphology and can be mistaken for it or obscure it (e.g., Notley et al, 2010). Rejecting eye movements minimizes drastically the confounding effects of eyeblink artifact on the response.

Table 9.1 Recommended Clinical Protocols for Obtaining and Evaluating Middle Latency Responses (MLRs)

Parameter	Recommendation	Comments
Stimulus type	Clicks, tone bursts	Depends on purpose of MLR
Stimulus duration	<10 msec	
Stimulus rate	7.1–17.1/s	Nb and Pb may be present more often with maximum length sequence
Stimulus intensity	70 dB nHL	
Stimulus mode	Monaural	
Time window	0–70 msec	
Signal averages	500–1000	May need more replications with lower number of responses averaged
High-pass cutoff	10 Hz	
Low-pass cutoff	300 Hz	
50- or 60-Hz notch filter	Off	
Number of electrode channels	2–4	Minimum of one electrode over each hemisphere for neural examination
Noninverting electrodes	Cz, C3, C4	
Inverting electrode	Ai/nose/nape	Earlobe better than mastoid
Artifact rejection	± 100 μV	Set to reject 10% of averages
Eyeblink rejection	Electrodes above/below eye	
Subject state	Awake, relaxed, and still	Light sleep okay
Latency measures	Na and Pa absolute latencies	
Amplitude measures	Na-Pa peak to peak (μV)	
Hemispheric differences	Na-Pa from C3-inverting vs C4-inverting	≥50% considered abnormal
Ear differences	Na-Pa from right ear vs left ear stimuli	≥50% considered abnormal

Abbreviations: MLR, middle latency response; nHL, normal hearing level.

Currently, many commercially available AEP systems do not allow for more than a two-channel electrode configuration. If using the MLR to estimate thresholds, one channel should be dedicated only to MLR data collection (Cz-Ai or Cz-nose) and the other to recording the electro-oculogram. However, if the MLR is being obtained for neuropathologic purposes, one should use both channels for MLR data collection to enable hemispheric and/or ear differences in Na-Pa amplitude to be examined. If two channels of MLR data are necessary for the testing of a given patient, one can also use the artifact rejection circuit to minimize eyeblink artifact in the electroencephalogram (EEG) response. To do this, after electrode placement but prior to testing, ask the listener to blink slowly and naturally each time he or she hears the stimulus, and then set the artifact rejection level so that it is below the amplitude levels of the eyeblink artifact.

Pearl

Although more commonly done with SCPs, placing electrodes for one channel above and below one eye to detect and reject electro-ocular activity (i.e., eyeblinks) is helpful with MLR recordings. If the number of channels available does not permit electro-ocular recordings, the artifact rejection levels can be set individually for each patient.

Participant State

Postauricular Muscle Artifact

Generally, participants should be reclined with their head and neck well supported. They should be instructed to relax, remain quiet and still with their eyes open, and not sleep. If, in their case history, participants report a tendency to grind their teeth (e.g., temporomandibular joint [TMJ] disorders), they should be reminded frequently to relax their jaw to avoid the confounding effects of PAM, which is located just behind the ear. Even individuals without TMJ disorders may have a PAM artifact in response to auditory stimuli, so it is important to ensure that PAM movement is minimized when obtaining MLRs. PAM will not average out of the

response like other noise because it is synchronized to the evoking stimulus (Bell, Smith, Allen, and Lutman, 2004). The latency, amplitude, and morphology of PAM artifact is similar to that of the Na-Pa components of the MLR and may push Na and Pa to a longer than normal latency and reduce their amplitudes (**Fig. 9.6**). For this reason, often PAM is mistaken for the MLR itself. However, although the PAM response is bipolar, it is consistently earlier in latency than Na and Pa, with a negative peak that occurs ~12 to 15 msec (versus a Na latency range of ~18 to 20 msec), a subsequent positive peak, and another large negative peak around 45 msec, which can be mistaken for Nb (which typically falls between 35 to 45 msec). Additionally, PAM artifact has an amplitude of ~5 µV, which is a bit larger than the neural response (e.g., Bell, Smith, Allen, and Lutman, 2004). It has been demonstrated that placing the electrodes on the earlobes, nose, or nape of the neck (Bell et al, 2004) rather than the mastoids will decrease the influence of PAM on the MLR (Matas et al, 2009). Additionally, using softer stimuli may reduce or eliminate PAM in some listeners (Notley et al, 2010), as will muscle relaxants and anesthesia (Bell et al, 2004; Notley et al, 2010).

Pearl

Placing the noninverting (reference) electrode on the earlobe, nose, or nape of the neck will help to minimize the likelihood of triggering the PAM artifact. In a clinic without medical personnel, clinicians may also be able to minimize the PAM artifact by simply decreasing the intensity level of the stimulus 5 to 10 dB.

Effects of Sleep and Sedation in Adults versus Infants/Young Children

The MLR can be obtained reliably in individuals of any age provided the response is recorded during wakefulness, light sleep, or rapid eye movement (REM) sleep (Collet et al, 1988; Kraus et al, 1985; McGee, Kraus, Killion, Rosenberg, and King, 1993). Sedated or deeply sleeping infants often do not produce an MLR (Collet et al, 1988; Kraus, McGee, and Comp-

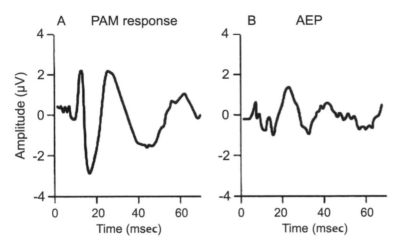

Fig. 9.6 A middle latency response (MLR) waveform with postauricular muscle (PAM) artifact preceding it in latency (*left panel*). An MLR with no PAM artifact (*right panel*). (From Bell, S. L., Smith, D. C., Allen, R., & Lutman, M. E. (2004). Recording the middle latency response of the auditory evoked potential as a measure of depth of aenesthesia: A technical note. *British Journal of Anesthesia, 92*(3), 444. Copyright 2004 by the Board of Management and Trustees of the *British Journal of Anesthesia*. Reprinted with permission.)

eratore, 1989), although it can be reliably recorded in adolescents or adults even in deep sleep stages. MLRs fluctuate with arousal state and are more labile during sleep versus passive wakefulness.

The MLR is difficult to obtain in infants or children under anesthesia or sedation (Gordon et al, 2005; McGee et al, 1993). In adults under anesthesia versus normal awake controls, the amplitude of the MLR components is reduced, although the myogenic and EEG noise levels are also reduced, improving the quality of the MLR. No change in latency with anesthesia has been noted (Notley et al, 2010). Some studies suggest that the MLR can be used to evaluate the depth of anesthesia (e.g., Bell et al, 2004; Bell, Smith, Allen, and Lutman, 2006), whereas others found too much within-subject variability for this purpose and suggest it may be more suitable as a measure of awareness during sedation (Notley et al, 2010). Consistent with this purpose, recent data demonstrate that in all cases where Pa was absent in MLRs obtained from severely comatose patients (**Fig. 9.7**), the outcome was death or progression to

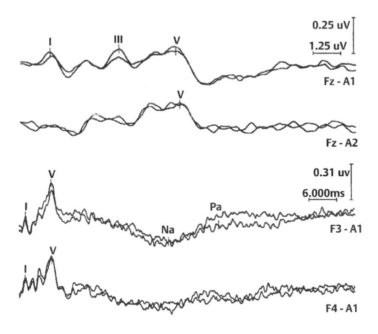

Fig. 9.7 Normal auditory brainstem response (ABR) and absent Pa of the middle latency response (MLR) consistent with poor negative outcome (death or lack of return to consciousness) in patients in persistent coma. The top two waveforms are ABRs only. The bottom two waveforms are ABRs and MLRs. (From Logi, F., Fischer, C., Murri, L., & Mauguière, F. (2003). The prognostic value of evoked responses from primary somatosensory and auditory cortex in comatose patients. *Clinical Neurophysiology, 114*(9), 1620. Copyright 2003 by Elsevier. Reprinted with permission.)

a permanently vegetative state (Fischer and Luauté, 2005; Logi, Fischer, Murri, and Mauguière, 2003).

Test Environment

Because of the overlap of spectral energy with MLRs and electrical noise, bandpass filtering will not eliminate 50 or 60 Hz electrical noise from an MLR response. All MLR testing should be conducted in a sound-treated room with the AEP equipment (e.g., computer) located outside. It may be necessary to turn off lights and unplug all unused electrical equipment (e.g., television or DVD player) inside the test suite to minimize confounding 50- or 60-Hz electrical energy. Additionally, keeping the electrode leads from the scalp to the pre-amplifier short will minimize electrical noise in the response. To avoid stimulus artifact, alternating polarity stimuli should be delivered via insert earphones, preferably with electrical shielding, and care should be taken to keep the electrode leads separate from the transducer cords.

◆ Summary

The MLR has been used in research since its discovery in the late 1950s. Interest in its use as a clinical tool has waxed and waned since. Recently, as recording and analysis protocols and commercially available equipment have become more refined, the clinical MLR has enjoyed a clinical rebirth. A quick search of the literature will demonstrate data that support its daily use in comprehensive test batteries for hearing and neurologic assessments in individuals of all ages.

References

Ahveninen, J., Jääskeläinen, I. P., Pekkonen, E., Hallberg, A., Hietanen, M., Näätänen, R., et al. (1999). Post-withdrawal changes in middle-latency auditory evoked potentials in abstinent human alcoholics. *Neuroscience Letters, 268*(2), 57–60. PubMed

Amenedo, E., & Díaz, F. (1998). Effects of aging on middle-latency auditory evoked potentials: A cross-sectional study. *Biological Psychiatry, 43*(3), 210–219. PubMed

Arehole, S., Augustine, L. E., & Simhadri, R. (1995). Middle latency response in children with learning disabilities: Preliminary findings. *Journal of Communication Disorders, 28*(1), 21–38. PubMed

Barajas, J. J., Exposito, M., Fernandez, R., & Martin, L. J. (1988). Middle latency response to a 500-Hz tone pip in normal-hearing and in hearing-impaired subjects. *Scandinavian Audiology, 17*(1), 21–26. PubMed

Bell, S. L., Allen, R., & Lutman, M. E. (2001). The feasibility of maximum length sequences to reduce acquisition time of the middle latency response. *Journal of the Acoustical Society of America, 109*(3), 1073–1081. PubMed

Bell, S. L., Allen, R., & Lutman, M. E. (2002). Optimizing the acquisition time of the middle latency response using maximum length sequences and chirps. *Journal of the Acoustical Society of America, 112*(5, Pt 1), 2065–2073. PubMed

Bell, S. L., Smith, D. C., Allen, R., & Lutman, M. E. (2004). Recording the middle latency response of the auditory evoked potential as a measure of depth of anaesthesia: A technical note. *British Journal of Anaesthesia, 92*(3), 442–445. PubMed

Bell, S. L., Smith, D. C., Allen, R., & Lutman, M. E. (2006). The auditory middle latency response, evoked using maximum length sequences and chirps, as an indicator of adequacy of anesthesia. *Anesthesia and Analgesia, 102*(2), 495–498. PubMed

Black, F. O., Lilly, D. J., Fowler, L. P., & Stypulkowski, P. H. (1987). Surgical evaluation of candidates for cochlear implants. *Annals of Otology, Rhinology, and Laryngology, 128*(Suppl), 96–99.

Borgmann, C., Ross, B., Draganova, R., & Pantev, C. (2001). Human auditory middle latency responses: influence of stimulus type and intensity. *Hearing Research, 158*(1–2), 57–64. PubMed

Buchwald, J. S., Erwin, R. J., Van Lancker, D., Guthrie, D., Schwafel, J., & Tanguay, P. (1992). Midlatency auditory evoked responses: P1 abnormalities in adult autistic subjects. *Electroencephalography and Clinical Neurophysiology/Evoked Potentials Section, 84*(2), 164–171. PubMed

Chermak, G. D., & Musiek, F. E. (1997). *Central Auditory Processing Disorders.* San Diego, CA: Singular.

Collet, L., Duclaux, R., Challamel, M. J., & Revol, M. (1988). Effect of sleep on middle latency response (MLR) in infants. *Brain and Development, 10*(3), 169–173. PubMed

Davids, T., Valero, J., Papsin, B. C., Harrison, R. V., & Gordon, K. A. (2008a). Effects of stimulus manipulation on electrophysiological responses in pediatric cochlear implant users: 1. Duration effects. *Hearing Research, 244*(1–2), 7–14. PubMed

Davids, T., Valero, J., Papsin, B. C., Harrison, R. V., & Gordon, K. A. (2008b). Effects of stimulus manipulation on electrophysiological responses of pediatric cochlear implant users: 2. Rate effects. *Hearing Research, 244*(1–2), 15–24. PubMed

Dietrich, S., Barry, S. J., & Parker, D. E. (1995). Middle latency auditory responses in males who stutter. *Journal of Speech, Language, and Hearing Research: JSLHR, 38*(1), 5–17. PubMed

Erwin, R. J., & Buchwald, J. S. (1986). Midlatency auditory evoked responses: Differential effects of sleep in the human. *Electroencephalography and Clinical Neurology, 65*(5), 383–392. PubMed

Fifer, R. C., & Sierra-Irizarry, B. (1988). Clinical applications of the auditory middle latency response. *American Journal of Otology, 9*(Suppl), 47–56. PubMed

Firszt, J. B., Chambers, R. D., & Kraus, N. (2002). Neurophysiology of cochlear implant users: 2. Comparison among speech perception, dynamic range, and physiological measures. *Ear and Hearing, 23*(6), 516–531. PubMed

Fischer, C., & Luauté, J. (2005). Evoked potentials for the prediction of vegetative state in the acute stage of coma. *Neuropsychological Rehabilitation, 15*(3–4), 372–380. PubMed

Fukushima, E. M., & Penteado de Castro, N., Jr. (2007). A study of logon-evoked middle latency responses in female subjects with normal hearing. *Brazilian Journal of Otorhinolaryngology, 73*(3), 308–314. PubMed

Game, C. J. A., Gibson, W. P. R., & Pauka, C. K. (1987). Electrically evoked brainstem auditory potentials. *Annals of Otology, Rhinology, and Laryngology, 128*(Suppl), 94–95.

Geisler, C. D., Frishkopf, L. S., & Rosenblith, W. A. (1958). Extracranial responses to acoustic clicks in man. *Science, 128*(3333), 1210–1211. PubMed

Gordon, K. A., Papsin, B. C., & Harrison, R. V. (2005). Effects of cochlear implant use on the electrically evoked middle latency response in children. *Hearing Research, 204*(1–2), 78–89. PubMed

Groenen, P., Snik, A., & van den Broek, P. (1997). Electrically evoked auditory middle latency responses versus perception abilities in cochlear implant users. *Audiology, 36*(2), 83–97. PubMed

Harkrider, A. W., & Champlin, C. A. (2001). Acute effect of nicotine on non-smokers: 2. MLRs and 40-Hz responses. *Hearing Research, 160*(1–2), 89–98. PubMed

Hashimoto, I. (1982). Auditory evoked potentials from the human midbrain: Slow brain stem responses. *Electroencephalography and Clinical Neurophysiology, 53*(6), 652–657. PubMed

Jacobson, G. P., Privitera, M., Neils, J. R., Grayson, A. S., & Yeh, H. S. (1990). The effects of anterior temporal lobectomy (ATL) on the middle-latency auditory evoked potential (MLAEP). *Electroencephalography and Clinical Neurophysiology, 75*(3), 230–241. PubMed

Jessen, F., Kucharski, C., Fries, T., Papassotiropoulos, A., Hoenig, K., Maier, W., et al. (2001). Sensory gating deficit expressed by a disturbed suppression of the P50 event-related potential in patients with Alzheimer's disease. *American Journal of Psychiatry, 158*(8), 1319–1321. PubMed

Kavanagh, K. T., Domico, W. D., Crews, P. L., & McCormick, V. A. (1988). Comparison of the intrasubject repeatability of auditory brain stem and middle latency responses elicited in young children. *Annals of Otology, Rhinology, and Laryngology, 97*(3, Pt 1), 264–271. PubMed

Kelly, A. S., Purdy, S. C., & Thorne, P. R. (2005). Electrophysiological and speech perception measures of auditory processing in experienced adult cochlear implant users. *Clinical Neurophysiology, 116*(6), 1235–1246. PubMed

Kileny, P. R., & Kemink, J. L. (1987). Electrically evoked middle-latency auditory potentials in cochlear implant candidates. *Archives of Otolaryngology—Head and Neck Surgery, 113*(10), 1072–1077. PubMed

Kileny, P. R., Kemink, J. L., & Miller, J. M. (1989). An intrasubject comparison of electric and acoustic middle latency responses. *American Journal of Otology, 10*(1), 23–27. PubMed

Kileny, P. R., Paccioretti, D., & Wilson, A. F. (1987). Effects of cortical lesions on middle-latency auditory evoked responses (MLR). *Electroencephalography and Clinical Neurophysiology, 66*(2), 108–120. PubMed

Kraus, N., & McGee, T. (1990). Clinical applications of the middle latency response. *Journal of the American Academy of Audiology, 1*(3), 130–133. PubMed

Kraus, N., McGee, T., & Comperatore, C. (1989). MLRs in children are consistently present during wakeful ness, stage 1, and REM sleep. *Ear and Hearing, 10*(6), 339–345. PubMed

Kraus, N., McGee, T., Littman, T., & Nicol, T. (1992). Reticular formation influences on primary and non-primary auditory pathways as reflected by the middle latency response. *Brain Research, 587*(2), 186–194. PubMed

Kraus, N., Smith, D. I., Reed, N. L., Stein, L. K., & Cartee, C. (1985). Auditory middle latency responses in children: Effects of age and diagnostic category. *Electroencephalography and Clinical Neurophysiology, 62*(5), 343–351. PubMed

Logi, F., Fischer, C., Murri, L., & Mauguière, F. (2003). The prognostic value of evoked responses from primary somatosensory and auditory cortex in comatose patients. *Clinical Neurophysiology, 114*(9), 1615–1627. PubMed

Makhdoum, M. J., Groenen, P. A., Snik, A. F., & van den Broek, P. (1998). Intra- and interindividual correlations between auditory evoked potentials and speech perception in cochlear implant users. *Scandinavian Audiology, 27*(1), 13–20. PubMed

Matas, C. G., Neves, I. F., Carvalho, F. M., & Leite, R. A. (2009). Post-auricular muscle reflex in the middle latency evoked auditory response. *Brazilian Journal of Otorhinolaryngology, 75*(4), 579–585. PubMed

Maurizi, M., Ottaviani, F., Paludetti, G., Rosignoli, M., Almadori, G., & Tassoni, A. (1984). Middle-latency auditory components in response to clicks and low- and middle-frequency tone pips (0.5–1 kHz). *Audiology, 23*(6), 569–580. PubMed

McGee, T., & Kraus, N. (1996). Auditory development reflected by middle latency response. *Ear and Hearing, 17*(5), 419–429. PubMed

McGee, T., Kraus, N., Killion, M., Rosenberg, R., & King, C. (1993). Improving the reliability of the auditory middle latency response by monitoring EEG delta activity. *Ear and Hearing, 14*(2), 76–84. PubMed

McPherson, D. L., Tures, C., & Starr, A. (1989). Binaural interaction of the auditory brain-stem potentials and middle latency auditory evoked potentials in infants and adults. *Electroencephalography and Clinical Neurophysiology*, *74*(2), 124–130. PubMed

Miyamoto, R. T. (1986). Electrically evoked potentials in cochlear implant subjects. *The Laryngoscope*, *96*(2), 178–185. PubMed

Munjal, S. K., Panda, N. K., & Pathak, A. (2010). Relationship between severity of traumatic brain injury (TBI) and extent of auditory dysfunction. *Brain Injury*, *24*(3), 525–532. PubMed

Musiek, F. E., Baran, J. A., & Shinn, J. (2004). Assessment and remediation of an auditory processing disorder associated with head trauma. *Journal of the American Academy of Audiology*, *15*(2), 117–132. PubMed

Musiek, F. E., Charette, L., Kelly, T., Lee, W. W., & Musiek, E. (1999). Hit and false positive rates for the middle latency response in patients with central nervous system involvement. *Journal of the American Academy of Audiology*, *10*(3), 124–132.

Musiek, F. E., Charette, L., Morse, D., & Baran, J. A. (2004). Central deafness associated with a midbrain lesion. *Journal of the American Academy of Audiology*, *15*(2), 133–151, quiz 172–173. PubMed

Musiek, F. E., & Geurkink, N. A. (1981, May-Jun). Auditory brainstem and middle latency evoked response sensitivity near threshold. *Annals of Otology, Rhinology, and Laryngology*, *90*(3, Pt 1), 236–240. PubMed

Nagle, S., & Musiek, F. E. (2009). Morphological changes in the middle latency response using maximum length sequence stimuli. *Journal of the American Academy of Audiology*, *20*(8), 492–502. PubMed

Nelson, M. D., Hall, J. W., & Jacobson, G. P. (1997). Factors affecting the recordability of auditory evoked response (AER) component Pb (P1). *Journal of the American Academy of Audiology*, *8*(2), 89–99. PubMed

Notley, S. V., Bell, S. L., & Smith, D. C. (2010). Auditory evoked potentials for monitoring during anaesthesia: A study of data quality. *Medical Engineering and Physics*, *32*(2), 168–173. PubMed

Nousak, J. K., & Stapells, D. R. (2005). Auditory brainstem and middle latency responses to 1 kHz tones in noise-masked normally-hearing and sensorineurally hearing-impaired adults. *International Journal of Audiology*, *44*(6), 331–344. PubMed

Osterhammel, P. A., Shallop, J. K., & Terkildsen, K. (1985). The effect of sleep on the auditory brainstem response (ABR) and the middle latency response (MLR). *Scandinavian Audiology*, *14*(1), 47–50. PubMed

Ozdamar, O., Bohórquez, J., & Ray, S. S. (2007). P(b) (P(1) resonance at 40 Hz: Effects of high stimulus rate on auditory middle latency responses (MLRs) explored using deconvolution. *Clinical Neurophysiology*, *118*(6), 1261–1273. PubMed

Praamstra, P., Hagoort, P., Maassen, B., & Crul, T. (1991, June). Word deafness and auditory cortical function: A case history and hypothesis. *Brain*, *114*(Pt 3), 1197–1225. PubMed

Purdy, S. C., Kelly, A. S., & Davies, M. G. (2002). Auditory brainstem response, middle latency response, and late cortical evoked potentials in children with learning dis-

abilities. *Journal of the American Academy of Audiology*, *13*(7), 367–382. PubMed

Ramkissoon, I., & Chambers, R. D. (2008). Effects of chronic and acute smoking on AMLRs in older and younger listeners. *International Journal of Audiology*, *47*(12), 715–723. PubMed

Rojas Sosa, M. C., Fraire Martínez, M. I., Olvera Gómez, J. L., & Jáuregui-Renaud, K. (2009). Early auditory middle latency evoked potentials correlates with recovery from aphasia after stroke. *Clinical Neurophysiology*, *120*(1), 136–139. PubMed

Scherg, M., Vasajar, J., & Picton, T. (1989). A source analysis of the late human auditory evoked potentials. *Journal of Cognitive Neuroscience*, *1*, 336–355.

Scherg, M., & Volk, S. A. (1983). Frequency specificity of simultaneously recorded early and middle latency auditory evoked potentials. *Electroencephalography and Clinical Neurophysiology*, *56*(5), 443–452. PubMed

Schochat, E., & Musiek, F. E. (2006). Maturation of outcomes of behavioral and electrophysiologic tests of central auditory function. *Journal of Communication Disorders*, *39*(1), 78–92. PubMed

Setzen, G., Cacace, A. T., Eames, F., Riback, P., Lava, N., McFarland, D. J., et al. (1999). Central deafness in a young child with moyamoya disease: Paternal linkage in a Caucasian family—two case reports and a review of the literature. *International Journal of Pediatric Otorhinolaryngology*, *48*(1), 53–76. PubMed

Shallop, J. K., Beiter, A. L., Goin, D. W., & Mischke, R. E. (1990). Electrically evoked auditory brain stem responses (EABR) and middle latency responses (EMLR) obtained from patients with the nucleus multichannel cochlear implant. *Ear and Hearing*, *11*(1), 5–15. PubMed

Sloan, T. B. (2002). Anesthetics and the brain. *Anesthesiology Clinics of North America*, *20*(2), 265–292. PubMed

Stach, V., & Hudson, M. (1990). Middle and late auditory evoked potentials in multiple sclerosis. *Seminars in Hearing*, *11*, 221–230.

Stapells, D. R., Galambos, R., Costello, J. A., & Makieg, S. (1988). Inconsistency of auditory middle latency and steady-state responses in infants. *Electroencephalography and Clinical Neurophysiology*, *71*(4), 289–295.

Suzuki, T., & Hirabayashi, M. (1987). Age-related morphological changes in auditory middle-latency response. *Audiology*, *26*(5), 312–320. PubMed

Tampas, J. W., & Harkrider, A. W. (2006). Auditory evoked potentials in females with high and low acceptance of background noise when listening to speech. *Journal of the Acoustical Society of America*, *119*(3), 1548–1561. PubMed

Tanaka, Y., Kamo, T., Yoshida, M., & Yamadori, A. (1991, December). 'So-called' cortical deafness: Clinical, neurophysiological and radiological observations. *Brain*, *114*(Pt 6), 2385–2401. PubMed

Tucker, D. A., Dietrich, S., Harris, S., & Pelletier, S. (2002). Effects of stimulus rate and gender on the auditory middle latency response. *Journal of the American Academy of Audiology*, *13*(3), 146–153, quiz 171–172. PubMed

Tucker, D. A., Dietrich, S., McPherson, D. L., & Salamat, M. T. (2001). Effect of stimulus intensity level on auditory middle latency response brain maps in human adults. *Journal of the American Academy of Audiology, 12*(5), 223–232. PubMed

Tucker, D. A., & Ruth, R. A. (1996). Effects of age, signal level, and signal rate on the auditory middle latency response. *Journal of the American Academy of Audiology, 7*(2), 83–91. PubMed

Versino, M., Bergamaschi, R., Romani, A., Banfi, P., Callieco, R., Citterio, A., et al. (1992). Middle latency auditory evoked potentials improve the detection of abnormalities along auditory pathways in multiple sclerosis patients. *Electroencephalography and Clinical Neurophysiology, 84*(3), 296–299. PubMed

Woods, D. L., & Clayworth, C. C. (1986). Age-related changes in human middle latency auditory evoked potentials. *Electroencephalography and Clinical Neurophysiology, 65*(4), 297–303. PubMed

Woods, D. L., Clayworth, C. C., Knight, R. T., Simpson, G. V., & Naeser, M. A. (1987, Mar). Generators of middle- and long-latency auditory evoked potentials: implications from studies of patients with bitemporal lesions. *Electroencephalography and Clinical Neurophysiology, 68*(2), 132–148. PubMed

Yvert, B., Crouzeix, A., Bertrand, O., Seither-Preisler, A., & Pantev, C. (2001). Multiple supratemporal sources of magnetic and electric auditory evoked middle latency components in humans. *Cerebral Cortex, 11*(5), 411–423. PubMed

Yvert, B., Fischer, C., Bertrand, O., & Pernier, J. (2005). Localization of human supratemporal auditory areas from intracerebral auditory evoked potentials using distributed source models. *NeuroImage, 28*(1), 140–153. PubMed

Chapter 10

Cortical Event–Related Potentials

Letitia White and Samuel R. Atcherson

Cortical event–related potentials (CERPs) comprise a broad category of auditory evoked potentials (AEPs), including several important sensory and cognitive types, with a wide variety of terminology with which to classify or group them. As described in Chapter 1, CERPs are classified by their latencies, general anatomical origin, and neural response behaviors to transient, steady-state, and sustained stimulus types. In this chapter, we cover information related to the late auditory evoked potential (P1/N1/P2 complex), the mismatch negativity (MMN), and the P300 component.

Pauline A. Davis (1939) is often credited with discovering the CERP when she observed changes in an electroencephalogram (EEG) recording in response to abrupt sounds. Her discovery came to be called "vertex potential" because of its maximum amplitude on the top center of the head. It was through this discovery that Pauline's husband, Hallowell Davis, and colleagues performed an impressive number of experiments from the 1930s through the 1960s. For several years, the "holy grail" of the vertex potential for H. Davis would be its eventual use as an objective means of estimating behavioral (audiogram) thresholds in infants and other difficult-to-test patients. Although CERPs can indeed be used to estimate behavioral thresholds (Lightfoot and Kennedy, 2006; Musiek, Froke, and Weihing, 2005), it has largely been replaced by the auditory brainstem response (ABR). CERP recordings generally require awake (eyes open), alert, and quiet patients, which can be challenging with younger children. However, the advantage over the ABR is that they can provide some functional information about the auditory cortex and other higher-order structures and processes. The MMN discovered by Näätänen, Gaillard, and Mäntysalo (1978) is another CERP that appears to reflect a preconscious discrimination processing of two or more different sounds, and it does not require patients to actively attend to the stimuli. Finally, the P300 component, discovered by Sutton and colleagues (Sutton, Braren, Zubin, and John, 1965; Sutton, Tueting, Zubin, and John, 1967), is a late (300–600 msec) positive CERP that is evoked by infrequent or unexpected (target) stimuli presented in a sequence of another, more repetitive and frequent (standard) stimulus (e.g., an oddball paradigm). The P300 appears to reflect both exogenous and endogenous characteristics. For example, as an exogenous potential, the listener must first be able to discriminate between the standard and deviant stimuli. In general, the more difficult the discrimination task, the longer the latency, and the smaller the amplitude will become (Polich, Howard, and Starr, 1985). The fact that the P300 can also arise to omitted stimuli demonstrates its role as an endogenous, cognitive potential (McCullagh, Weihing, and Musiek, 2009). **Figure 10.1** shows an example of CERP components within an oddball paradigm recording in a clinical case example.

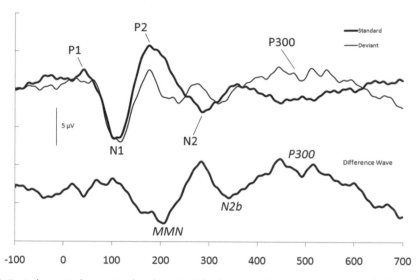

Fig. 10.1 Typical cortical event–related potential (CERP) components. These waveforms were derived using an oddball paradigm with 1000-Hz (standard) and 2000-Hz (deviant) tone bursts. The patient was asked to mentally count the number of deviant stimuli heard. Following the oddball recordings, the difference wave was calculated by subtracting the standard waveform from the deviant waveform, which allows better visualization of the mismatch negativity (MMN) and N2b. (*Note:* The patient had a history of several motor vehicle accident–related head injuries with complaints of difficulty hearing despite normal hearing sensitivity. The P300 component exhibited a small amplitude and longer than expected latency.)

In contrast to early latency potentials (e.g., ABR), CERPs exhibit latencies of 50 msec or greater, requiring slower stimulation rates, and they exhibit larger voltages at the scalp, requiring fewer stimulus presentations. In addition, CERPs have a longer maturational time course, they are generally influenced by subject state, and they are more amenable to the effects of training. A wide variety of speech and nonspeech stimuli can be used with trials containing either a single stimulus or two or more different stimuli. Oddball paradigms involving relatively fewer unexpected (deviant or target) stimuli within a sequence of different but more frequent (standard) stimuli are utilized in MMN and P300 recordings. Unlike the P300, the MMN is best visualized when subtracting the deviant averaged waveform from the standard averaged waveform. The P1/N1/P2 complex is an obligatory response that does not require an oddball paradigm or separate averaging of different stimuli. However, when the evoking stimulus contains a discriminable change within its duration, a second, usually smaller P1/N1/P2 complex can be evoked, which has been termed the *acoustic change complex (ACC)*, or the C complex. Although all CERPs represent activity through the level of the cortex, pinpointing the precise neuro-anatomical generators for each component is difficult at best, mainly because of numerous temporally and spatially overlapping contributions. All these variables are described briefly in the following section.

◆ Late Auditory Evoked Potential

Description of the Waveform

The late auditory evoked potentials (LAEPs) were among the first to be recorded long before signal averaging was available (Davis, 1939). With signal averaging, components P1, N1, P2, and N2 could be identified that occur in succession between 50 and 250 msec post-stimulus onset (Hay and Davis, 1971). The letters P and N refer to positive and negative voltages, respectively. The P1 component is the earliest of the LAEPs occurring at ~50 msec, and it is assumed to be the same as the Pb component of the middle latency response (MLR) (e.g., Ponton, Eggermont, Khosla, Kwong, and Don, 2002). The N1 and P2 components occur with latencies of 100 msec (range, 90–150 msec) and

180 msec (range, 160–200 msec), respectively (Williams, Tepas, and Morlock, 1962). The N1-P2 complex is considered the most stable and salient feature of the LAEP as it is elicited by virtually any stimulus with a relatively abrupt onset or change, including stimulus offsets and interruptions in ongoing stimuli (Atcherson, Gould, Mendel, and Ethington, 2009; Davis and Zerlin, 1966; Dimitrijevic, Michalewski, Zeng, Pratt, and Starr, 2008; Martin and Boothroyd, 1999). The N2 component is the last of the LAEP components with a latency of 300 to 350 msec. Sometimes N2 is rather prominent in the waveforms (perhaps tied to stimulus intensity), but other times it is barely distinguishable from background activity. Although N2 has largely been ignored in the field of audiology because of the use of relatively awake and alert patients, its amplitude actually becomes larger with the onset of sleep (Näätänen and Picton, 1987). However, this component is not to be confused with the N2b component, which is often associated with the MMN and P300 in oddball paradigm recordings (e.g., Patel and Azzam, 2005). With moderately high-level stimuli, N1 and P2 components can reach amplitudes of up to 5 µV independently and have peak-to-peak amplitudes of around 10 µV. Generally, LAEP components are larger in amplitude compared with earlier potentials because of the more superficial location of their generators within the cortex. Finally, latencies and amplitudes appear to exhibit good test–retest reliability using both tone bursts and natural speech stimuli (Atcherson, Gould, Pousson, and Prout, 2006; Tremblay, Friesen, Martin, and Wright, 2003).

Neural Generators

P1 appears to arise from sources from the primary auditory cortex, specifically Heschl's gyrus, but may have thalamic and auditory association area contributions as well (Buchwald, Erwin, Van Lancker, Guthrie, Schwafel, and Tanguay, 1992; Liégeois-Chauvel, Musolino, Badier, Marquis, and Chauvel, 1994; McGee and Kraus, 1996; Ponton and Eggermont, 2001). N1 appears to have multiple temporally overlapping, spatially distributed cortical sources. These sources include activation of Heschl's gyri and the planum temporale (resulting in radially and tangentially oriented dipoles) with contributions from frontocentral sources, the cingulate gyrus, and other auditory association areas in the lateral temporal and parietal lobe (Atcherson et al, 2006; Alcaini, Giard, Thévenet, and Pernier, 1994; Anderer, Pascual-Marqui, Semlitsch, and Saletu, 1998; Giard, Perrin, Echallier, Thévenet, Froment, and Pernier, 1994; McCallum and Curry, 1980; Näätänen and Picton, 1987; Pascual-Marqui, Michel, and Lehmann, 1994; Picton, Alain, Woods, John, Scherg, Valdes-Sosa, et al, 1999; Scherg and Von Cramon, 1985; 1986; Wolpaw and Penry, 1975a). P2 appears to be generated in the vicinity of the primary auditory cortex within the temporal lobe (Hari, Hämäläinen, Ilmoniemi, Kaukoranta, Reinikainen, Salminen, et al, 1984; Vaughan and Ritter, 1970). N2 probably arises from the frontal lobes, limbic system, or other obscure subcortical structures (Kiehl, Laurens, Duty, Forster, and Liddle, 2001; Näätänen, 1982).

Pitfall

It cannot be assumed that electrode placement on the scalp over the temporal lobe (or any other site) will reflect activity only at that site. Recall that there are likely numerous generators that are temporally overlapping and synchronously activated. Also, the magnitude of an LAEP component will be determined to a large extent on the orientation and strength of the generators' dipoles, as well as the location of the reference electrode which may or may not also be picking up activity.

Stimulus and Recording Parameters

As stated earlier, the LAEP components can be elicited by virtually any acoustic change. Although LAEPs can be elicited with clicks, they are more commonly elicited with short-duration tone bursts and both speech and speech-like stimuli. Most clinical systems are able to record LAEPs with some minor test protocol adjustments. **Table 10.1** shows commonly used stimulus and recording parameters for LAEPs.

Special Consideration

Although P1/N1/P2, or N1-P2, is often grouped together as a complex, the majority of LAEP studies have focused on the N1 component as evidenced by several extensive literature reviews on this component alone (e.g., Eggermont and Ponton, 2002; Näätänen and Picton, 1987; Hyde, 1997; Woods, 1995). However, the P1 component has received substantial attention in the past 15 years because it can serve as a developmental or maturational marker for central auditory nervous system development (e.g., Eggermont, Ponton, Don, Waring, and Kwong, 1997; Sharma, Martin, Roland, Bauer, Sweeney, Gilley, et al., 2005).

Because LAEPs are transient responses, they respond well to stimuli with relatively fast rise/fall times of up to ~50 msec (Alain, Woods, and Covarrubias, 1997; Onishi and Davis, 1968). Stimuli with long overall durations are not necessary, however, they might be useful in threshold estimation studies (grimes and Feldman, 1971). The clinician should be aware that N1 and P2 have been shown to decrease in latency and increase in amplitude as the toneburst stimulus plateau increased from 9-128 msec (Eddins and Peterson, 1999). When stimulus durations are long (several hundred milliseconds or more), an offset LAEP can also be observed that mimics the onset LAEP. However, the neural generators that give rise to the onset and offset LAEPs may be slightly different (Mittelman, Bleich, and Pratt, 2005). In addition, long-duration stimuli can produce a sustained negativity potential that persists for as long as the stimulus is on (Picton, Woods, and Proulx, 1978). To produce a clean-onset LAEP, tone burst stimuli with rise/fall times of 10 to 20 msec and a plateau of 50 to 80 msec work reasonably well. The effects of stimulus envelope shaping on tone bursts may be irrelevant at the cortical level because of longer rise times and plateaus, but linear or Blackman ramps are generally applied. The stimulus polarity also appears to be irrelevant for all CERPs. However, McPherson et al (2007) suggest that rarefaction polarity be

Table 10.1 Suggested Stimulus Parameters and Recording Considerations for Late Auditory Evoked Potentials

Stimulus Parameters	
Type	Tone bursts (audiogram frequencies) and other nonlinguistic stimuli (10–20 msec rise/fall time, 20–60 msec plateau, linear, or Blackman ramp) Speech or speechlike (words, consonant-vowel, or vowel stimuli) Clicks (though generally not recommended)
Intensity	60–70 dB peSPL (peak equivalent sound pressure level, suprathreshold) Variable in 5–10 dB step decrements (threshold estimation)
Polarity	Rarefaction, but generally not relevant (see text)
Rate	0.7 to 1.7/s (will depend on stimulus duration and time window)
Presentations	500 per trial (as few as 50 to as many as 1000 may be needed, depending on the patient characteristics during the test and amount of noise)
Transducer	ER-3A (or loudspeaker with hearing aids and cochlear implants)
Recording Considerations	
Electrodes	Cz (noninverting), ipsilateral or contralateral earlobe (inverting and not linked), and Fpz (ground) Above or below one eye (with two-channel system, and if more channels are available an electrode lateral to one eye)
Amplification	50,000 to 75,000 times
Artifact rejection	± 100 µV
Data points	256 points (~426 samples/s) or 512 points (~853 samples/s)
Time window	−100 to 500 msec or longer (will depend on stimulation rate and desired component latencies)
Filters	0.1 to 100 Hz during acquisition and offline digital filtering of 1 to 20 Hz or 1 to 40 Hz
Replications	A minimum of two

used with tone bursts and to consider reversing the polarity if rarefaction polarity waveforms are poor in morphology. The intensity level at which stimuli are presented will vary depending on the type of stimulus used and the purpose of the assessment. For suprathreshold applications, an intensity level that would be perceived as "comfortable" is usually more than sufficient (usually 60–70 dB peSPL). Calibrated intensity levels, however, will vary depending on certain stimulus parameters and proper instrumentation (see Chapter 22).

Minimally, a two-channel electrode system is needed, with one noninverting electrode placed on the site of interest (usually Cz) and the other noninverting electrode placed above or below one eye to detect and reject eyeblink activity. A single inverting electrode can be placed on the ipsilateral or contralateral earlobe. Finally, the ground electrode can be placed on either the high forehead or the unused earlobe. Because the two noninverting electrodes will share the same inverting electrode site, the references are linked with a jumper cable. The preceding electrode montage, again, is the minimum. Ideally, four or more channels would be preferable to add at least one more electrode lateral to one eye and one or more additional electrodes on the head (e.g., C3-Cz-C4 recordings). With multichannel recordings, such as C3 and C4 recordings, a linked earlobe setup can be used. That is, each earlobe will have an inverting electrode but will be electrically linked together by plugging both electrodes into the same jumper cable.

Measurement Parameters

Latency

The measurement of latencies is rather easy and straightforward, with P1 occurring at 50 msec, N1 occurring anywhere between 90 and 150 msec, P2 occurring anywhere between 160 and 200 msec, and N2 occurring between 300 and 350 msec. In general, the maximum or centermost point on the broad wave is selected. With wide-acquisition filter settings (e.g., 0.1–100 Hz), the waveforms may appear to be "noisier" and may make novice clinicians uncertain about which peaks to select if several are nearby. After the recordings, additional digital filtering can be applied to "smooth out" the waveform. Spectrally, the LAEP components are low in frequency (**Fig. 10.2**), such that the low-pass cutoff can be set to as low

as 15 Hz. However, a low-pass filter of 30 to 40 Hz is recommended to avoid distorting the waveform. The high-pass cutoff could be left at 0.1 Hz but should not be raised higher than 1 Hz, above which some waveform distortion can occur. If the option is available, a 12 dB/octave filter slope is recommended. Another technique that can help with latency measures is the smoothing function (Chapter 3). In general, the smoothing function can be applied numerous times with little alteration to latency; however, the overall amplitude may be affected (Hall, 2007). It is always best to obtain the cleanest waveforms possible during the actual recording and to rely on additional filtering or smoothing as needed or as defined by protocols.

Amplitude

Amplitude measures can be obtained in one of two ways: peak-to-peak (or peak-to-trough) such as with N1-P2, or baseline-to-peak measures. In some cases, the N1-P2 peak-to-peak amplitude measurement may be more stable than individual component baseline-to-peak measurement (Zhang, Eliassen, Anderson, Scheifele, and Brown, 2009). To obtain baseline-to-peak measures, a relatively flat prestimulus period is helpful. Wherever the peak latency is measured, the amplitude measure would also be taken. Because amplitude is susceptible to the effects of the amount of noise in the recordings, the state of the listener, and even habituation of responses in

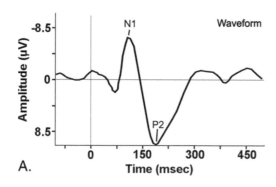

A.

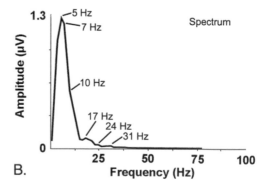

B.

Fig. 10.2 Illustration of fast Fourier transform (FFT) on a late auditory evoked potential (LAEP) waveform. (**A**) Averaged LAEP waveform represented in the time domain (msec). (**B**) Applying FFT on the waveform, the

spectral energy is represented in the frequency domain (Hz), with energy up to ~50 Hz. The greatest spectral energy occurs at about 5 Hz.

long recording sessions, it is helpful to obtain two replications, and the morphology ought to appear "repeatable." Although statistical methods are available for determining the presence or absence of a component, a general rule of thumb is to check to make sure that the component of interest is at least 2 to 3 times larger than the activity in the prestimulus period. McPherson et al (2007) recommend that the prestimulus period be at least 10% of the desired analysis window.

Subject Effects

Eyes Open

In contrast to earlier potentials, LAEPs are highly susceptible to the influence of several electroencephalogram (EEG) brain states. For example, when a patient is awake but relaxed with eyes closed, a large, continuous α wave with EEG frequencies between 8 and 12 Hz is produced, which can overlap in time and amplitude with certain components of the LAEP. To keep patients alert, they can quietly read a book (magazines are not recommended) or watch a subtitled movie with the audio kept at a minimum.

Eyeblinks

With the requirement of having eyes open for LAEP recordings comes the potential problem of eyeblinks. Eyeblinks can be quite large in amplitude, completely obscuring the LAEP, particularly if the patient synchronizes eyeblinks with stimuli. Avoiding or minimizing eyeblink activity in the recorded LAEP can come in several forms. First, the patient can be instructed to relax and to minimize all forms of

movement, including eyeblinks. Unfortunately, some patients may go to great lengths to keep from blinking (introducing unwanted myogenic activity), they may increase the frequency of their eyeblinks (due to perceived dry eye), or they may introduce an unwanted variable on the LAEP where eyeblink avoidance becomes an attentional task. Simply telling the patient to relax and pay no attention to the stimulus may be all that is needed. An effective method for dealing with eyeblinks is to use electrodes around the eye so that eyeblinks that reach artifact rejection levels are not included in the average. The artifact rejection levels should be set low enough to reject any large, unwanted artifact but high enough so that the ongoing EEG is untouched. Watching a subtitled video will help to encourage relaxation and minimize eyeblink activity for most patients.

Attention

The effects of attention on the LAEP are broad and varied, but in general N1 tends to become larger in amplitude (Hillyard, Hink, Schwent, and Picton, 1973), whereas P2 becomes smaller (Hansen and Hillyard, 1980). P2 is believed to decrease in amplitude because of the increase in a processing negativity (called Nd) that arises during selective attention (Hansen and Hillyard, 1980).

Hearing Sensitivity

Data are significantly lacking in the area of hearing sensitivity effects on the LAEP. On the one hand, some studies demonstrate no differences in N1 and P2 components between those with normal hearing and those with hearing loss (Adler and Adler, 1991; Wall, Dalebout, Davidson, and Fox, 1991), whereas others have demonstrated latency delays in those with hearing loss (Martin and Boothroyd, 1999; Oates, Kurtzberg, and Stapells, 2002). In a preliminary investigation of auditory deprivation in young to middle-aged adults with and without hearing loss, Buckley (2003) demonstrated that although latencies were not different between groups, P1, N1, and P2 amplitudes were significantly different between groups when stimuli were presented based on SL rather than on at fixed intensity level. Because hearing loss is also associated with advancing age, more research is needed on the effects of all these variables for greater clarity and understanding.

Development and Maturation

Because of the generator locations within the cortex, LAEP components have a much longer maturational time course than would be expected for ABR (~2 years to adultlike morphology) and MLR (~10–12 years to adultlike morphology). Although the LAEPs will undergo great developmental changes throughout childhood, the underlying generators are functional at birth (Kushnerenko, Ceponiene, Balan, Fellman, Huotilaine, and Näätänen, 2002). LAEP components are thought to reach adultlike morphology during puberty (Eggermont and Ponton, 2003; Wunderlich, Cone-Wesson, and Shepherd, 2006). Bishop et al (2007), however, suggest that there are three steplike and clearly distinguishable developmental periods for LAEPs: 5 to 12 years, 13 to 16 years, and adulthood. Because LAEP components can be recorded in infants (Kushnerenko, Ceponiene, Balan, Fellman, Huotilaine, and Näätänen, 2002; Wunderlich and Cone-Wesson, 2006),

Sharma et al (2005) have used the P1 component as a biomarker of auditory development. With proper auditory stimulation, P1 latency is expected to decrease with age. Using the P1 in this way may have clinical applications in assessing the efficacy of hearing aid and cochlear implant fittings and even as an objective tool in the decision to switch from hearing aids to a cochlear implant. **Figure 10.3** illustrates the maturational difference in the LAEP for an 18-month-old child and a young adult. Notice the prominence of P1 in the child with a latency of ~120 msec. On reaching puberty, all LAEPs are expected to appear and shift in latency to be more adultlike.

Clinical Applications

There are several potential clinical applications for LAEPs. In some cases, a standard clinical evoked potential system is all that is needed. In other cases, more sophisticated equipment (e.g., Compumedics Neuroscan), stimulation, or analysis techniques may be required above and beyond the capabilities of the standard clinical system. LAEPs can be recorded in a variety of patient populations including individuals with hearing loss, auditory neuropathy spectrum disorder (ANSD), and hearing aid or cochlear implant users. Thus, in the brief review of some of the clinical applications that follow, readers should be aware that the techniques described may have broad clinical applications with many factors and patient groups that have yet to be examined.

Neurodiagnostics

Although clinicians are more likely to use ABR and MLR, LAEPs still have an important place in neurodiagnostics. Although high intersubject variability and lack of normative data are current limitations, as various auditory disorders are better understood, LAEPs may aid in differential diagnosis. Already LAEPs have demonstrated some abnormal patterns in patients with tinnitus (Santos Filha and Matas, 2010), ANSD (Michalewski, Starr, Nguyen, Kong, and Zeng, 2005), cortical lesions (Knight, Hillyard, Woods, and Neville, 1980), diffuse brain injury (Kileny and Berry, 1983), and auditory processing and language/learning problems (Jirsa and Clontz, 1990; Tonnquist-Uhlén, 1996; Warrier,

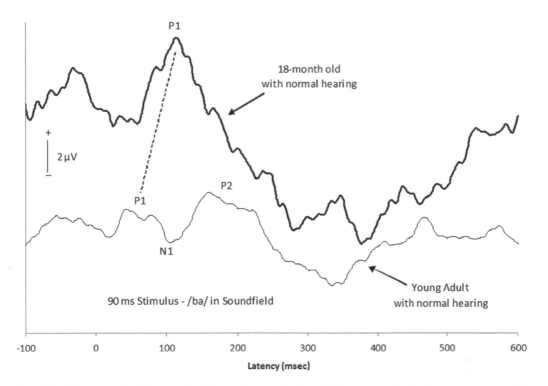

Fig. 10.3 Maturational differences in late auditory evoked potentials (LAEPs). Notice the differences in waveform morphology between the 18-month-old child and the young adult, both of whom have normal hearing. The prominent P1 component at 100 msec for the child is expected to shorten in latency, and N1 and P2 are expected to emerge and develop through puberty. The stimulus presentations (/ba/) were made through a loudspeaker for the child, and ER-3A insert earphones for the adult.

Johnson, Hayes, Nicol, and Kraus, 2004). Although not the focus on this textbook, LAEPs have been shown to be abnormal in a variety of psychiatric disorders.

Cortical Evoked Response Audiometry

The attempt at using LAEPs to estimate (or validate) hearing thresholds has been around since the days of Hallowell Davis (1965). However, clinicians had largely abandoned LAEPs for this application in favor of the ABR because of its ease of use and because the ABR can be performed while the patient is asleep (ideal for newborns). The major limitation of the ABR is that it does not provide any functional information beyond the brainstem. Thus, the ABR falls short in helping with medical-legal cases of nonorganic or exaggerated hearing loss (see, e.g., Hone, Norman, Keogh, and Kelly, 2003; Hyde, Alberti, Matsumoto, and Li, 1986; Lightfoot and Kennedy, 2006). LAEP thresholds have been shown to be within 10 dB of behavioral thresholds more than 80% of the time in patient populations with Meniere's disease and noise induced hearing loss (Prasher, Mula, and Luxon, 1993; Lightfoot and Kennedy, 2006). Readers interested in using cortical evoked response audiometry (CERA) would benefit from Dr. Lightfoot's Web site (http://www.corticalera.com/). Recently, however, there has been some renewed interest in using LAEPs to estimate hearing thresholds in infants with objective, statistical techniques such as Hotelling's T^2 (Carter, Golding, Dillon, aned Seymour, 2010; Golding, Pearce, Seymour, Cooper, Ching, and Dillon, 2007;). Software and measurement techniques, as described by Lightfoot and Kennedy (2006), Golding et al (2007), and Carter et al (2010), have yet to be implemented in commercial evoked potential systems.

Hearing Devices

There is great interest among researchers and clinicians in studying the effects of acoustic (air and bone conduction) and electric forms of auditory stimulation on the central auditory nervous system. Such studies may be useful for determining cochlear implant candidacy, for determining treatment efficacy, and for showing continued auditory development or plasticity. As hearing aids and cochlear implants introduce yet another element to the processing of acoustic signals, studies have been conducted (e.g., Billings, Tremblay, Souza, and Binns, 2007; Friesen and Picton, 2010; Rahne, Ehelebe, Rasinski, and Götze, 2010; Tremblay, Billings, Friesen, and Souza, 2006; Zhang, Samy, Anderson, and Houston, 2009) or are currently under way to study signal-processing effects before LAEPs can be used in a meaningful way clinically. Some cochlear implant users exhibit a large stimulus-related artifact that obscures the LAEP components (**Fig. 10.4**). Numerous techniques have been suggested in the literature to counteract this problem (Atcherson, Damji, and Upson, 2011; Friesen and Picton, 2010; Gilley, Sharma, Dorman, Finley, Panch, and Martin, 2006; Sharma, Martin, Roland, Bauer, Sweeney, Gilley, et al, 2005).

Auditory Training

The neurons of the cortex appear to have tremendous capacity for change. Not only are they influenced by the environment and experience (Eggermont and Ponton, 2002; Gilbert, Sigman, and Crist, 2001;), but they are also affected by impairments of the peripheral auditory system (Ponton and Eggermont, 2001) and training (Tremblay, Kraus, McGee, Ponton, and Otis, 2001; Tremblay, Shahin, Picton, and Ross, 2009). In general, N1 and P2 amplitudes can be modified with auditory training. In children with auditory-processing deficits or learning impairments, the efficacy of formal auditory-based training (e.g., Earobics, Cognitive Concepts, Cambridge, MA) may also be assessed using LAEP (Warrier, Johnson, Hayes, Nicol, and Kraus, 2004). Warrier et al (2004) found that some children with learning impairments had abnormal N2 response-timing patterns in noise, but they improved to within normal limits following training.

◆ Mismatch Negativity

Description of the Waveform

As previously mentioned, the MMN was discovered by Risto Näätänen and colleagues in 1978. It is a component of the AEP that peaks ~100 to 250 msec post-stimulus onset and is thought to represent the detection of stimulus change (Kraus and McGee, 1994; Kraus, McGee, Micco, Sharma, Carrell, and Nicol, 1993; Kujala, Kallio, Tervaniemi, and Näätänen, 2001; Näätänen, 1992; Näätänen, Gaillard, and Män-

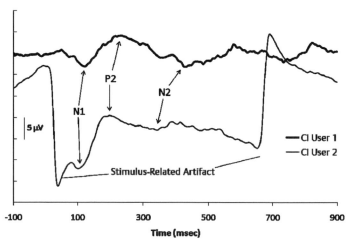

Fig. 10.4 Stimulus-related artifact is present in some cochlear implant users. Waveforms in this figure were elicited with a 656- msec tone burst (1 kHz) presented at 80-dB SPL (sound pressure level) in the sound field with Cz (noninverting) and nonimplant earlobe (inverting) electrodes. A third electrode placed on the infraorbital ridge below one eye (on the nonimplant side) was used to pick up eyeblink activity. Both adult patients with cochlear implants were Advanced Bionics CII (Advanced Bionics Corp., Valencia, CA) users with Auria Harmony behind-the-ear processors and T-mics. Notice the differences in late auditory evoked potentials (LAEPs) waveforms, with CI user 2 having a large stimulus-related artifact at onset and offset of the 656 msec tone.

tysalo, 1978). Kraus (1999) described the MMN as a "central sensory representation" occurring after peripheral encoding. In a very general sense, it can be thought of as a physiologic difference limen. It has been elicited to a wide variety of sound attributes using both speech and nonspeech stimuli. These attributes include changes in intensity, frequency, and duration. MMNs have also been recorded to sound omissions, gaps in stimuli, spatial changes, and changes in stimulus onset asynchrony.

Because elicitation of the MMN does not require attention on the part of the listener (Novak, Ritter, Vaughan, and Wiznitzer, 1990), it is considered a preattentive response. It has been recorded in infants at birth (Alho, Sainio, Sajaniemi, Reinikainen, and Näätänen, 1990), in sleeping adults (Nielsen-Bohlman, Knight, Woods, and Woodward, 1991), and in some comatose patients (Kane, Curry, Butler, and Cummins, 1993). Because of its preattentive nature and the fact that it can be recorded in newborns as well as sleeping and comatose patients, one might predict a high degree of clinical popularity. Unfortunately, that is not currently the case. The MMN lacks clinical utility because of time-intensive recording techniques, poor signal-to-noise ratios (SNRs) that make response identification challenging, and a lack of consistency between behavioral and electrophysiologic findings at the individual level (Dalebout and Fox, 2000, 2001). A great deal of literature about the MMN exists, and researchers continue to search for ways to improve its clinical utility.

The MMN is evoked using an oddball paradigm (Hall, 1992; McPherson, 1996), in which an occasional "deviant" stimulus (also known as a target or rare stimulus) is intermingled among a series of standard stimuli (also known as frequent stimuli). For ease of response identification and evaluation, the standard and deviant stimuli are averaged separately, and a difference wave is obtained. Three techniques have been developed to extract the MMN from the EEG recording. For the first procedure, the waveform elicited by the standard stimulus in the oddball paradigm is subtracted from the waveform elicited by the deviant stimulus. For the second technique, recordings are obtained for a standard oddball paradigm, as well as for a train of deviant stimuli presented alone. The response from the deviant stimuli alone is then subtracted from the response to the same deviant stimuli when they are presented as part of the oddball. The third extraction technique involves recording responses to two separate oddball sequences. The standard stimulus in one test run becomes the deviant stimulus in the second test run. The response to the stimulus when it was a standard in the first run is then subtracted from the response to the same stimulus when it was a deviant in the second test run. The third procedure lacks popularity because of the time constraints involved in obtaining responses to two oddball sequences. Generally speaking, it does not matter which extraction technique is used to elicit the MMN so long as care has been taken to control for refractory effects in the second condition—the deviant alone condition (Walker, Carpenter, Downs, Cranford, Stuart, and Pravica, 2001).

Neural Generators

There are multiple presumed generator sites for the MMN. The major generators in adults are located on the superior surface of the temporal lobe in the primary and secondary auditory cortices. Frontal and subcortical sources may also be involved (Alho, Sams, Paavilainen, and Näätänen, 1986; Näätänen, 1990). A magnetoencephalographic (MEG) study by Hari et al (1984) provided the first direct evidence for the role of the auditory cortex in the generation of the MMN. Subsequent MEG studies have supported the finding that the auditory cortex is involved in MMN generation (Alho, 1995), with responses being largest over the frontocentral electrode sites in adults. Feature-specific processing of a stimulus, known as parallel processing, is thought to occur during MMN generation (Schairer, Gould, and Pousson, 2001). By looking at the relationship between processes activated by different types of deviants, researchers have found that the processes by which the different features elicit an MMN are at least partly independent of each other (Levänen, Hari, McEvoy, and Sams, 1993; Schröger, 1995, 1996; Takegata, Paavilainen, Näätänen, and Winkler, 1999; Wolff and Schröger, 1995).

Stimulus/Recording Parameters

The MMN can be elicited by minimal stimulus differences, even those that approximate behavioral discrimination thresholds (Kraus et al, 1993; Sams, Paavilainen, Alho, and Näätänen, 1985; Tiitinen, May, Reinikainen, and Näätänen, 1994). In general, as the magnitude of difference between the standard and target stimuli increases, the MMN response amplitude increases and latency decreases (Näätänen, Gaillard, and Mäntysalo, 1978; Näätänen, Paavilainen, and Reinikainen, 1989; Picton, 1995; Sams, Paavilainen, Alho, and Näätänen, 1985). This is true only to a point. Because the MMN is overlapped by N1, if the magnitude of difference between deviant and standard stimuli is too large, MMN latency may approach the latency range of the N1 response, creating possible overlap and difficulty in interpretation (Sinkkonen and Tervaniemi, 2000). Also, if the difference between standard and deviant stimuli is too great, it will be more difficult for listeners to ignore the stimuli. If listener attention shifts to the deviant when it occurs, a P3a response may be elicited, which could reduce or eliminate the MMN. Deviances of up to 10% are thought to produce MMNs that are minimally impacted by overlapping N1 and P3 responses (Lang, Nyrke, Ek, Aaltonen, Raimo, and Näätänen, 1990).

Suggested recording parameters can be found in **Table 10.2**. This table illustrates a paradigm in which a single deviant is used. Pakarinen, Takegata, Rinne, Huotilainen, and Näätänen (2007) suggested a multifeature paradigm in which multiple deviants along different dimensions are used to obtain an auditory discrimination profile. In the aforementioned study, the authors suggest use of four different types of deviants (i.e., frequency, intensity, duration, and gap) at three deviation magnitudes for use in a clinical setting. In other words, three separate stimulus sequences would be presented. Each sequence would contain all deviance types. The sequences would differ from each other in the magnitude of difference between standard and deviant stimuli. For example, one sequence might contain deviants that are easily discriminable from the standard. The other sequences would be made more difficult by decreasing the magnitude of difference between the standard and deviant stimuli. The deviants would all be presented in the same oddball sequence with the standard tone occurring at a probability of 60 percent. Each different deviant type would occur with a

Table 10.2 Summary of Recording Parameters for the Mismatch Negativity Using a Single Deviant Paradigm

Recording and Stimulus Parameters	
Filter (Hz)	0.1–10 or 0.1–30[a]
Window	−50 to 500 msec
Noninverting electrodes	Fz, Cz, C3, C4, 1 bipolar channel to monitor eyeblinks
Inverting electrode	Mastoid or nose[b]
Deviant probability	5–20 percent
ISI	50–4000 msec[c]
Total number of sweeps	At least 1400 (see Deviant probability)

[a] Sinkkonen and Tervaniemi (2000) recommend an upper cutoff of 10 Hz to optimize quantification of latency measures. Duncan et al (2009) recommend a more conventional upper cutoff of 30 Hz.

[b] Walker-Black and Stuart (2008) found best waveform morphology/response presence using a mastoid reference, as compared with nose or linked mastoid references. Duncan et al (2009) recommend a nose reference so response reversal at the mastoid can be visualized. Nose reference was recommended by Näätänen (1992), but it can be difficult clinically because of high artifact (Lang, Eerola, Korpilahti, Holopainen, Salo, and Aaltonen, 1995).

[c] Stimulation rate depends on deviance type (Näätänen and Picton, 1987). For short-duration, simple stimuli, 300 msec is adequate (Lang et al, 995).

probability of 10 percent. In this paradigm, the stimuli alternate with every other tone being either the standard or one of the deviants. The authors suggest that a multi-feature paradigm would allow clinicians to construct an auditory discrimination profile, which could give information on auditory system development, plasticity, and response to auditory training. For further detail on stimulus parameters that are appropriate for different types of stimuli (i.e., frequency vs intensity vs temporal variants), the reader is referred to Duncan et al (2009).

Measurement Parameters

Determining whether an MMN is present or absent in individual listeners can be very challenging for many reasons. Primarily, the amplitude of the response is small, and it is embedded in a great deal of background noise, creating a poor SNR. In the early days of MMN recording, the response was identified through visual inspection of the waveforms. The inherent difficulty in identifying the MMN visually, researchers have recently moved away from visual inspection and toward other means, including area under the curve measurement, integrated MMN analysis, and principal component analysis. Because the MMN is not a commonly used clinical tool, these methods will not be described in depth here. (For an in-depth review of other methods of quantifying the MMN, the reader is referred to McGee, Kraus, and Nicol, 1997; Petermann, Kummer, Burger, Lohscheller, Eysholdt, and Döllinger, 2009). It should be noted that there is no clear consensus on the best clinical approach to quantifyng the MMN.

Latency and Amplitude

When evaluating and quantifying the MMN, latency and amplitude are among the parameters that are commonly measured. These parameters are thought to reflect the magnitude of physical difference between the deviant and standard stimuli (Tervaniemi, 1999). The MMN typically occurs between 100 and 250 msec. Because it is a wide, negative deflection from the baseline, there may not be a clear peak in the response. When visual inspection was a common means of response identification, latency onset and offset were often measured. MMN amplitudes range from ~0.5 to 5 μV, with common values of 1 to 2 μV. Again, in studies that used visual inspection to identify the response, often the amplitude of the most negative peak in the latency range was chosen.

Topography

In addition to looking at latency and amplitude, it is useful to look at scalp topography when evaluating whether an MMN is present. The response is typically larger over the frontocentral regions. Furthermore, when using a recording montage in which the nose serves as the inverting electrode, a reversal in response polarity can be observed at the mastoid electrodes (relative to the noninverting electrodes).

Subject Effects

Development/Maturation Effects

In general, significant maturational changes are seen in the topography of MMN from infancy through adulthood, particularly over left and frontal electrode sites. Based on this, it seems that the MMN generators may not be mature in childhood (Korpilahti and Lang, 1994; Kurtzberg, Vaughan, Kreuzer, and Fliegler, 1995; Morr, Shafer, Kreuzer, and Kurtzberg, 2002). However, it is consistently present in children to frequency (Ceponiene, Cheour, and Näätänen, 1998; Kurtzberg, Vaughan, Kreuzer, and Fliegler, 1995), duration (Korpilahti and Lang, 1994), and speech-stimulus contrasts (Csépe, 1995).

In addition to topographical changes, latency changes are seen with maturation. Decreases in latency during infancy and childhood have been reported (Korpilahti and Lang, 1994; Morr, Shafer, Kreuzer, and Kurtzberg, 2002; Shafer, Morr, Kreuzer, and Kurtzberg, 2000). One could suggest that the speed of the processes underlying discrimination decreases from infancy through childhood. Although compelling, these results have not been demonstrated consistently (Kraus et al, 1993). Additionally, some researchers have found that children have larger MMN amplitudes than adults (Kraus, McGee, Sharma, Carrell, and Nicol, 1992). Not surprisingly, an examination of data from children leads to an appreciation of the considerable variability in MMN amplitudes within age groups and within a single participant (Kurtzberg, Vaughan, Kreuzer, and Fliegler, 1995).

Aging Effects

Not only does the MMN change as the underlying neural centers supporting it mature, but it may also provide information regarding the natural aging process, as a neural index of the plasticity of the auditory system (Kraus, McGee, Carrell, and Sharma, 1995). Researchers have found that with advancing age, the duration of the auditory sensory memory trace declines (Pekkonen, Rinne, Reinikainen, Kujala, Alho, and Näätänen, 1996), suggesting reduced neural plasticity.

Neurologic Abnormalities

The MMN might serve as an indicator of the functional state of the cortex, as well as sensory and/or perceptual potential. In addition, disorders of automatic processing or neural plasticity may be investigated using the MMN (Näätänen, 1995). As an indicator of the functional state of the cortex, MMN amplitude is larger when task vigilance is increased (Lang, Eerola, Korpilahti, Holopainen, Salo, and Aaltonen, 1995). The MMN is attenuated in the presence of sedatives (Duncan and Kaye, 1987; Pietrowsky, Fehm, and Born, 1990) and alcohol (Jääskeläinen, Pekkonen, Alho, Sinclair, Sillanaukee, and Näätänen, 1995). Based on this line of thought, Kane, Curry, Butler, and Cummins (1993) suggested the use of the MMN in the prognosis of comatose patients (for a review, see Daltrozzo, Wioland, Mutschler, and Kotchoubey, 2007). The MMN may also serve as a tool for the evaluation of aural rehabilitation for cochlear implantees (Kraus and McGee, 1994; Ponton and Don, 1995).

Auditory discrimination skills have also been studied using the MMN in several neurologic disorders, including dyslexia (Baldeweg, Richardson, Watkins, Foale, and Gruzelier, 1999; Kujala, Kallio, Tervaniemi, and Näätänen, 2001), schizophrenia (for a review, see Michie, 2001), Parkinson disease (Pekkonen, Jousmäki, Reinikainen, and Partanen, 1995), Alzheimer disease (Pekkonen, Jousmäki, Könönen, Reinikainen, and Partanen, 1994),

aphasia (Aaltonen, Tuomainen, Laine, and Niemi, 1993), dysphasia (Korpilahti and Lang, 1994), and learning disabilities in pediatrics (Kraus and McGee, 1994). Generally speaking, evaluation of group grand-averaged waveforms indicates that MMN amplitudes are attenuated in these pathologic populations.

Clinical Applications

Clinical application for the purposes of evaluating auditory discrimination in individual listeners is limited at this time because of concerns regarding methods and test-operating characteristics. Research continues with efforts directed toward improving the SNR of the response and making recording times shorter. Many studies in the MMN literature report on group-averaged waveforms and report that for overall group data, averaged MMN responses are smaller for different patient populations, but there is a lack of data regarding the ability of the MMN to identify pathology in individual listeners (i.e., sensitivity). Finally, test–retest reliability has been reported to be between $r = 0.3$ and 0.6, suggesting that the MMN is useful at the group level but not at the individual level (Escera and Grau 1996; Frodl-Bauch, Kathmann, Möller, and Hegerl, 1997; Joutsiniemi, Ilvonen, Sinkkonen, Huotilainen, Tervaniemi, Lehtokoski, et al, 1998; Schröger, 1998).

♦ P300

Description of the Waveform

The P300, discovered by Sutton, Braren, Zubin, and John (1965), is an LAEP that usually occurs between 250 and 500 msec but may peak as late as 600 msec. It is elicited when a listener consciously discriminates an infrequent target stimulus in a chain of frequent standard stimuli (i.e., oddball paradigm). Because conscious discrimination and attention are required, the P300 is often referred to as a cognitive response. As described earlier in the chapter, the P300 is influenced by both exogenous and endogenous factors. It has been demonstrated in the auditory (Sutton, Braren, Zubin, and John, 1965), somatosensory (Yamaguchi and Knight, 1991), and visual

(Courchesne, Hillyard, and Galambos, 1975) modalities. In the auditory modality, stimulus frequency, intensity, and duration are among the many parameters that can be varied to elicit the response. Because of the vast nature of the P300 literature, this chapter provides an introduction and a brief overview of the response and its clinical application.

The P300 is referred to as such because it follows the P1 and P2 components of the LAEP and peaks at ~300 msec. The response can be divided into two waves or components: P3a and P3b. The P3a occurs in response to large stimulus differences and does not depend on attention, whereas the P3b is thought to reflect discrimination, which occurs only when the listener is actively attending (Polich, 1989; Squires, Squires, and Hillyard, 1975;). The focus of this chapter is on the P3b.

To obtain the response, listeners are asked to count or push a button when target sounds occur (Courchesne, 1978; Kurtzberg, Vaughan, and Kreuzer, 1979). Because it is a robust response, the P300 is typically visible with 20 to 30 averages of the target stimuli (Polich and Starr, 1984), with maximal responses occurring over the central parietal region of the scalp (Polich and Starr, 1983). The P300 is thought to be a neural index of the timing of cognitive processes, specifically succession and speed of mental processes (Kutas, McCarthy, and Donchin, 1977; Sutton, Braren, Zubin, and John, 1965). Additionally, short-term memory and decision making are reflected by the P300 (Donchin, 1981; Harrison, Buchwald, and Kaga, 1986; Squires, Wickens, Squires, and Donchin, 1976). Endogenous factors that influence the P300 include state of arousal and attention (Picton and Hillyard, 1974). Exogenous factors that influence the P300 include the probability of a target presentation, as well as the level of difficulty of the discrimination task. (Donchin and Coles, 1988).

Neural Generators

The precise neural generators of the P300 are unclear; however, multiple sources have been suggested, both cortical and subcortical (Anderer, Pascual-Marqui, Semlitsch, and Saletu, 1998; Hruby and Marsalek, 2003). The hippocampus, which is part of the limbic system, is thought to play a role in generating the P300 (Halgren, Squires, Wilson, Rohrbaugh, Babb, and Crandall, 1980; McCarthy, Wood, Alison, Goff, Williamson, and Spencer, 1982). Additionally, thalamic contributions have been suggested (Wood, Allison, Goff, Williamson, and Spencer, 1980). Furthermore, because selective attention is an underlying process involved in the P300 response, pathways such as the mesencephalic reticular formation, medial thalamus, and prefrontal cortex may also be involved (Yingling and Hosobuchi, 1984; Yingling and Skinner, 1977). Cortically, the frontal region of the brain (Courchesne, 1978; Desmedt and Debecker, 1979), centroparietal regions (Goff, Allison, and Vaughan, 1978; Simson, Vaughn, and Ritter, 1977), and auditory cortex (Richer, Johnson, and Beatty, 1983) are indicated in response generation.

Stimulus/Recording Parameters

By virtue of the fact that the P300 is primarily an endogenous response, it is less influenced by stimulus parameters than the earlier, more exogenous potentials (Picton and Fitzgerald, 1983), but it is not completely independent of stimulus parameters. The listener must be able to distinguish between the target and the frequent stimulus, and the easier the discrimination task, the more robust the P300 response. For example, if a listener is asked to identify a 1000-Hz target tone in an oddball sequence with 2000-Hz frequent tones, the resulting response will be more robust and earlier in latency than if the 1000-Hz target were presented among a series of 1200-Hz frequent tones.

The effects of stimulus frequency (Cass and Polich, 1997; Vesco, Bone, Ryan, and Polich, 1993), intensity (Cass and Polich, 1997; Polich, Ellerson, and Cohen, 1996), and duration (O'Brien and Stuart, 2001; Polich, 1989) on the P300 have been extensively studied. Researchers have looked at how different the target and frequent stimuli must be to evoke a P300 response. Generally, latency decreases and amplitude increases as differences between the target and standard stimuli become more discriminable. See **Table 10.3** for a suggested P300 paradigm.

Table 10.3 Sample P300 Paradigm

Stimulus Parameters	
Type	Tone burst with long onset/offset times and extended plateau (10-50-10). Tones should vary in one dimension and be easily distinguishable (i.e., 1000 Hz frequent versus 2000 Hz target).
Intensity	Stimuli should be easily heard, so moderate levels are recommended. Softer presentation levels will require more averages and thus, longer recording time.
Target probability	20%; Target presentation is "pseudorandom" with the constraints that a target should never immediately follow another target – there should always be at least 2 standard stimuli between targets and the target should never be presented first in the sequence.
Rate	1/s
Recording Parameters	
Time window	–100 to 700 msec if tonal stimuli are used; if speech stimuli are used, extend the time window out to 800 msec.
Filters	0.1 to 100 Hz
Electrode sites	Minimally, noninverting electrodes at Fz, Cz, and Pz. If hemispheric information is desired, use additional noninverting electrodes. Inverting electrode at linked earlobes or mastoids. Ocular electrodes above and below the eye to monitor and correct eyeblink artifacts.

Measurement Parameters

Latency and amplitude are important indices when quantifying and evaluating P300 responses. Both indices vary depending on the stimulus parameters employed, as well as subject factors, such as memory and speed of processing. P300 latency is thought to reflect stimulus classification time and may serve as an index of neural activity underlying the speed of attention allocation and immediate memory operations (Duncan-Johnson, 1981; Magliero, Bashore, Coles, and Donchin, 1984; Polich, 1986, 1987). Interestingly, the more confident the listener is about the discrimination, the earlier the latency will be. Latency is measured from the stimulus onset to the point of largest amplitude (peak) of the P300 response. In many instances, there are multiple peaks in the P300 latency range. Different strategies have been suggested, including the intersect method (Dalebout and Robey, 1997), where latency is calculated as the midpoint of the P300 positivity, measured from the initial point at which the waveform crosses the baseline at the beginning of the response to the point at the end of the response where the waveform crosses the baseline. Another

method would be to pick the latency of the most positive peak in the P300 window.

Amplitude reflects attention resource allocation (Sommer, Matt, and Leuthold, 1990). There are two common methods for determining P300 amplitude. The first involves measuring the amplitude from the peak of the P300 to either the preceding or following trough. Another method is to measure from the P300 peak to the baseline. The latter method allows quantification of the P300 amplitude independent of the preceding or following troughs.

Subject Effects

Maturation Effects

Myelination occurs for several years after birth in the higher auditory pathways in humans (Schochat and Musiek, 2004). According to Buchwald (1990), the P300 is not mature until the early teen years. Latency decreases systematically with development (Goodin, Squires, Henderson, and Starr, 1978; Goodin, Squires, and Starr, 1978; Kurtzberg, Vaughan, and Kreuzer, 1979) until adulthood, when it begins to increase. The P300 can be recorded in infants and children, but delayed latencies resulting from increased processing time would be expected. In addition, because of the attention and task vigilance required, challenges could be expected in recording the response in the pediatric population.

Aging Effects

The effects of aging on the P300 have been demonstrated by many authors. Polich (1996) provided a meta-analysis of this research. There is a great deal of variation in the reported findings as a result of differences in research methods. In general, the latency of the P300 increases with age by a few msec/year. It has been estimated that beyond young adulthood, latency increases ~1.25 to 1.4 msec/year (Barajas, 1990; Picton, Stuss, Champagne, and Nelson, 1984). Amplitude reductions are also seen. In addition to changes in amplitude and latency, the reliability of the P300 declines with age (Stenklev and Laukli, 2004).

Auditory Processing Disorders

Jirsa and Clontz (1990) studied the P300 in children with auditory processing disorders (APDs). They found that children with APD exhibited longer response latencies and reduced amplitudes relative to an age-matched normal control group. Although not statistically significant, the children with APD who performed best on the behavioral test battery also exhibited the shortest P300 latencies. Additionally, there was a high degree of variability in the responses of both the children with APD and in a normal age-matched control group, though variability was highest for the APD group.

Jirsa (1992) further investigated the use of the P300 in children with APD when he evaluated the clinical utility of the use of the P300 as an electrophysiologic index of behavioral change after intervention. Jirsa reported decreased response latencies and increased amplitudes in children who received intervention. The measures did not change in APD control subjects who did not receive intervention or in a normal control group. Jirsa suggested that P300 latency and amplitude measures are sensitive to changes in clinical status following a treatment program but recommended that results be interpreted with caution.

Clinical Applications

Clinically, the P300 has been used to evaluate a variety of pathological conditions, including schizophrenia, Parkinson disease (Hansch, Syndulko, Cohen, Goldberg, Potvin, and Tourtellotte, 1982), chronic renal failure (Cohen, Syndulko, Rever, Kraut, Coburn, and Tourtellotte, 1983), chronic alcoholism (Pfefferbaum, Horvath, Roth, and Kopell, 1979) senile dementia (Goodin, Squires, Henderson, and Starr, 1978, Goodin, Squires, and Starr, 1978; Pfefferbaum, Ford, Roth, and Kopell, 1980) Alzheimer disease (Brown, Marsh, and LaRue, 1982), cerebrovascular lesions, head trauma, brain tumors (Ebner, Haas, Lücking, Schily, Wallesch, and Zimmermann, 1986; Michalewski, Rosenberg, and Starr, 1986; Musiek, Baran, and Pinheiro, 1989), and aphasia (Selinger, Prescott, and Shucard, 1989). A fair amount of variability has been reported between subjects in latency and amplitude measures, prompting Picton and Hillyard (1988) to suggest that the P300 may correlate more with the degree of overall cognitive dysfunction than with any specific disorder. It has been proposed that the P300 could be useful in monitoring progress during and after therapy, as it is stable within listeners, and a decrease in latency would imply an increase in cognitive capacity (Polich and Starr, 1983).

◆ Summary

CERPs are a broad class of both sensory and cognitive types with a rich history across numerous disciplines. Some CERPs have made their way into routine neurodiagnostic use by some clinicians (e.g., P1/N1/P2 complex) and can easily be recorded using standard clinical equipment. Others, however, remain well within the confines of a laboratory or specialized clinics for the study of speech perception, attention, and other higher-order processes. In auditory-based fields, it is expected that we will come to rely more and more on CERPs as new knowledge is gained about the brain and as techniques are more refined and made more accessible to clinicians.

References

Aaltonen, O., Tuomainen, J., Laine, M., & Niemi, P. (1993). Discrimination of speech and non-speech sounds by brain damaged subjects: Electrophysiological evidence for distinct memory processes. *Brain and Language, 44*, 139–152. PubMed

Adler, G., & Adler, J. (1991). Auditory stimulus processing at different stimulus intensities as reflected by auditory evoked potentials. *Biological Psychiatry, 29*(4), 347–356. PubMed

Alain, C., Woods, D. L., & Covarrubias, D. (1997). Activation of duration-sensitive auditory cortical fields in humans. *Electroencephalography and Clinical Neurophysiology, 104*(6), 531–539. PubMed

Alcaini, M., Giard, M. H., Thévenet, M., & Pernier, J. (1994). Two separate frontal components in the N1 wave of the human auditory evoked response. *Psychophysiology, 31*(6), 611–615. PubMed

Alho, K. (1995). Cerebral generators of mismatch negativity (MMN) and its magnetic counterpart (MMNm) elicited by sound changes. *Ear and Hearing, 16*(1), 38–51. PubMed

Alho, K., Sainio, K., Sajaniemi, N., Reinikainen, K., & Näätänen, R. (1990). Event-related brain potential of human newborns to pitch change of an acoustic stimulus. *Electroencephalography and Clinical Neurophysiology, 77*(2), 151–155. PubMed

Alho, K., Sams, M., Paavilainen, P., & Näätänen, R. (1986). Small pitch separation and the selective-attention effect on the ERP. *Psychophysiology, 23*(2), 189–197. PubMed

Anderer, P., Pascual-Marqui, R. D., Semlitsch, H. V., & Saletu, B. (1998). Differential effects of normal aging on sources of standard N1, target N1 and target P300 auditory event-related brain potentials revealed by low resolution electromagnetic tomography (LORETA). *Electroencephalography and Clinical Neurophysiology, 108*(2), 160–174. PubMed

Atcherson, S. R., Gould, H. J., Pousson, M. A., & Prout, T. M. (2006). Long-term stability of N1 sources using low-resolution electromagnetic tomography. *Brain Topography, 19*(1–2), 11–20. PubMed

Atcherson, S. R., Gould, H. J., Mendel, M. I., & Ethington, C. A. (2009). Auditory N1 component to gaps in continuous narrowband noises. *Ear and Hearing, 30*(6), 687–695. PubMed

Atcherson, S. R., Damji, Z., & Upson, S. (2011). Applying a subtraction technique to minimize cochlear implant artifact with soundfield and direct audio input stimulations. *Cochlear Implants International, 12*(4), 234–237. PubMed

Baldeweg, T., Richardson, A., Watkins, S., Foale, C., & Gruzelier, J. (1999). Impaired auditory frequency discrimination in dyslexia detected with mismatch evoked potentials. *Annals of Neurology, 45*(4), 495–503. PubMed

Barajas, J. J. (1990). The effects of age on human P3 latency. *Acta Oto-Laryngologica, 476*(Suppl), 157–160. PubMed

Billings, C. J., Tremblay, K. L., Souza, P. E., & Binns, M. A. (2007). Effects of hearing aid amplification and stimulus intensity on cortical auditory evoked potentials. *Audiology and Neuro-Otology, 12*(4), 234–246. PubMed

Bishop, D. V., Hardiman, M., Uwer, R., & Von Suchodoletz, W. (2007). Maturation of the long-latency auditory ERP: Step function changes at start and end of adolescence. *Developmental Science, 10*(5), 565–575.

Brown, W. S., Marsh, J. T., & LaRue, A. (1982). Event-related potentials in psychiatry: differentiating depression and dementia in the elderly. *Bulletin of the Los Angeles Neurological Societies, 47*, 91–107. PubMed

Buchwald, J. S. (1990). Comparison of plasticity in sensory and cognitive processing systems. *Clinics in Perinatology, 17*(1), 57–66. PubMed

Buchwald, J. S., Erwin, R., Van Lancker, D., Guthrie, D., Schwafel, J., & Tanguay, P. (1992). Midlatency auditory evoked responses: P1 abnormalities in adult autistic subjects. *Electroencephalography and Clinical Neurophysiology, 84*(2), 164–171. PubMed

Buckley, K. A. (2003). Effects of auditory deprivation on cortical processing. *Hearing Journal, 56*(6), 16–18.

Carter, L., Golding, M., Dillon, H., & Seymour, J. (2010). The detection of infant cortical auditory evoked potentials (CAEPs) using statistical and visual detection techniques. *Journal of the American Academy of Audiology, 21*(5), 347–356. PubMed

Cass, M., & Polich, J. (1997). P300 from a single-stimulus paradigm: Auditory intensity and tone frequency effects. *Biological Psychology, 46*(1), 51–65. PubMed

Ceponiene, R., Cheour, M., & Näätänen, R. (1998). Interstimulus interval and auditory event-related potentials in children: Evidence for multiple generators. *Electroencephalography and Clinical Neurophysiology, 108*(4), 345–354. PubMed

Charles C. Wood, Truett Allison, William R. Goff, Peter D. Williamson, Dennis D. Spencer, On the Neural Origin of P300 in Man, In: H.H. Kornhubek and L. Deecke, Editor(s), Progress in Brain Research, Elsevier, 1980, Volume 54, Pages 51–56, ISSN 0079-6123, ISBN 9780444801968,10.1016/S0079-6123(08)61605-2. (http://www.sciencedirect.com/science/article/pii/S0079612308616052)

Cohen, S. N., Syndulko, K., Rever, B., Kraut, J., Coburn, J., & Tourtellotte, W. W. (1983). Visual evoked potentials and long latency event-related potentials in chronic renal failure. *Neurology, 33*(9), 1219–1222. PubMed

Courchesne, E. (1978). Neurophysiological correlates of cognitive development: changes in long-latency event-related potentials from childhood to adulthood. *Electroencephalography and Clinical Neurophysiology, 45*(4), 468–482. PubMed

Courchesne, E., Hillyard, S. A., & Galambos, R. (1975). Stimulus novelty, task relevance and the visual evoked potential in man. *Electroencephalography and Clinical Neurophysiology, 39*(2), 131–143. PubMed

Csépe, V. (1995). On the origin and development of the mismatch negativity. *Ear and Hearing, 16*(1), 91–104. PubMed

Dalebout, S. D., & Fox, L. G. (2001). Reliability of the mismatch negativity in the responses of individual listeners. *Journal of the American Academy of Audiology, 12*(5), 245–253. PubMed

Dalebout, S. D., & Fox, L. G. (2000). Identification of the mismatch negativity in the responses of individual listeners. *Journal of the American Academy of Audiology, 11*(1), 12–22. PubMed

Dalebout, S. D., & Robey, R. R. (1997). Comparison of the intersubject and intrasubject variability of exogenous and endogenous auditory evoked potentials. *Journal of the American Academy of Audiology, 8*(5), 342–354. PubMed

Daltrozzo, J., Wioland, N., Mutschler, V., & Kotchoubey, B. (2007). Predicting coma and other low responsive patients outcome using event-related brain potentials: A meta-analysis. *Clinical Neurophysiology, 118*(3), 606–614. PubMed

Davis, H. (1965). Slow cortical responses evoked by acoustic stimuli. Acta Oto-laryngologica, 59(2-6), 179-185.

Davis, H., & Zerlin, S. (1966). Acoustic relations of the human vertex potential. *Journal of the Acoustical Society of America, 39*(1), 109–116. PubMed

Davis, P. A. (1939). Effects of acoustic stimuli on the waking human brain. *Journal of Neurophysiology, 2*(2), 494–499.

Desmedt, J. E., & Debecker, J. (1979). Wave form and neural mechanism of the decision P350 elicited without pre-stimulus CNV or readiness potential in random sequences of near-threshold auditory clicks and finger stimuli. *Electroencephalography and Clinical Neurophysiology, 47*(6), 648–670. PubMed

Dimitrijevic, A., Michalewski, H. J., Zeng, F. G., Pratt, H., & Starr, A. (2008). Frequency changes in a continuous tone: Auditory cortical potentials. *Clinical Neurophysiology, 119*(9), 2111–2124. PubMed

Donchin, E. (1981). Presidential address, 1980. Surprise! ... Surprise? *Psychophysiology, 18*(5), 493–513. PubMed

Donchin, E., & Coles, M. G. H. (1988). Is the P300 component a manifestation of context updating? *Behavioral and Brain Sciences, 11*(3), 357–374.

Duncan-Johnson, C. C. (1981, May). Young Psychophysiologist Award address, 1980. P300 latency: a new metric of information processing. *Psychophysiology, 18*(3), 207–215. PubMed

Duncan, C. C., Barry, R. J., Connolly, J. F., Fischer, C., Michie, P. T., Näätänen, R., et al. (2009). Event-related potentials in clinical research: Guidelines for eliciting, recording, and quantifying mismatch negativity, P300, and N400. *Clinical Neurophysiology, 120*(11), 1883–1908. PubMed

Duncan, C. C., & Kaye, W. H. (1987). Effects of clonidine on event-related potential measures of information processing. In R. Johnson, Jr., J. W. Rohrbaugh, & R. Parasuraman (Eds.), *Current trends in event-related potential research* (pp. 527–531). Amsterdam: Elsevier.

Ebner, A., Haas, J. C., Lücking, C. H., Schily, M., Wallesch, C. W., & Zimmermann, P. (1986). Event-related brain potentials (P300) and neuropsychological deficit in patients with focal brain lesions. *Neuroscience Letters, 64*(3), 330–334. PubMed

Eddins, A. C., & Peterson, J. R. (1999). Time-intensity trading in the late auditory evoked potential. *Journal of Speech, Language, and Hearing Research: JSLHR, 42*(3), 516–525. PubMed

Eggermont, J. J., & Ponton, C. W. (2002). The neurophysiology of auditory perception: From single units to evoked potentials. *Audiology and Neuro-Otology, 7*(2), 71–99. PubMed

Eggermont, J. J., & Ponton, C. W. (2003). Auditory-evoked potential studies of cortical maturation in normal hearing and implanted children: Correlations with changes in structure and speech perception. *Acta Oto-Laryngologica, 123*(2), 249–252. PubMed

Eggermont, J. J., Ponton, C. W., Don, M., Waring, M. D., & Kwong, B. (1997). Maturational delays in cortical evoked potentials in cochlear implant users. *Acta Oto-Laryngologica, 117*(2), 161–163. PubMed

Escera, C., & Grau, C. (1996). Short-term replicability of the mismatch negativity. *Electroencephalography and Clinical Neurophysiology, 100*(6), 549–554. PubMed

Friesen, L. M., & Picton, T. W. (2010. A method for removing cochlear implant artifact. *Hearing Research, 259*(1–2), 95–106. PubMed

Frodl-Bauch, T., Kathmann, N., Möller, H. J., & Hegerl, U. (1997). Dipole localization and test-retest reliability of frequency and duration mismatch negativity generator processes. *Brain Topography, 10*(1), 3–8. PubMed

Giard, M. H., Perrin, F., Echallier, J. F., Thévenet, M., Froment, J. C., & Pernier, J. (1994). Dissociation of temporal and frontal components in the human auditory N1 wave: A scalp current density and dipole model analysis. *Electroencephalography and Clinical Neurophysiology, 92*(3), 238–252. PubMed

Gilbert, C. D., Sigman, M., & Crist, R. E. (2001). The neural basis of perceptual learning. *Neuron, 31*(5), 681–697. PubMed

Gilley, P. M., Sharma, A., Dorman, M., Finley, C. C., Panch, A. S., & Martin, K. (2006). Minimization of cochlear implant stimulus artifact in cortical auditory evoked potentials. *Clinical Neurophysiology, 117*(8), 1772–1782. PubMed

Goff, E. R., Allison, T., & Vaughan, H. G., Jr. (1978). The functional neuroanatomy of event related potentials. In E. Callway, P. Tueting, & S. H. Koslow (Eds), *Event-related potentials in man* (pp. 1–79). New York: Academic Press.

Golding, M., Pearce, W., Seymour, J., Cooper, A., Ching, T., & Dillon, H. (2007). The relationship between obligatory cortical auditory evoked potentials (CAEPs) and functional measures in young infants. *Journal of the American Academy of Audiology, 18*(2), 117–125. PubMed

Goodin, D. S., Squires, K. C., Henderson, B. H., & Starr, A. (1978). Age-related variations in evoked potentials to auditory stimuli in normal human subjects. *Electroencephalography and Clinical Neurophysiology, 44*(4), 447–458. PubMed

Goodin, D. S., Squires, K. C., & Starr, A. (1978). Long latency event-related components of the auditory evoked potential in dementia. *Brain, 101*(4), 635–648. PubMed

Grimes, C. T., & Feldman, A. S. (1971). Evoked response thresholds for long and short duration tones. *Audiology, 10*(5), 358–364. PubMed

Halgren, E., Squires, N. K., Wilson, C. L., Rohrbaugh, J. W., Babb, T. L., & Crandall, P. H. (1980). Endogenous potentials generated in the human hippocampal formation and amygdala by infrequent events. *Science, 210*(4471), 803–805. PubMed

Hall, J. W., III. (1992). *Handbook of auditory evoked responses*. Needham Heights, MA: Allyn & Bacon.

Hall, J. W., III. (2007). *New handbook of auditory evoked responses*. Boston: Pearson Allyn & Bacon.

Hansen, J. C., & Hillyard, S. A. (1980). Endogenous brain potentials associated with selective auditory attention. *Electroencephalography and Clinical Neurophysiology, 49*(3–4), 277–290. PubMed

Hansch, E. C., Syndulko, K., Cohen, S. N., Goldberg, Z. I., Potvin, A. R., & Tourtellotte, W. W. (1982). Cognition in Parkinson disease: An event-related potential perspective. *Annals of Neurology, 11*(6), 599–607. PubMed

Hari, R., Hämäläinen, M., Ilmoniemi, R., Kaukoranta, E., Reinikainen, K., Salminen, J., et al. (1984). Responses of the primary auditory cortex to pitch changes in a sequence of tone pips: Neuromagnetic recordings in man. *Neuroscience Letters, 50*(1–3), 127–132. PubMed

Harrison, J., Buchwald, J., & Kaga, K. (1986). Cat P300 present after primary auditory cortex ablation. *Electroencephalography and Clinical Neurophysiology, 63*(2), 180–187. PubMed

Hay, I. S., & Davis, H. (1971). Slow cortical evoked potentials: Interactions of auditory, vibro-tactile and shock stimuli. *Audiology, 10*(1), 9–17. PubMed

Hillyard, S. A., Hink, R. F., Schwent, V. L., & Picton, T. W. (1973). Electrical signs of selective attention in the human brain. *Science, 182*(108), 177–180. PubMed

Hone, S. W., Norman, G., Keogh, I., & Kelly, V. (2003). The use of cortical evoked response audiometry in the assessment of noise-induced hearing loss. *Otolaryngology–Head and Neck Surgery, 128*(2), 257–262. PubMed

Hruby, T., & Marsalek, P. (2003). Event-related potentials—the P3 wave. *Acta Neurobiologiae Experimentalis, 63*(1), 55–63. PubMed

Hyde, M. (1997). The N1 response and its applications. *Audiology and Neuro-Otology, 2*(5), 281–307. PubMed

Hyde, M., Alberti, P., Matsumoto, N., & Li, Y. L. (1986). Auditory evoked potentials in audiometric assessment of compensation and medicolegal patients. *Annals of Otology, Rhinology, and Laryngology, 95*(5, Pt 1), 514–519. PubMed

Jääskeläinen, I. P., Pekkonen, E., Alho, K., Sinclair, J. D., Sillanaukee, P., & Näätänen, R. (1995). Dose-related effect of alcohol on mismatch negativity and reaction time performance. *Alcohol (Fayetteville, N.Y.), 12*(6), 491–495. PubMed

Jirsa, R. E. (1992). The clinical utility of the P3 AERP in children with auditory processing disorders. *Journal of Speech and Hearing Research, 35*(4), 903–912. PubMed

Jirsa, R. E., & Clontz, K. B. (1990). Long latency auditory event-related potentials from children with auditory processing disorders. *Ear and Hearing, 11*(3), 222–232. PubMed

Joutsiniemi, S. L., Ilvonen, T., Sinkkonen, J., Huotilainen, M., Tervaniemi, M., Lehtokoski, A., et al. (1998). The mismatch negativity for duration decrement of auditory stimuli in healthy subjects. *Electroencephalography and Clinical Neurophysiology, 108*(2), 154–159. PubMed

Kane, N. M., Curry, S. H., Butler, S. R., & Cummins, B. H. (1993). Electrophysiological indicator of awakening from coma. *Lancet, 341*(8846), 688. PubMed

Kiehl, K. A., Laurens, K. R., Duty, T. L., Forster, B. B., & Liddle, P. F. (2001). Neural sources involved in auditory target detection and novelty processing: An event-related fMRI study. *Psychophysiology, 38*(1), 133–142. PubMed

Kileny, P., & Berry, D. A. (1983). Selective impairment of late vertex and middle latency auditory evoked responses. In G. T. Mencher and S. E. Gerber (Eds.). *The multiply handicapped hearing impaired child*. New York: Grune & Stratton.

Knight, R. T., Hillyard, S. A., Woods, D. L., & Neville, H. J. (1980). The effects of frontal and temporal-parietal lesions on the auditory evoked potential in man. *Electroencephalography and Clinical Neurophysiology, 50*(1–2), 112–124. PubMed

Korpilahti, P., & Lang, H. A. (1994). Auditory ERP components and mismatch negativity in dysphasic children. *Electroencephalography and Clinical Neurophysiology, 91*(4), 256–264. PubMed

Kraus, N. (1999). Speech sound perception, neurophysiology, and plasticity. *International Journal of Pediatric Otorhinolaryngology, 47*(2), 123–129. PubMed

Kraus, N., & McGee, T. (1994). Mismatch negativity in the assessment of central auditory function. *American Journal of Audiology, 3*(2), 39–51.

Kraus, N., McGee, T., Carrell, T. D., Sharma, A. (1995). Neurophysiologic bases of speech discrimination. *Ear and Hearing, 16*(1), 19–37. PubMed

Kraus, N., McGee, T., Micco, A., Sharma, A., Carrell, T., & Nicol, T. (1993). Mismatch negativity in school-age children to speech stimuli that are just perceptibly different. *Electroencephalography and Clinical Neurophysiology, 88*(2), 123–130. PubMed

Kraus, N., McGee, T., Sharma, A., Carrell, T., & Nicol, T. (1992). Mismatch negativity event-related potential elicited by speech stimuli. *Ear and Hearing, 13*(3), 158–164. PubMed

Kujala, T., Kallio, J., Tervaniemi, M., & Näätänen, R. (2001). The mismatch negativity as an index of temporal processing in audition. *Clinical Neurophysiology, 112*(9), 1712–1719. PubMed

Kurtzberg, D., Vaughan, H. G., Jr, & Kreuzer, J. A. (1979). Task related cortical potentials in children. *Progress in Clinical Neurophysiology, 6*, 216–223.

Kurtzberg, D., Vaughan, H. G., Jr, Kreuzer, J. A., & Fliegler, K. Z. (1995). Developmental studies and clinical application of mismatch negativity: Problems and prospects. *Ear and Hearing, 16*(1), 105–117. PubMed

Kushnerenko, E., Ceponiene, R., Balan, P., Fellman, V., Huotilaine, M., & Näätäne, R. (2002). Maturation of the auditory event-related potentials during the first year of life. *Neuroreport, 13*(1), 47–51. PubMed

Kutas, M., McCarthy, G., & Donchin, E. (1977). Augmenting mental chronometry: the P300 as a measure of stimulus evaluation time. *Science, 197*(4305), 792–795. PubMed

Lang, A. H., Nyrke, T., Ek, M., Aaltonen, O., Raimo, Y., & Näätänen, R. (1990). Pitch discrimination performance and auditory event related potentials. In C. H. M. Brunia, A. W. K. Gaillard, & A. Kok (Eds.), *Psychophysiological brain research* (pp. 294–298). Tillburg, the Netherlands: University Press.

Lang, A. H., Eerola, O., Korpilahti, P., Holopainen, I., Salo, S., & Aaltonen, O. (1995). Practical issues in the clinical application of mismatch negativity. *Ear and Hearing, 16*(1), 118–130. PubMed

Levänen, S., Hari, R., McEvoy, L., & Sams, M. (1993). Responses of the human auditory cortex to changes in one versus two stimulus features. *Experimental Brain Research, 97*(1), 177–183. PubMed

Liégeois-Chauvel, C., Musolino, A., Badier, J. M., Marquis, P., & Chauvel, P. (1994). Evoked potentials recorded from the auditory cortex in man: Evaluation and topography of the middle latency components. *Electroencephalography and Clinical Neurophysiology, 92*(3), 204–214. PubMed

Lightfoot, G., & Kennedy, V. (2006, Oct). Cortical electric response audiometry hearing threshold estimation: Accuracy, speed, and the effects of stimulus presentation features. *Ear and Hearing, 27*(5), 443–456. PubMed

Magliero, A., Bashore, T. R., Coles, M. G. H., & Donchin, E. (1984). On the dependence of P300 latency on stimulus evaluation processes. *Psychophysiology, 21*(2), 171–186. PubMed

Martin, B. A., & Boothroyd, A. (1999). Cortical, auditory, event-related potentials in response to periodic and aperiodic stimuli with the same spectral envelope. *Ear and Hearing, 20*(1), 33–44. PubMed

McArthur, G. M., Bishop, D. V., & Proudfoot, M. (2003). Do video sounds interfere with auditory event-related potentials? *Behavior Research Methods, Instruments, and Computers, 35*(2), 329–333. PubMed

McCallum, W. C., & Curry, S. H.(1980). The form and distribution of auditory evoked potentials and CNVS when stimuli and responses are lateralized. In H. H. Kornhuber & L. Deecke (Eds.), *Progress in brain research: Motivation, motor and sensory processes of the brain. Electrical potentials, behavior and clinical use* (Vol. 54, pp. 767–775). New York: Elsevier.

McCullagh, J., Weihing, J., & Musiek, F. (2009). Comparisons of P300s from standard oddball and omitted paradigms: implications to exogenous/endogenous contributions. *Journal of the American Academy of Audiology, 20*(3), 187–195, quiz 219. PubMed

McCarthy, G., Wood, C. C., Alison, T., Goff, W. R., Williamson, P. D., & Spencer, D. D. (1982). Intracranial recordings of event related potentials in humans engaged in cognitive tasks. *Society for Neuroscience Abstracts, 8,* 976.

McGee, T., & Kraus, N. (1996). Auditory development reflected by middle latency response. *Ear and Hearing, 17*(5), 419–429. PubMed

McGee, T., Kraus, N., & Nicol, T. (1997). Is it really a mismatch negativity? An assessment of methods for determining response validity in individual subjects. *Electroencephalography and Clinical Neurophysiology, 104*(4), 359–368. PubMed

McPherson, D. L. (1996). *Late potentials of the auditory system.* San Diego, CA: Singular.

McPherson, D. L., Ballachanda, B. B., & Kaf, W. (2007). Middle and long latency auditory evoked potentials. In R. J. Roeser, M. Valente, & H. Hosford-Dunn (Eds.), *Audiology: Diagnosis* (pp. 443–477). New York: Thieme.

Michalewski, H., Rosenberg, C., & Starr, A. (1986). Event-related potentials in dementia. In R. Cracco &

I. Bodis-Wollner (Eds.), *Evoked potentials* (pp. 521–528). New York: Alan R. Liss.

Michalewski, H. J., Starr, A., Nguyen, T. T., Kong, Y. Y., & Zeng, F. G. (2005). Auditory temporal processes in normal-hearing individuals and in patients with auditory neuropathy. *Clinical Neurophysiology, 116*(3), 669–680. PubMed

Michie, P. T. (2001). What has MMN revealed about the auditory system in schizophrenia? *International Journal of Psychophysiology, 42*(2), 177–194. PubMed

Mittelman, N., Bleich, N., & Pratt, H. (2005). Early ERP components to gaps in white noise: Onset and offset responses. *International Congress Series, 1278,* 3–6.

Morr, M. L., Shafer, V. L., Kreuzer, J. A., & Kurtzberg, D. (2002). Maturation of mismatch negativity in typically developing infants and preschool children. *Ear and Hearing, 23*(2), 118–136. PubMed

Musiek, F. E., Gollegly, K., Kibbe, K. & Verkest, S. P-300 Results in Patients with Lesions of the Auditory Areas of the Cerebrum. American Auditory Society, 16th Annual Meeting, New Orleans, LA, September 24, 1989.

Musiek, F. E., Froke, R., & Weihing, J. (2005). The auditory P300 at or near threshold. *Journal of the American Academy of Audiology, 16*(9), 698–707. PubMed

Näätänen, R. (1995). The mismatch negativity: A powerful tool for cognitive neuroscience. *Ear and Hearing, 16*(1), 6–18. PubMed

Näätänen, R. (1992). *Attention and brain function.* Hillsdale, NJ: Lawrence Erlbaum.

Näätänen, R., Gaillard, A. W., & Mäntysalo, S. (1978). Early selective-attention effect on evoked potential reinterpreted. *Acta Psychologica, 42*(4), 313–329. PubMed

Näätänen, R., Paavilainen, P., & Reinikainen, K. (1989). Do event-related potentials to infrequent decrements in duration of auditory stimuli demonstrate a memory trace in man? *Neuroscience Letters, 107*(1–3), 347–352. PubMed

Näätänen, R., & Picton, T. (1987). The N1 wave of the human electric and magnetic response to sound: A review and an analysis of the component structure. *Psychophysiology, 24*(4), 375–425. PubMed

Näätänen, R. (1982). Processing negativity: An evoked-potential reflection of selective attention. *Psychological Bulletin, 92*(3), 605–640. PubMed

Näätänen, R. (1990). The role of attention in auditory information processing as revealed by event related potentials and other brain measures of cognitive function. *Behavioral and Brain Sciences, 13*(2), 201–288.

Nielsen-Bohlman, L., Knight, R. T., Woods, D. L., & Woodward, K. (1991). Differential auditory processing continues during sleep. *Electroencephalography and Clinical Neurophysiology, 79*(4), 281–290. PubMed

Novak, G. P., Ritter, W., Vaughan, H. G., Jr, & Wiznitzer, M. L. (1990). Differentiation of negative event-related potentials in an auditory discrimination task. *Electroencephalography and Clinical Neurophysiology, 75*(4), 255–275. PubMed

Oates, P. A., Kurtzberg, D., & Stapells, D. R. (2002). Effects of sensorineural hearing loss on cortical event-related potential and behavioral measures of speech-sound processing. *Ear and Hearing, 23*(5), 399–415. PubMed

O'Brien, P. J., & Stuart, A. (2001). The effect of auditory stimulus duration on the P300 response. *Journal of Speech-Language Pathology and Audiology, 10*(1), 19–23.

Onishi, S., & Davis, H. (1968). Effects of duration and rise time of tone bursts on evoked V potentials. *Journal of the Acoustical Society of America, 44*(2), 582–591. PubMed

Pakarinen, S., Takegata, R., Rinne, T., Huotilainen, M., & Näätänen, R. (2007). Measurement of extensive auditory discrimination profiles using the mismatch negativity (MMN) of the auditory event-related potential (ERP). *Clinical Neurophysiology, 118*(1), 177–185. PubMed

Pascual-Marqui, R. D., Michel, C. M., & Lehmann, D. (1994,). Low resolution electromagnetic tomography: A new method for localizing electrical activity in the brain. *International Journal of Psychophysiology, 18*(1), 49–65. PubMed

Patel, S. H., & Azzam, P. N. (2005). Characterization of N200 and P300: Selected studies of the event-related potential. *International Journal of Medical Sciences, 2*(4), 147–154. PubMed

Pekkonen, E., Jousmäki, V., Könönen, M., Reinikainen, K., & Partanen, J. (1994). Auditory sensory memory impairment in Alzheimer's disease: An event-related potential study. *Neuroreport, 5*(18), 2537–2540. PubMed

Pekkonen, E., Jousmäki, V., Reinikainen, K., & Partanen, J. (1995). Automatic auditory discrimination is impaired in Parkinson's disease. *Electroencephalography and Clinical Neurophysiology, 95*(1), 47–52. PubMed

Pekkonen, E., Rinne, T., Reinikainen, K., Kujala, T., Alho, K., & Näätänen, R. (1996). Aging effects on auditory processing: An event-related potential study. *Experimental Aging Research, 22*(2), 171–184. PubMed

Petermann, M., Kummer, P., Burger, M., Lohscheller, J., Eysholdt, U., & Döllinger, M. (2009, Jan). Statistical detection and analysis of mismatch negativity derived by a multi-deviant design from normal hearing children. *Hearing Research, 247*(2), 128–136. PubMed

Pfefferbaum, A., Ford, J. M., Roth, W. T., & Kopell, B. S. (1980). Age-related changes in auditory event-related potentials. *Electroencephalography and Clinical Neurophysiology, 49*(3–4), 266–276. PubMed

Pfefferbaum, A., Horvath, T. B., Roth, W. T., & Kopell, B. S. (1979). Event-related potential changes in chronic alcoholics. *Electroencephalography and Clinical Neurophysiology, 47*(6), 637–647. PubMed

Picton, T. W. (1995). The neurophysiological evaluation of auditory discrimination. *Ear and Hearing, 16*(1), 1–5. PubMed

Picton, T. W., Alain, C., Woods, D. L., John, M. S., Scherg, M., Valdes-Sosa, P., *et al.* (1999). Intracerebral sources of human auditory-evoked potentials. *Audiology and Neuro-Otology, 4*(2), 64–79. PubMed

Picton, T. W., & Fitzgerald, P. G. (1983). A general description of the human auditory evoked potentials. In E. J. Moore (Ed.), Bases of auditory brain-stem evoked responses (pp. 141–156). New York: Grune & Stratton.

Picton, T. W., & Hillyard, S. A. (1974). Human auditory evoked potentials: 2. Effects of attention.

Electroencephalography and Clinical Neurophysiology, 36(2), 191–199. PubMed

Picton, T. W., & Hillyard, S. A. (1988). Endogenous event-related potentials. In T. W. Picton (Ed.), *Human event-related potentials: EEG handbook* (rev., Vol. 3) (p. 361–426). Amsterdam: Elsevier.

Picton, T. W., Stuss, D. T., Champagne, S. C., & Nelson, R. F. (1984). The effects of age on human event-related potentials. *Psychophysiology, 21*(3), 312–325. PubMed

Picton, T. W., Woods, D. L., & Proulx, G. B. (1978). Human auditory sustained potentials. I. The nature of the response. *Electroencephalography and Clinical Neurophysiology, 45*(2), 186–197. PubMed

Pietrowsky, R., Fehm, H. L., & Born, J. (1990). An analysis of the effects of corticotrophin releasing hormone (h-CRH), adrenocoroticotropin (ATCH), and beta-endrophin on ERPs in humans. In C.M. H. Brunia, A. W. K. Gaillard, & A. Kok (Eds.), *Psychophysical brain research*, (pp. 106–110). Tilburg, the Netherlands: Tilburg University Press.

Polich, J. (1986). Attention, probability, and task demands as determinants of P300 latency from auditory stimuli. *Electroencephalography and Clinical Neurophysiology, 63*(3), 251–259. PubMed

Polich, J. (1987). Task difficulty, probability, and inter-stimulus interval as determinants of P300 from auditory stimuli. *Electroencephalography and Clinical Neurophysiology, 68*(4), 311–320. PubMed

Polich, J. (1989). Frequency, intensity, and duration as determinants of P300 from auditory stimuli. *Journal of Clinical Neurophysiology, 6*(3), 277–286. PubMed

Polich, J. (1996). Meta-analysis of P300 normative aging studies. *Psychophysiology, 33*(4), 334–353. PubMed

Polich, J., Ellerson, P. C., & Cohen, J. (1996). P300, stimulus intensity, modality, and probability. *International Journal of Psychophysiology, 23*(1–2), 55–62. PubMed

Polich, J., Howard, L., & Starr, A. (1985). Stimulus frequency and masking as determinants of P300 latency in event-related potentials from auditory stimuli. *Biological Psychology, 21*(4), 309–318. PubMed

Polich, J., & Starr, A. (1983). Middle, late and long latency auditory evoked potentials. In B. E. Moore (Ed.), *Bases of auditory brainstem evoked responses* (pp. 345–361). New York: Grune & Stratton.

Polich, J., & Starr, A. (1984). Evoked potentials in aging. In J. L. Alpert (Ed.), *Clinical neurology of aging* (pp. 49–177). New York: Oxford University Press.

Ponton, C. W., & Don, M. (1995). The mismatch negativity in cochlear implant users. *Ear and Hearing, 16*(1), 131–146. PubMed

Ponton, C. W., & Eggermont, J. J. (2001). Of kittens and kids: Altered cortical maturation following profound deafness and cochlear implant use. *Audiology and Neuro-Otology, 6*(6), 363–380. PubMed

Ponton, C., Eggermont, J. J., Khosla, D., Kwong, B., & Don, M. (2002). Maturation of human central auditory system activity: Separating auditory evoked potentials by dipole source modeling. *Clinical Neurophysiology, 113*(3), 407–420. PubMed

Prasher, D., Mula, M., & Luxon, L. (1993). Cortical evoked potential criteria in the objective assessment of auditory threshold: A comparison of noise induced hearing loss with Ménière's disease. *Journal of Laryngology and Otology, 107*(9), 780–786. PubMed

Rahne, T., Ehelebe, T., Rasinski, C., & Götze, G. (2010). Auditory brainstem and cortical potentials following bone-anchored hearing aid stimulation. *Journal of Neuroscience Methods, 193*(2), 300–306. PubMed

Richer, F., Johnson, R. A., & Beatty, J. (1983). Sources of late components of the brain magnetic response. *Society for Neuroscience Abstracts, 9*, 656.

Sams, M., Paavilainen, P., Alho, K., & Näätänen, R. (1985). Auditory frequency discrimination and event-related potentials. *Electroencephalography and Clinical Neurophysiology, 62*(6), 437–448. PubMed

Santos Filha, V. A., & Matas, C. G. (2010). Late auditory evoked potentials in individuals with tinnitus. *Brazilian Journal of Otorhinolargyngology, 76*(2), 263–270. PubMed

Schairer, K. S., Gould, H. J., & Pousson, M. A. (2001). Source generators of mismatch negativity to multiple deviant stimulus types. *Brain Topography, 14*(2), 117–130. PubMed

Scherg, M., & Von Cramon, D. (1986). Evoked dipole source potentials of the human auditory cortex. *Electroencephalography and Clinical Neurophysiology, 65*(5), 344–360. PubMed

Scherg, M., & Von Cramon, D. (1985). Two bilateral sources of the late AEP as identified by a spatio-temporal dipole model. *Electroencephalography and Clinical Neurophysiology, 62*(1), 32–44. PubMed

Schochat, E., & Musiek, F. (2004). Maturation of outcomes of behavioral and electrophysiologic test of central auditory function. *Journal of Communication Disorders, 39*(1), 78–92.

Schröger, E. (1995). Processing of auditory deviants with changes in one versus two stimulus dimensions. *Psychophysiology, 32*(1), 55–65. PubMed

Schröger, E. (1996). Interaural time and level differences: Integrated or separated processing? *Hearing Research, 96*(1–2), 191–198. PubMed

Schröger, E. (1998). Measurement and interpretation of the mismatch negativity. *Behavior Research Methods, Instruments, and Computers, 30*, 131–145.

Selinger, M., Prescott, T. E., & Shucard, D. W. (1989). Auditory event-related potential probes and behavioral measures of aphasia. *Brain and Language, 36*(3), 377–390. PubMed

Shafer, V. L., Morr, M. L., Kreuzer, J. A., & Kurtzberg, D. (2000). Maturation of mismatch negativity in school-age children. *Ear and Hearing, 21*(3), 242–251. PubMed

Sharma, A., Martin, K., Roland, P., Bauer, P., Sweeney, M. H., Gilley, P., et al. (2005). P1 latency as a biomarker for central auditory development in children with hearing impairment. *Journal of the American Academy of Audiology, 16*(8), 564–573. PubMed

Simson, R., Vaughn, H. G., Jr, & Ritter, W. (1977). The scalp topography of potentials in auditory and visual discrimination tasks. *Electroencephalography and Clinical Neurophysiology, 42*(4), 528–535. PubMed

Sinkkonen, J., & Tervaniemi, M. (2000). Towards optimal recording and analysis of the mismatch negativity. *Audiology and Neuro-Otology, 5*(3–4), 235–246. PubMed

Sommer, W., Matt, J., & Leuthold, H. (1990). Consciousness of attention and expectancy as reflected in event-related potentials and reaction times. *Journal of Experimental Psychology: Learning, Memory, and Cognition, 16*(5), 902–915. PubMed

Squires, N. K., Squires, K. C., & Hillyard, S. A. (1975). Two varieties of long-latency positive waves evoked by unpredictable auditory stimuli in man. *Electroencephalography and Clinical Neurophysiology, 38*(4), 387–401. PubMed

Squires, K. C., Wickens, C., Squires, N. K., & Donchin, E. (1976). The effect of stimulus sequence on the waveform of the cortical event-related potential. *Science, 193*(4258), 1142–1146. PubMed

Stenklev, N. C., & Laukli, E. (2004). Cortical cognitive potentials in elderly persons. *Journal of the American Academy of Audiology, 15*(6), 401–413. PubMed

Sutton, S., Braren, M., Zubin, J., & John, E. R. (1965). Evoked-potential correlates of stimulus uncertainty. *Science, 150*(700), 1187–1188. PubMed

Sutton, S., Tueting, P., Zubin, J., & John, E. R. (1967). Information delivery and the sensory evoked potential. *Science, 155*(768), 1436–1439. PubMed

Takegata, R., Paavilainen, P., Näätänen, R., & Winkler, I. (1999). Independent processing of changes in auditory single features and feature conjunctions in humans as indexed by the mismatch negativity. *Neuroscience Letters, 266*(2), 109–112. PubMed

Tervaniemi, M. (1999). Pre-attentive processing of musical information in the human brain. *Journal of New Music Research, 28*(3), 237–245.

Tiitinen, H., May, P., Reinikainen, K., & Näätänen, R. (1994). Attentive novelty detection in humans is governed by pre-attentive sensory memory. *Nature, 372*(6501), 90–92. PubMed

Tonnquist-Uhlén, I. (1996). Topography of auditory evoked cortical potentials in children with severe language impairment. *Scandinavian Audiology, 44*(Suppl), 1–40. PubMed

Tremblay, K. L., Billings, C. J., Friesen, L. M., & Souza, P. E. (2006). Neural representation of amplified speech sounds. *Ear and Hearing, 27*(2), 93–103. PubMed

Tremblay, K. L., Friesen, L., Martin, B. A., & Wright, R. (2003). Test-retest reliability of cortical evoked potentials using naturally produced speech sounds. *Ear and Hearing, 24*(3), 225–232. PubMed

Tremblay, K. L., Kraus, N., McGee, T., Ponton, C., & Otis, B. (2001). Central auditory plasticity: changes in the N1-P2 complex after speech-sound training. *Ear and Hearing, 22*(2), 79–90. PubMed

Tremblay, K. L., Shahin, A. J., Picton, T., & Ross, B. (2009). Auditory training alters the physiological detection of stimulus-specific cues in humans. *Clinical Neurophysiology, 120*(1), 128–135. PubMed

Vaughan, H. G., Jr, & Ritter, W. (1970). The sources of auditory evoked responses recorded from the human scalp. *Electroencephalography and Clinical Neurophysiology, 28*(4), 360–367. PubMed

Vesco, K. K., Bone, R. C., Ryan, J. C., & Polich, J. (1993). P300 in young and elderly subjects: Auditory frequency and intensity effects. *Electroencephalography and Clinical Neurophysiology, 88*(4), 302–308. PubMed

Walker, L. J., Carpenter, M., Downs, C. R., Cranford, J. L., Stuart, A., & Pravica, D. (2001). Possible neuronal refractory or recovery artifacts associated with recording the mismatch negativity response. *Journal of the American Academy of Audiology, 12*(7), 348–356. PubMed

Walker-Black, L., & Stuart, A. (2008). Effect of inverting electrode on mismatch negativity presence for perceptible/imperceptible tonal frequency contrasts. *International Journal of Audiology, 47*(11), 708–714.

Wall, L. G., Dalebout, S. D., Davidson, S. A., & Fox, R. A. (1991). Effect of hearing impairment on event-related potentials for tone and speech distinctions. *Folia Phoniatrica, 43*(6), 265–274. PubMed

Warrier, C. M., Johnson, K. L., Hayes, E. A., Nicol, T., & Kraus, N. (2004). Learning impaired children exhibit timing deficits and training-related improvements in auditory cortical responses to speech in noise. *Experimental Brain Research, 157*(4), 431–441. PubMed

Williams, H. L., Tepas, D. I., & Morlock, H. C., Jr (1962). Evoked responses to clicks and electroencephalographic stages of sleep in man. *Science, 138*, 685–686. PubMed

Wolff, C., & Schröger, E. (1995). MMN elicited by one-, two-, and three-dimensional deviants. *Journal of Psychophysiology, 9*, 384–385.

Wolpaw, J. R., & Penry, J. K. (1975). A temporal component of the auditory evoked response. *Electroencephalography and Clinical Neurophysiology, 39*(6), 609–620. PubMed

Woods, D. L. (1995). The component structure of the N1 wave of the human auditory evoked potential. *Electroencephalography and Clinical Neurophysiology, 44*(Suppl), 102–109. PubMed

Wunderlich, J. L., & Cone-Wesson, B. K. (2006). Maturation of CAEP in infants and children: A review. *Hearing Research, 212*(1–2), 212–223. PubMed

Wunderlich, J. L., Cone-Wesson, B. K., & Shepherd, R. (2006). Maturation of the cortical auditory evoked potential in infants and young children. *Hearing Research, 212*(1–2), 185–202. PubMed

Yamaguchi, S., & Knight, R. T. (1991). Age effects on the P300 to novel somatosensory stimuli. *Electroencephalography and Clinical Neurophysiology, 78*(4), 297–301. PubMed

Yingling, C. D., & Hosobuchi, Y. (1984). A subcortical correlate of P300 in man. *Electroencephalography and Clinical Neurophysiology, 59*(1), 72–76. PubMed

Yingling, C. D., & Skinner, J. E. (1977). Gating of thalamic input to cerebral cortex by nucleus reticularis thalami. In J. E. Desmedt (Ed.), *Progress in clinical neurophysiology: Attention, voluntary contraction, and event-related cerebral potentials* (pp. 70–96). Basel: Karger.

Zhang, F., Eliassen, J., Anderson, J., Scheifele, P., & Brown, D. (2009). The time course of the amplitude and latency in the auditory late response evoked by repeated tone bursts. *Journal of the American Academy of Audiology, 20*(4), 239–250. PubMed

Zhang, F., Samy, R. N., Anderson, J. M., & Houston, L. (2009). Recovery function of the late auditory evoked potential in cochlear implant users and normal-hearing listeners. *Journal of the American Academy of Audiology, 20*(7), 397–408. PubMed

Chapter 11

Development of Vestibular Evoked Myogenic Potentials

Tina M. Stoody and Yell Inverso

The discovery of the vestibular evoked myogenic potential (VEMP) response dates back to the 1950s. During this time, the research community was actively looking for ways to estimate behavioral thresholds using auditory evoked potentials (AEPs). Geisler, Frishkopf and Rosenblith (1958) published the first study using new computer averaging technology and reported a new auditory evoked waveform they believed to be of cortical origin. In 1964, Bickford, Jacobson, and Cody argued that these responses were myogenic, or muscular, in origin, based on their ability to record similar waveforms from various electrode locations placed over muscle regions in the neck. Bickford and colleagues also noted that when relaxation of the neck was accomplished, the response disappeared. In addition, this response was recorded from patients with known hearing loss, but it could not be obtained from patients with known vestibular lesions (Ackley, Tamaki, Oliszewski, and Inverso, 2004; Colebatch, Rothwell, Bronstein, and Ludman, 1994). This discovery led to speculation that this myogenic response was of a vestibular origin (Bickford et al, 1964). In 1971, Townsend and Cody further differentiated two different myogenic responses, the postauricular muscle response and the inion response. They also established that the inion response was of saccular origin by analyzing responses recorded from participants with various well-known vestibular lesions. Additional studies using animal models (Didier, Cazals, and Aurousseau, 1987; Young, Fernández, and Goldberg, 1977) and later humans (Murofushi, Matsuzaki, and Wu, 1999) further solidified that this response originated in the otolith organs rather than the auditory system.

Early on, the inion response and what it represented were not well understood. The presence of an inion response to visual (light) and somatosensory (peripheral nerve) stimulation led researchers to believe that it was a nonspecific response (Bickford et al, 1964; Cody and Bickford, 1969). Therefore, vestibular evoked potentials did not generate much clinical interest until the 1990s (Colebatch, Halmagyi, and Skuse, 1994; Zhou and Cox, 2004). Colebatch et al (1994) recorded the inion response from the sternocleidomastoid (SCM) muscle. Consistent responses obtained from participants with normal hearing and vestibular function, as well as recordings from participants with known lesions, confirmed the vestibular origin and usefulness of the inion response for assessment of the saccule (Colebatch et al, 1994). This work spurred further research into the clinical utility of the VEMP. The term *vestibular evoked myogenic potentials*, which is used today, was coined by Robertson and Ireland in 1995. Today's VEMP reflects activity from the vestibular system that is elicited by high-intensity sound stimulation, and the potential is detected as an alteration in the tonic status of the SCM muscle.

◆ Description

Morphology, Amplitude, and Spectrum

The VEMP response is a biphasic waveform. The peaks are named after their mean latencies in milliseconds, p13 and n23 (Colebatch and Halmagyi, 1992). Akin and Murnane (2001) reported a mean latency of 10.9 msec for the positive peak and 17.7 msec for the negative peak. In addition to the p13 and n23 nomenclature, many individuals have reported on the peak components as P1 and N2. Later potentials are present in the VEMP waveform, termed n34 and p44. These later occuring peaks are not always present in normal responses, but occur bilaterally and at lower thresholds, and appear to arise from the cochlea rather than the vestibular mechanism (Colebatch, Rothwell, Bronstein, and Ludman, 1994; Welgampola and Colebatch, 2005).

The VEMP is predominantly an ipsilateral response (Kushiro et al, 2000; Murofushi, Halmagyi, Yavor, and Colebatch, 1996; Uchino et al, 1997; Wilson et al, 1995). Colebatch and colleagues (1994) demonstrated that the response occurred over the SCM muscle ipsilateral to the acoustic stimulus. Akin and Murnane (2001) also showed that in normal subjects, a VEMP response was present only from the activated SCM muscle ipsilateral to the stimulated ear. Murofushi, Ochiai, Ozeki, and Iwasaki (2004) investigated the laterality of VEMP responses using clicks and tone bursts and concluded that the responses to both stimuli are ipsilateral-dominant.

Amplitude

There is a large amount of variability in VEMP amplitudes within normal responses. The amplitude of the response peaks is measured in microvolts and is often described as a peak-to-peak amplitude. Variations in amplitudes have been reported to range from several microvolts to several hundred microvolts (Colebatch et al, 1994; Li, Houlden, and Tomlinson, 1999). Welgampola and Colebatch (2005) reported peak-to-peak amplitudes of 25 to 297 µV in normal subjects. Amplitude can vary between individuals, as well as between ears within an individual. The variations in amplitude are due in large part to

SCM muscle tension and the intensity of the stimulus (Zhou and Cox, 2004). It is common for normal responses to be asymmetric when comparing sides. This asymmetry can occur from differences in tonic electromyographic (EMG) levels, muscular effort, structural differences in SCM muscles, the thickness of subcutaneous tissue layers, and the location of electrode placement (Chang, Yang, Wang, and Young, 2007; Sheykholeslami, Murofushi, and Kaga, 2001). Controlling EMG levels is an important factor in VEMP measurement and will be discussed later in this chapter. Although differences in amplitude are expected for the reasons mentioned already, it is suggested that the asymmetry is significant if the VEMP response on one side is three times larger than the other (Brantberg and Fransson, 2001).

Latency

In contrast to amplitude measures, test–retest reliability studies reveal that the latencies of p13 and n23 remain fairly constant regardless of SCM tension and stimulus intensity (Li et al, 1999). Latencies do not differ significantly from the right to left side in a normal VEMP response (Zhou and Cox, 2004). Response latencies are similar when either a click or a tone burst is used as the acoustic stimulus; however, low-frequency tone bursts will have slightly longer latencies. In addition, the latencies are minimally affected by the duration and rise/fall time of a tone burst such that longer tone burst durations will produce slightly increased latencies of p13 and n23 (Akin and Murnane, 2008; Akin, Murnane, and Proffitt, 2003).

◆ Neural Generators

VEMP Pathway

The VEMP response has been found to be originate in the saccule. Bickford and colleagues (1964) studied patients with auditory and vestibular lesions, and after noting that the VEMP was present in patients with profound hearing losses but absent in those with loss of labyrinthine function, they concluded that the VEMP had a vestibular origin.

Later studies by Colebatch and Halmagyi (1992) also demonstrated vestibular origins by comparing responses in individuals with peripheral audiovestibular lesions. Townsend and Cody (1971) noted the preservation of a VEMP response in patients with semicircular canal ablation and benign paroxysmal positional vertigo (BPPV). These findings led to the conclusion that the VEMP response is mediated by the otolithic organs (Rauch, 2006). Todd, Cody, and Banks (2000) reported that the VEMP has a well-defined tuning response with a maximum response frequency ~300 to 350 Hz, which is consistent with the acoustic sensitivity of the saccule.

Findings from both animal and human studies indicate that the VEMP is an ipsilateral response with a pathway that begins in the saccular macula continues to the afferent inferior vestibular nerve, the brainstem vestibular nuclei, the descending medial vestibulospinal tract, and then to the motor neurons of the SCM muscle (Akin and Murnane, 2008).

Although a thorough understanding of vestibular neuroanatomy and physiology is integral for a complete understanding of the generation and interpretation of the VEMP response, it is beyond the scope of this chapter, and the reader is encouraged to rely on a combination of the many published journal articles, book chapters, and reputable Web sites dedicated to this topic.

The vestibular organs are connected to a complex network of neural pathways, including the superior vestibular, inferior vestibular, and auditory branch of the eighth cranial nerve (CN VIII), which course upward to various nuclei in the brainstem. These pathways are made up of both motor and sensory neurons. The sensory neurons convey information to the brain about the body's position in space, while the motor neurons control muscular movement for balance. Contained within these pathways are several reflexes, including the vestibulocollic and vestibulospinal reflexes. When information about head movement is detected by the vestibular organs, such as the saccule, the neck muscles are reflexively stimulated to stabilize the head during the movement (Jones, 2000). The saccule is located medially and just posterior to the footplate of the stapes in the endolymph-filled membranous labyrinth. It is thought that when an acoustic stimulus of sufficient intensity is introduced to the inner ear, the saccule is stimulated by the pressure changes in the endolymph fluid from the movement of the stapes. This saccular stimulation in turn activates the vestibulocollic and vestibulospinal reflexes (Zhou and Cox, 2004), which aid in maintaining postural control.

Central Vestibular Pathways

A closer examination of the neurologic pathways of the vestibular system is warranted for a better understanding of the VEMP response. The peripheral vestibular system includes the three semicircular canals and the two otolith organs (utricle and saccule). The semicircular canals are responsible for detection of angular acceleration of the head. The hair cells of the sensory organs located within the semicircular canals, known as the cristae ampularis, send neural impulses up the superior vestibular branch of CN VIII. From there, the impulses are transmitted to the vestibular nuclei of the brainstem. Meanwhile, the otolith organs send neural impulses up the inferior vestibular branch of CN VIII, which also travels to the vestibular nuclei (Akin and Murnane, 2001; Iwasaki, Takai, Ito, and Murofushi, 2005). There are four vestibular nuclei on each side of the pons of the brainstem: the medial, lateral, superior, and inferior vestibular nuclei. Each nucleus has different connections to different neural pathways, including the thalamus, oculomotor nuclei, cerebellum, contralateral vestibular nuclei, reticular formation, and spinal cord (Haque and Dickman, 2008). Impulses from both the semicircular canals and the otolith organs are sent to all four of these vestibular nuclei on the ipsilateral side; however, the semicircular canals primarily connect to the superior and medial nuclei, and the otolith organs send connections primarily to the lateral, medial, and inferior nuclei. The saccule has unique innervations to another group of cells located in the brainstem called the y group, which then innervates the contralateral vertical muscle motor groups of the eye (Haque and Dickman, 2008). This connection has led to research on the use of the muscles of the eye as a recording site for the VEMP (Sauter, 2008).

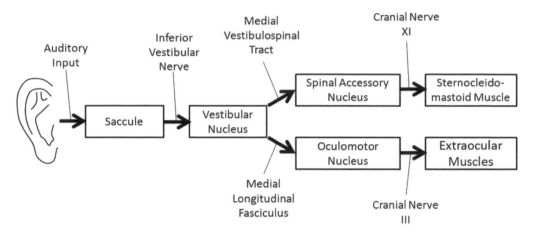

Fig. 11.1 A simple illustration of the two vestibular evoked myogenic pathways (VEMPs). Although both pathways begin with the saccule, inferior vestibular nerve, and vestibular nucleus, the cervical (cVEMP) pathway is on top, and the ocular (oVEMP) pathway is on the bottom.

This method is referred to as the ocular VEMP (or oVEMP). The presumed pathway for the oVEMP from the saccule to extraocular muscles is still under investigation, but Rosengren, Welgampola, and Colebatch (2010) suggested that the vestibular nuclei have outputs to the medial longitudinal fasciculus (MLF) and from the MLF to the oculomotor nuclei, associated cranial nerve, and muscle fibers of the extraocular muscles. A schematic of the central vestibular pathways as they relate to both cervical (cVEMP) and oVEMP responses is found in **Fig. 11.1**.

♦ Stimulus Effects

Stimulus parameters of primary interest are frequency spectrum, intensity, duration, and repetition rate. Alterations to these acoustic characteristics has been shown to elicit VEMP responses of varying amplitude, reproducibility, and diagnostic value (Cheng and Murofushi, 2001a,b; Huang, Su, and Cheng, 2005; Sheykholeslami, Habiby Kermany, and Kaga, 2001; Sheykholeslami et al, 2001; Takegoshi and Murofushi, 2003; Tamaki, 2007; Wu and Murofushi, 1999).

The earliest studies of the VEMP response (inion response) used short-duration click stimuli for elicitation. More recent studies have examined the use of various intensity levels of the click as well as more frequency-specific tone bursts. Akin and colleagues (2003) found that the intensity of the stimulus had a direct effect on the amplitude of the response for both the click and the tone burst stimuli. This finding was also supported by research by Lim and colleagues (1995). No effect was observed on latency in relation to the intensity of the click stimulus (Akin et al, 2003). The effects of the tone burst stimuli were related to the frequency and duration of the toneburst. VEMP responses were obtained at 250-, 500-, 750-, 1000-, 1500-, and and 2000 Hz, with the best responses being obtained at 500 and 750 Hz (Akin et al, 2003). Frequency-related differences in latency were noted such that lower frequencies resulted in longer latencies. However, this effect was noted only when a 2-msec rise/fall cycle was used. When a 4-msec cycle was used, the effect was not seen (Akin et al, 2003). Click stimuli have been found to produce waveforms with shorter latencies than the tone burst stimuli (Sauter, 2008). The sensitivity of the response to the frequency and duration of the stimulus must be taken into account when interpreting or comparing VEMP results. The amplitudes of the VEMP responses are more consistent across the different stimuli, allowing for more ease of interpretation.

Researchers have investigated stimulus parameters to evaluate which are optimal for VEMP recording. For both clicks and tone bursts, a loud and abrupt stimulus is needed. A level of 90 dB nHL (normal hearing level) is usually sufficient to evoke a VEMP (Zhou and Cox, 2004), but stimulus levels of 95 to 100 dB nHL are typically used to ensure adequate stimulation (Welgampola and Colebatch, 2005). In an examination of repetition rate, Wu and Murofushi (1999) compared rates of 1, 5, 10, 15, and 20 Hz and found that 1 and 5 Hz produced the highest amplitudes and the lowest variance for latencies. However, 1 Hz required more sweeps to obtain the desired signal-to-noise ratios (SNRs), so they concluded that 5 Hz was the optimal rate. The duration of the click used in AEP protocols is typically 0.1 msec (Colebatch, 1995; Colebatch et al, 1994; Halmagyi and Colebatch, 1995; Rauch, 2006; Robertson and Ireland, 1995; Welgampola and Colebatch, 2005), although Huang, Su, and Cheng (2005) found that a click duration of 0.5 msec produced superior VEMP morphology with increased amplitudes.

Murofushi, Matsuzaki, and Wu (1999) evaluated the frequency effect for tone burst stimuli. After comparing 0.5, 1, and 2 kHz, the greatest responses came from 0.5 kHz. This finding was confirmed by subsequent research (Akin and Murnane, 2001; Akin et al, 2003; Welgampola and Colebatch, 2001b). Todd, Cody, and Banks (2000) also investigated the tuning response of VEMPs and found that the maximum response is between 300 and 350 Hz. As mentioned, tone burst stimulus effects can also depend on rise/fall time parameters. A 1-msec rise/fall time is seen most often in the literature and has been found to produce the most consistent responses (Cheng and Murofushi, 2001a). In addition to rise/fall time, duration may have an effect on VEMP components. A decrease in amplitudes and an increase in latencies have been reported for stimulus durations of 7 msec and longer, possibly because of the activation of the stapedial reflex (Akin and Murnane, 2008; Cheng and Murofushi, 2001b; Welgampola and Colebatch, 2005). The suggestion of an evidence-based clinical protocol is beyond the scope of this chapter; please refer to Chapter 19 for more details on protocol.

♦ Subject Effects

Normal Hearing Processes

Aging Effects

As the body ages, significant changes such as deterioration of cells and tissues essential to the structure and function of visual, proprioceptive, and vestibular systems begin to occur. This results in decreased ability to process stimulus information from the environment. Change in only one of the three systems may not result in visible difficulties; however, a decline in at least two of these systems will have an impact on an individual's ability to maintain balance during everyday tasks. Decreases in function may include slowed neural impulses, narrowing of the visual field, and reduced muscle tone (Rose, 2003a). In the vestibular system, the number of hair cells located in each sensory organ, including the saccule, decreases. The reduced number of hair cells leads to reduced information about the individual's location in space being sent to the central nervous system (Rose, 2003a; Welgampola and Colebatch, 2001a). In addition to normal age-related changes, certain diseases that are common among older adults can impair balance. Visual impairments such as glaucoma, macular degeneration, and cataracts severely reduce the amount and quality of visual information being interpreted. Systemic diseases such as diabetes, hypertension, heart disease, and arthritis affect the muscular and proprioceptive systems. Neurogenic diseases such as stroke and Parkinson disease affect the brain's ability to process or send signals from and to the systems important for balance (Rose, 2003b).

Physiologic changes that occur with aging have an impact on the recording of VEMPs. Reduced muscle tone and strength affect an older adult's ability to maintain the constant contraction or the amount of contraction necessary to obtain a clear response (Akin and Murnane, 2007; Sauter, 2008). Welgampola and Colebatch (2001a) demonstrated a consistent trend in reduction of VEMP amplitude response with increases in age after accounting for the amount of muscle contraction. Although obtaining VEMP responses may be difficult because of decreased muscle contraction, assessing the saccular function in older adults may provide valuable information while assessing an individual's fall risk.

Gender Effects

There is not much evidence of a gender effect on the VEMP response. Researchers report no significant difference in amplitude or threshold between male and female subjects (Basta, Todt, and Ernst, 2005; Ochi and Ohashi, 2003). It is a little more unclear as to whether gender affects the latencies of p13-n23. Brantberg and Fransson (2001) reported that the p13 peak was significantly earlier in female patients and suggested that this could be caused by women having smaller heads and thus a shorter distance to the brainstem. However, subsequent research (Basta et al, 2005) did not reveal gender-related differences in latencies.

Hearing Loss

Vestibular disorders and auditory disorders may have comorbidity in patients; thus, evaluating the impact of sensorineural hearing loss on the VEMP is important for establishing the validity of its use as a tool. Although loud acoustic signals are used to generate a response, the signal produces a pressure wave that initiates hydrodynamic stimulation of vestibular hair cells. According to research completed by Ackley, Tamaki, Oliszewski, and Inverso (2004), clinical applications of VEMP indicate that this test is useful in assessing balance function in deaf/hard-of-hearing patients. Sazgar, Dortaj, Akrami, Akrami, and Karimi Yazdi (2006) looked specifically at the effects of high-frequency sensorineural hearing loss on VEMPs for the purpose of making the VEMP more useful in the diagnosis of vestibular disorders. Their study consisted of two main groups of patients, a control group of individuals with normal hearing and an experimental group composed of individuals with high-frequency hearing loss. The experimental group was further broken down into subgroups based on the severity of the hearing loss. There were some differences between the participants with normal hearing and those with hearing loss in the mean peak latencies of the VEMP responses, but a comparison between the subgroups showed fewer significant differences.

The authors concluded that the same causes of high-frequency sensorineural hearing loss may cause damage to the saccule as well. More research is needed to confirm these findings.

A significant stimulus intensity level within the inner ear is required to elicit the VEMP, therefore, a conductive hearing loss will significantly impact the ability to measure a VEMP response. Conductive hearing loss reduces the amount of sound energy that is transferred to the inner ear, thereby reducing the amount of energy reaching the saccule (Wang and Lee, 2007). VEMP results are often absent or have longer latencies when recorded in patients with conductive hearing loss (Akin and Murnane, 2007). Wang and Lee (2007) conducted a study using participants with middle ear effusion. VEMPs were recorded in 21 participants before and after fluid aspiration and drainage. Pure-tone audiometry confirmed recovery of hearing after fluid aspiration. Six of seven participants who had absent VEMP responses before aspiration had VEMP responses after aspiration. All participants with middle ear effusion showed significant improvement in asymmetry ratios after aspiration compared with ratios obtained before aspiration and when compared with VEMP measures in a control group of participants with normal hearing (Wang and Lee, 2007).

◆ Measurement Parameters

Electrode Placement

As with all other AEPs, the placement of recording electrodes is important in the recording of VEMPs. For a single-channel recording, there are three electrodes to be placed: the active (noninverting), reference (inverting), and ground. The active electrode may be placed over the belly or near the center of the muscle from which the response is being recorded (Sauter, 2008; Sheykholeslami et al, 2001). The reference electrode may be placed on the area of either origin or insertion of the muscle being recorded (Sauter, 2008). The sternum is a suitable reference location. The ground electrode is placed at any location on the body, away from the muscle being recorded. Commonly used locations include the forehead and the contralateral SCM. At times, another electrode is placed on the SCM next to the active electrode so as to allow for active monitoring of the EMG activity of the SCM during VEMP recording.

Recording Locations

As VEMPs have developed into a useful clinical tool, researchers have tried using different muscles as recording locations, such as the inion, trapezius muscle, muscles of the arms and legs, and SCM. For example, Ferber-Viart, Soulier, Dubreuil, and Duclaux (1998) recorded myogenic responses from the trapezius muscle to click stimuli from four different groups of patients based on their cochlear and vestibular function. Groups included individuals with complete unilateral cochleovestibular nerve damage, unilateral cochlear damage with preserved vestibular function, unilateral vestibular damage with preserved cochlear function of the neural pathways, and a control group of normal participants. The response of the trapezius muscle was bilateral to monaural stimulation. The authors found that in patients with no cochleovestibular function, the VEMP response was absent in the affected ear, whereas the response in the healthy ear was present but decreased in amplitude. Patients with intact cochlear function but absent vestibular function showed a response in the affected ear with decreased amplitudes, whereas the healthy ear had normal responses. Patients with cochlear damage also had reduced amplitudes of response in the pathologic ear and normal responses in the healthy ear. A limitation to this study is that it is difficult to assess whether or not patients with cochlear abnormalities also have otolith dysfunction (Ferber-Viart et al, 1998). The results suggest that there is a cochlear component to the VEMP response when measured from the trapezius muscle. Further study is needed on using the trapezius muscle as a location for VEMP responses to determine whether the response is of vestibular origin. Although the SCM provides the most robust and reliable VEMP data, the use of this muscle requires patients to extend and strain their necks. Therefore, assessing otolithic function with the trapezius muscle could be useful with

patients who may not be able to maintain the proper posture or positioning required to record from the SCM (described in the following section). The use of the trapezius muscle only requires patients to sit up and tuck their chins to the chests, a much easier position for most individuals (Ferber-Viart et al, 1998).

Patient Position

Several patient positions have been explored for optimal recording from the SCM. Some researchers have suggested having the patient sit or recline in a semirecumbent position and lift the head off the chair while the stimuli are presented. Participants could either be instructed to lift the head straight off the chair or to lift and then turn the head to one side (Sauter, 2008; Zapala, 2007). This method, though effective in obtaining a good contraction of the SCM, can be difficult to maintain by some individuals. Another method for obtaining contraction of the SCM is to have the patient sit upright and tilt the head slightly forward while turning to one side (Ochi, Ohashi, and Nishino, 2001; Sauter, 2008; Zapala, 2007). This method is not quite as tiring for most participants. Both methods require some means of ensuring a consistent contraction to each side for each presentation of the stimulus, as the amount of contraction has been shown to affect the amplitude of the results. Because analysis primarily depends on finding a difference in amplitude between sides, consistent amounts of contraction are necessary (Akin and Murnane, 2007; Ochi et al, 2001; Vanspauwen, Wuyts, and Van de Heyning, 2006; Zapala, 2007). Methods for controlling and maintaining this consistent muscle contraction are discussed later. Some patients, such as those with abnormal muscle weakness caused by age, cancer therapy, or muscular diseases, may not be able to maintain the needed contraction long enough to record accurate responses.

An emerging method for recording VEMPs involves recording the potentials of the inferior oblique muscle of the eye, referred to as the "oVEMP" (Rosengren, McAngus Todd, and Colebatch, 2005; Sauter, 2008). Active and reference electrodes are placed below the eye contralateral to the ear being stimulated, and a ground electrode is placed on either the forehead or the sternum. Patients are instructed to gaze upward and fixate on a point in the room while the stimuli are presented (Sauter, 2008). Further research on the reliability of this method is needed, but it may be an alternative for testing populations that have difficulty with the SCM methods. The oVEMP is associated with the vestibulo-ocular reflex (VOR). Clinically, the VOR will involve a recorded response from contracted extraocular muscles. Specifically, the contraction of the inferior oblique and rectus muscles (with upward eye gaze) has had the most success (Rosengren et al, 2005; Welgampola, Migliaccio, Myrie, Minor, and Carey, 2009).

Air Conduction versus Bone Conduction

VEMPs elicited via bone conduction or skull taps have also been examined. Taps can be delivered to the forehead or lateral skull, with some differences in polarity and sidedness of the resulting potential (Sheykholeslami, Murofushi, Kermany, and Kaga, 2000). VEMPs can also be evoked by using bone-conducted tone bursts at frequencies of ~200 Hz. VEMPs are typically larger for air-conducted tone bursts as a result of frequency tuning and because the stimuli have more sound energy because of longer durations (Akin et al, 2003; Todd, Cody, and Banks, 2000; Welgampola and Colebatch, 2001b). Sheykholeslami and colleagues (2000) recorded VEMPs using a clinical bone oscillator, although clinical bone vibrators generally require additional amplification to produce strong enough stimuli for VEMP testing. Although bone-conducted VEMPs are not as well lateralized as click-evoked VEMPs because the bone-conducted stimuli stimulate both ears at once, if the vibrator is placed over the mastoid, the VEMP ipsilateral to that mastoid tends to be larger (Welgampola, Rosengren, Halmagyi, and Colebatch, 2003).

SCM Contraction Controls/EMG Monitoring

The importance of maintaining a constant level of muscle contraction or EMG activity for accurate VEMP response analysis has been clearly established (Akin and Murnane, 2007; Akin et al, 2003; Colebatch, Halmagyi, and Skuse, 1994; Sauter, 2008; Vanspauwen et al, 2006). A diverse selection of methods for controlling the EMG or accounting for baseline EMG activity is available. One method is the monitoring and recording of the baseline EMG levels before the presentation of the stimulus. The baseline activity is then subtracted from the response waveform, and the remainder is considered the response. This method is known as rectification of the response (Akin and Murnane, 2007). Not all equipment used to measure VEMP responses has rectification features or capabilities. Another method is the use of a biofeedback mechanism in which the patient is given a visual representation of the EMG level and instructed to keep the same EMG level by keeping the visual object in a specified area. Some machines use a simple bar that moves up and down with the amount of contraction, whereas others use happy and sad face symbols to give patients feedback on their level of muscle contraction (Akin and Murnane, 2007; Sauter, 2008). Although these methods are effective and useful, they are costly and require the placement of extra electrodes for EMG monitoring. Vanspauwen et al (2006) devised a simpler, more cost-effective method with the use of a blood pressure cuff and sphygmomanometer in which the patient is instructed to push against the cuff to achieve a specified level of pressure that translates into the amount of contraction (**Fig. 11.2**). No single method has been shown in studies to be better than another, but emphasis on the use of some method for monitoring EMG or contraction levels is encouraged (Akin and Murnane, 2007; Sauter, 2008; Zapala, 2007).

Pearl

Consistency is key. When evaluating the amplitude of a myogenic response, the contraction of the SCM muscle must be consistent. It is often very difficult to determine visually whether a patient has maintained the same level of contraction throughout the testing process. This is especially important when comparing response amplitudes between ears. If you do not have a test system that monitors muscle contraction and gives visual feedback to the patient, you ay wish to purchase a blood pressure cuff and sphygmomanometer to control SCM contraction. Just be sure that the patient is pushing the cuff with their chin rather than with their arm/hand.

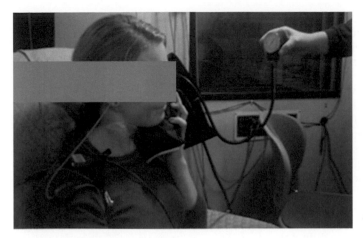

Fig. 11.2 Use of a blood pressure cuff sphygmomanometer to monitor the amount of muscle contraction during VEMP testing. Note that the electrode montage used in this example was the belly of the sternocleidomastoid (SCM) muscle referenced to the sternoclavicular joint, with the contralateral SCM serving as the ground.

♦ Clinical Interpretation

Since the discovery of the VEMP as an evaluative tool, there has been a focus on defining applications of VEMP procedures for diagnosing conditions that cause dizziness, such as superior canal dehiscence (SCD) (Brantberg et al, 2001; Brantberg, Bergenius, and Tribukait, 1999; Colebatch et al, 1994; Minor, Solomon, Zinreich, and Zee, 1998), Meniere disease (Magliulo, Cianfrone, Gagliardi, Cuiuli, and D'Amico, 2004; Rauch et al, 2004; Rauch, Zhou, Kujawa, Guinan, and Herrmann, 2004; Shojaku, Takemori, Kobayashi, and Watanabe, 2001), and acoustic neuroma or vestibular schwannoma (Chen, Young, and Wu, 2000; Patko, Vidal, Vibert, Tran Ba Huy, and de Waele, 2003; Tsutsumi, Tsunoda, Noguchi, and Komatsuzaki, 2000). Several VEMP measures have been suggested for use in interpreting VEMP waveforms. These include p13 and n23 latencies, p13-n23 amplitude, threshold, and an amplitude asymmetry ratio (Akin and Murnane, 2008). Latencies are affected by some central pathologies, including multiple sclerosis. Because of the large variability in absolute peak amplitudes, both between and within subjects, the use of absolute amplitudes as a diagnostic tool is limited. The p13-n23 peak-to-peak amplitude can be larger or reduced, along with certain vestibular pathologies, but reliable normative data are not available for definitive findings (Hall, 2007). VEMP threshold, or the lowest stimulus level able to elicit a VEMP response, is often reduced for people with Tullio phenomenon and SCD (Akin and Murnane, 2008). Among response abnormalities, Akin and Murnane (2008) reported that an absent response and an interaural amplitude difference are the most common findings in vestibular pathologies.

Side-to-side amplitude differences are measured to aid in the detection of a unilateral vestibular disorder. An asymmetry ratio (AR) is used to calculate the amplitude difference, which is expressed as a percentage. The AR is as follows:

$$AR = 100 (A_L - A_S)/(A_L + A_S),$$

where A_L equals the larger p13-n23 amplitude, and A_S equals the smaller amplitude. In normal VEMP responses, asymmetry ratios range from ~0% to 40% (Akin and Murnane, 2008). Others put the cutoff for a normal AR at 37% (Li et al, 1999) and at 35% (Welgampola and Colebatch, 2005). An AR over these percentages would usually indicate a unilateral hypofunction on the side with the smaller p13- n23 amplitude, though it may be also due to a unilateral hyperfunction on the side with the larger p13-n23 amplitude.

♦ Clinical Applications

The most commonly used assessment tools for diagnosing pathologies of the vestibular system, such as videonystagmography (VNG) and dynamic platform posturography (DPP), do not evaluate the function of the otolithic organs (Zhou and Cox, 2004). VEMP testing is therefore a valuable addition to the differential diagnosis of vestibular pathologies. The literature regarding VEMP has been rapidly growing, and it appears that there is considerable value in VEMP as a diagnostic measure. The following section introduces this topic; however, further inspection of this topic is covered in Chapter 19.

Zapala and Brey (2004) suggest three reasons why the VEMP is such a potentially important test in the evaluation of patients with vestibular pathologies. First, it is the only current test that evaluates the function of the saccule. Second, the neural pathway that is evaluated is significantly different from those that are evaluated in other vestibular tests, such as the VOR in VNG testing. The VOR pathway is organized from the level of the vestibular nuclei through the midbrain, and any lesions within that area may be detected during VNG evaluation. The VEMP pathway proceeds caudally from the vestibular nuclei down through cervical portions of the spinal cord, reflecting activation of the vestibulospinal tract. Another important difference in the VEMP pathway is that it includes the inferior branch of the vestibular nerve, and it is sensitive and more specific to pathologies that affect it. Third, VEMPs can add to our understanding of pathologic conditions that involve the vestibulospinal system. It may lead to the identification of additional treatable pathologies that are not currently recognized.

Through research and clinical experience, the VEMP has been shown to be useful in the diagnosis of several disorders. VEMP testing can provide valuable information in identifying Meniere disease, vestibular neuritis, Tullio phenomenon, SCD, ototoxicity, vestibular schwannomas, and otosclerosis (Welgampola and Colebatch, 2005; Zapala and Brey, 2004; Zhou and Cox, 2004). Because severe-profound sensorineural hearing loss (cochlear origin) does not preclude VEMP measurement, it is also of value during cochlear implant candidacy assessment.

Pearl

There is a need for evidence-based practice in VEMP testing. The use of VEMP testing in clinical audiology practice is still in its infancy when compared with other electrophysiologic measures (e.g., auditory brainstem response). Therefore, it is imperative that audiologists using VEMP for diagnostic purposes keep up-to-date on all emerging literature and should be prepared to evaluate how the results should be incorporated into their clinical protocols.

♦ Summary

VEMPs have gained in recognition and importance since the mid-1990s when the term was coined. The purpose of the VEMP test is to determine whether the otolithic organ, the saccule, and the inferior vestibular nerve and central connections are intact and working properly. It has long been believed that the saccule maintains a slight yet measurable sound sensitivity. This sensitivity is thought to be residual from the saccule's use as an organ of hearing in lower animals. VEMP testing, though rapidly evolving, appears to be beneficial. It is important to note that as with any test in its relative infancy, you must continue to seek up-to-date research and clinical reporting. Just as changes have occurred since the test's inception, it is possible (if not likely) that there will be many more alterations to both the VEMP parameters and the test's clinical utility.

References

Ackley, R. S., Tamaki, C., Oliszewski, C. N., & Inverso, Y. (2004). Vestibular evoked myogenic potential assessment of deaf and hard of hearing patients. In *Insights in practice: Clinical topics in otoneurology*. GN Otometrics, 2004.

Akin, F. W., & Murnane, O. D. (2001). Vestibular evoked myogenic potentials: Preliminary report. *Journal of the American Academy of Audiology, 12*(9), 445–452, quiz 491. PubMed

Akin, F. W., Murnane, O. D., & Proffitt, T. M. (2003). The effects of click and tone-burst stimulus parameters on the vestibular evoked myogenic potential (VEMP). *Journal of the American Academy of Audiology, 14*(9), 500–509, quiz 534–535. PubMed

Akin, F. W., & Murnane, O. (2007, April 18). *Advanced techniques in vestibular assessment: Tests of otolith function.* Paper presented at the American Academy of Audiology, Denver, CO.

Akin, F., & Murnane, O. (2008). Vestibular evoked myogenic potentials. In G. P. Jacobsen & N. T. Shepard (Eds.), *Balance function assessment and management* (pp. 405–434). San Diego: Plural Publishing.

Basta, D., Todt, I., & Ernst, A. (2005). Normative data for P1/N1-latencies of vestibular evoked myogenic potentials induced by air- or bone-conducted tone bursts. *Clinical Neurophysiology, 116*(9), 2216–2219. PubMed

Bickford, R. G., Jacobson, J. L., & Cody, D. T. R. (1964). Nature of averaged evoked potentials to sound and other stimuli in man. *Annals of the New York Academy of Sciences, 112,* 204–223. PubMed

Brantberg, K., Bergenius, J., & Tribukait, A. (1999). Vestibular-evoked myogenic potentials in patients with dehiscence of the superior semicircular canal. *Acta Oto-Laryngologica, 119*(6), 633–640. PubMed

Brantberg, K., & Fransson, P. A. (2001). Symmetry measures of vestibular evoked myogenic potentials using objective detection criteria. *Scandinavian Audiology, 30*(3), 189–196. PubMed

Brantberg, K., Bergenius, J., Mendel, L., Witt, H., Tribukait, A., & Ygge, J. (2001). Symptoms, findings and treatment in patients with dehiscence of the superior semicircular canal. *Acta Oto-Laryngologica, 121*(1), 68–75. PubMed

Chang, C. H., Yang, T. L., Wang, C. T., & Young, Y. H. (2007). Measuring neck structures in relation to vestibular evoked myogenic potentials. *Clinical Neurophysiology, 118*(5), 1105–1109. PubMed

Chen, C. W., Young, Y. H., & Wu, C. H. (2000). Vestibular neuritis: Three-dimensional videonystagmography and vestibular evoked myogenic potential results. *Acta Oto-Laryngologica, 120*(7), 845–848. PubMed

Cheng, P.-W., & Murofushi, T. (2001a). The effect of rise/fall time on vestibular-evoked myogenic potential triggered by short tone bursts. *Acta Oto-Laryngologica, 121*(6), 696–699. PubMed

Cheng, P. W., & Murofushi, T. (2001b). The effects of plateau time on vestibular-evoked myogenic potentials triggered by tone bursts. *Acta Oto-Laryngologica, 121*(8), 935–938. PubMed

Cody, D. T. R., & Bickford, R. G. (1969). Averaged evoked myogenic responses in normal man. *The Laryngoscope, 79*(3), 400–416. PubMed

Colebatch, J. G., & Halmagyi, G. M. (1992). Vestibular evoked potentials in human neck muscles before and after unilateral vestibular deafferentation. *Neurology, 42*(8), 1635–1636. PubMed

Colebatch, J. G., Rothwell, J. C., Bronstein, A., & Ludman, H. (1994). Click-evoked vestibular activation in the Tullio phenomenon. *Journal of Neurology, Neurosurgery, and Psychiatry, 57*(12), 1538–1540. PubMed

Didier, A., Cazals, Y., & Aurousseau, C. (1987). Brainstem connections of the anterior and posterior parts of the saccule in the guinea pig. *Acta Oto-Laryngologica, 104*(5–6), 385–391. PubMed

Ferber-Viart, C., Soulier, N., Dubreuil, C., & Duclaux, R. (1998). Cochleovestibular afferent pathways of trapezius muscle responses to clicks in human. *Acta Oto-Laryngologica, 118*(1), 6–10. PubMed

Geisler, C. D., Frishkopf, L. S., & Rosenblith, W. A. (1958). Extracranial responses to acoustic clicks in man. *Science, 128*(3333), 1210–1211. PubMed

Hall, J. W. (2007). Electrically evoked and myogenic responses. In *New handbook of auditory evoked responses* (pp. 581–628). Boston: Pearson.

Halmagyi, G., & Colebatch, J. (1995). Vestibular evoked myogenic potentials in the sternomastoid muscle are not of lateral canal origin. *Acta otolaryngologica Supplementum, 520 Pt 1*(S520), 1–3.

Haque, A., & Dickman, J. D. (2008). Vestibular system function: From physiology to pathology. In W. Clark & K. K. Ohlemiller (Eds.), *Anatomy and physiology of hearing for audiologists* (pp. 284–310). St. Louis: Thompson Delmar Learning.

Huang, T. W., Su, H. C., & Cheng, P. W. (2005). Effect of click duration on vestibular-evoked myogenic potentials. *Acta Oto-Laryngologica, 125*(2), 141–144. PubMed

Iwasaki, S., Takai, Y., Ito, K., & Murofushi, T. (2005). Abnormal vestibular evoked myogenic potentials in the presence of normal caloric responses. *Otology and Neurotology, 26*(6), 1196–1199. PubMed

Jones, G. M. (2000). Posture. In E. R. Kandel, J. H. Schwartz, and T. M. Jessell (Eds.), *Principles of neural science* (4th ed., pp. 816–828). New York: McGraw-Hill.

Kushiro, K., Zakir, M., Sato, H., Ono, S., Ogawa, Y., Meng, H., et al. (2000). Saccular and utricular inputs to single vestibular neurons in cats. *Experimental Brain Research, 131*(4), 406–415. PubMed

Li, M. W., Houlden, D., & Tomlinson, R. D. (1999). Click evoked EMG responses in sternocleidomastoid muscles: Characteristics in normal subjects. *Journal of Vestibular Research: Equilibrium Orientation, 9*(5), 327–334. PubMed

Lim, C. L., Clouston, P., Sheean, G., & Yiannikas, C. (1995). The influence of voluntary EMG activity and click intensity on the vestibular click evoked myogenic potential. *Muscle and Nerve, 18*(10), 1210–1213. PubMed

Magliulo, G., Cianfrone, G., Gagliardi, M., Cuiuli, G., & D'Amico, R. (2004). Vestibular evoked myogenic potentials and distortion-product otoacoustic emissions combined with glycerol testing in endolymphatic hydrops: Their value in early diagnosis. *The Annals of Otology, Rhinology, and Laryngology, 113*(12), 1000–1005. PubMed

Minor, L. B., Solomon, D., Zinreich, J. S., & Zee, D. S. (1998). Sound- and/or pressure-induced vertigo due to bone dehiscence of the superior semicircular canal. *Archives of Otolaryngology—Head & Neck Surgery, 124*(3), 249–258. PubMed

Murofushi, T., Halmagyi, G. M., Yavor, R. A., & Colebatch, J. G. (1996). Absent vestibular evoked myogenic potentials in vestibular neurolabyrinthitis. An indicator of inferior vestibular nerve involvement? *Archives of Otolaryngology—Head and Neck Surgery, 122*(8), 845–848. PubMed

Murofushi, T., Matsuzaki, M., & Wu, C. H. (1999). Short tone burst-evoked myogenic potentials on the sternocleidomastoid muscle: Are these potentials also of vestibular origin? *Archives of Otolaryngology–Head & Neck Surgery*, 125(6), 660–664. PubMed

Murofushi, T., Ochiai, A., Ozeki, H., & Iwasaki, S. (2004). Laterality of vestibular evoked myogenic potentials. *International Journal of Audiology*, 43(2), 66–68. PubMed

Ochi, K., Ohashi, T., & Nishino, H. (2001). Variance of vestibular-evoked myogenic potentials. *The Laryngoscope*, 111(3), 522–527. PubMed

Ochi, K., & Ohashi, T. (2003). Age-related changes in the vestibular-evoked myogenic potentials. *Otolaryngology–Head and Neck Surgery*, 129(6), 655–659. PubMed

Patko, T., Vidal, P. P., Vibert, N., Tran Ba Huy, P., & de Waele, C. (2003). Vestibular evoked myogenic potentials in patients suffering from an unilateral acoustic neuroma: A study of 170 patients. *Clinical Neurophysiology*, 114(7), 1344–1350. PubMed

Rauch, S. D. (2006). Vestibular evoked myogenic potentials. *Current Opinion in Otolaryngology–Head and Neck Surgery*, 14(5), 299–304. PubMed

Rauch, S. D., Silveira, M. B., Zhou, G., Kujawa, S. G., Wall, C., III, Guinan, J. J., et al. (2004). Vestibular evoked myogenic potentials versus vestibular test battery in patients with Meniere's disease. *Otology and Neurotology*, 25(6), 981–986. PubMed

Rauch, S. D., Zhou, G., Kujawa, S. G., Guinan, J. J., & Herrmann, B. S. (2004). Vestibular evoked myogenic potentials show altered tuning in patients with Ménière's disease. *Otology and Neurotology*, 25(3), 333–338. PubMed

Robertson, D. D., & Ireland, D. J. (1995Feb). Vestibular evoked myogenic potentials. *Journal of Otolaryngology*, 24(1), 3–8. PubMed

Rose, D. J. (2003a). Understanding balance and mobility. In *Fall proof! A comprehensive balance and mobility training program*. (pp. 3–27). Champaign, IL: Human Kinetics.

Rose, D. J. (2003b). Why do many older adults fall? In *Fall proof! A comprehensive balance and mobility training program*. (pp. 29–46). Champaign, IL: Human Kinetics.

Rosengren, S. M., McAngus Todd, N. P., & Colebatch, J. G. (2005). Vestibular-evoked extraocular potentials produced by stimulation with bone-conducted sound. *Clinical Neurophysiology*, 116(8), 1938–1948. PubMed

Rosengren, S. M., Welgampola, M. S., & Colebatch, J. G. (2010). Vestibular evoked myogenic potentials: Past, present and future. *Clinical Neurophysiology*, 121(5), 636–651. PubMed

Sauter, T. B. (2008). Vestibular evoked myogenic potentials: 2008 update. *Audiology Online*.

Sazgar, A. A., Dortaj, V., Akrami, K., Akrami, S., & Karimi Yazdi, A. R. (2006). Saccular damage in patients with high-frequency sensorineural hearing loss. *European Archives of Oto-Rhino-Laryngology*, 263(7), 608–613. PubMed

Sheykholeslami, K., Habiby Kermany, M., & Kaga, K. (2001). Frequency sensitivity range of the saccule to bone-conducted stimuli measured by vestibular evoked myogenic potentials. *Hearing Research*, 160(1–2), 58–62. PubMed

Sheykholeslami, K., Murofushi, T., & Kaga, K. (2001). The effect of sternocleidomastoid electrode location on vestibular evoked myogenic potential. *Auris, Nasus, Larynx*, 28(1), 41–43. PubMed

Sheykholeslami, K., Murofushi, T., Kermany, M. H., & Kaga, K. (2000). Bone-conducted evoked myogenic potentials from the sternocleidomastoid muscle. *Acta Oto-Laryngologica*, 120(6), 731–734. PubMed

Shojaku, H., Takemori, S., Kobayashi, K., & Watanabe, Y. (2001). Clinical usefulness of glycerol vestibular-evoked myogenic potentials: Preliminary report. *Acta Oto-Laryngologica Supplementum*, 545, 65–68. PubMed

Takegoshi, H., & Murofushi, T. (2003). Effect of white noise on vestibular evoked myogenic potentials. *Hearing Research*, 176(1–2), 59–64. PubMed

Tamaki, C. (2007). *Variations of threshold, amplitude and latencies of vestibular-evoked myogenic potentials (VEMP)*. Unpublished dissertation, Gallaudet University, Washington, DC.

Todd, N. P. M., Cody, F. W. J., & Banks, J. R. (2000). A saccular origin of frequency tuning in myogenic vestibular evoked potentials? Implications for human responses to loud sounds. *Hearing Research*, 141(1–2), 180–188. PubMed

Townsend, G. L., & Cody, D. T. (1971, Feb). The averaged inion response evoked by acoustic stimulation: its relation to the saccule. *Annals of Otology, Rhinology, and Laryngology*, 80(1), 121–131. PubMed

Tsutsumi, T., Tsunoda, A., Noguchi, Y., & Komatsuzaki, A. (2000). Prediction of the nerves of origin of vestibular schwannomas with vestibular evoked myogenic potentials. *American Journal of Otology*, 21(5), 712–715. PubMed

Uchino, Y., Sato, H., Sasaki, M., Imagawa, M., Ikegami, H., Isu, N., et al. (1997). Sacculocollic reflex arcs in cats. *Journal of Neurophysiology*, 77(6), 3003–3012. PubMed

Vanspauwen, R., Wuyts, F. L., & Van de Heyning, P. H. (2006). Improving vestibular evoked myogenic potential reliability by using a blood pressure manometer. *Laryngoscope*, 116(1), 131–135. PubMed

Wang, M. C., & Lee, G. S. (2007). Vestibular evoked myogenic potentials in middle ear effusion. *Acta Oto-Laryngologica*, 127(7), 700–704. PubMed

Welgampola, M. S., & Colebatch, J. G. (2001a). Vestibulocollic reflexes: Normal values and the effect of age. *Clinical Neurophysiology*, 112(11), 1971–1979. PubMed

Welgampola, M. S., & Colebatch, J. G. (2001b). Characteristics of tone burst-evoked myogenic potentials in the sternocleidomastoid muscles. *Otology and Neurotology*, 22(6), 796–802. PubMed

Welgampola, M. S., & Colebatch, J. G. (2005, May). Characteristics and clinical applications of vestibular-evoked myogenic potentials. *Neurology*, 64(10), 1682–1688. PubMed

Welgampola, M. S., Migliaccio, A. A., Myrie, O. A., Minor, L. B., & Carey, J. P. (2009). The human sound-evoked vestibulo-ocular reflex and its electromyographic correlate. *Clinical Neurophysiology*, 120(1), 158–166. PubMed

Welgampola, M. S., Rosengren, S. M., Halmagyi, G. M., & Colebatch, J. G. (2003). Vestibular activation by bone conducted sound. *Journal of Neurology, Neurosurgery, and Psychiatry*, 74(6), 771–778. PubMed

Wilson, V. J., Boyle, R., Fukushima, K., Rose, P. K., Shinoda, Y., Sugiuchi, Y., *et al.* (1995). The vestibulocollic reflex. *Journal of Vestibular Research*, *5*(3), 147–170. PubMed

Wu, C. H., & Murofushi, T. (1999). The effect of click repetition rate on vestibular evoked myogenic potential. *Acta Oto-Laryngologica*, *119*(1), 29–32. PubMed

Young, E. D., Fernández, C., & Goldberg, J. M. (1977). Responses of squirrel monkey vestibular neurons to audio-frequency sound and head vibra-tion. *Acta Oto-Laryngologica*, *84*(5–6), 352–360. PubMed

Zapala, D. A. (2007). The VEMP: Ready for the clinic. *Hearing Journal*, *60*(3), 10–20.

Zapala, D. A., & Brey, R. H. (2004). Clinical experience with the vestibular evoked myogenic potential. *Journal of the American Academy of Audiology*, *15*(3), 198–215. PubMed

Zhou, G., & Cox, L. C. (2004). Vestibular evoked myogenic potentials: History and overview. *American Journal of Audiology*, *13*(2), 135–143. PubMed

Chapter 12

Electrocochleography: Clinical Applications

Cathy C. Henderson

Electrocochleography (ECochG) is a test of early latency evoked potentials associated with the inner ear and the auditory nerve. Ruth (1989) described these potentials as follows: cochlear microphonic (CM), a graded alternating current (AC) potential generated by hair cells; summating potential (SP), a complex direct current (DC) potential generated by hair cells that appears to reflect distortion of the cochlear transduction process; and action potential (AP), a compound action potential of the auditory nerve that represents the synchronous discharge of a large number of neurons arising from the distal portion of the eighth cranial nerve (CN VIII). ECochG can be used in the diagnosis and monitoring of Meniere disease, the enhancement of wave I of the auditory brainstem response (ABR), and intraoperative monitoring (Ruth, Lambert, and Ferraro, 1988). It has also been suggested for the diagnosis of auditory neuropathy spectrum disorder (ANSD) (Hall, 2007). **Figure 12.1** illustrates examples of a normal and an abnormal ECochG, the latter of which may be seen in Meniere disease. A more comprehensive review of the literature for ECochG can be found in Chapter 5. Subsequently, this chapter will serve more as a clinical guide or "how to" on the process of performing an ECochG.

◆ Recording the ECochG: Different Electrodes

In contrast to most other auditory evoked potentials (AEPs), ECochG involves electrodes that are placed within the ear canal or on the promontory of the cochlea. The type of electrode used for measurement will directly influence the amplitude of the ECochG tracing. Electrodes can be transtympanic (TT) or extratympanic (ET). The most robust response is obtained from the TT electrode, which is a needle electrode placed through the tympanic membrane (TM) and resting on the promontory wall near the round window. A silver ball electrode placed near the round window during surgery may also be used for this type of recording. Recordings using TT electrodes are "near-field" in that they are much closer to the source of activity and provide very large responses and may require very little averaging. Use of TT electrodes is considered invasive, requiring physician involvement, and are not covered further in this chapter.

Good clinical results can be achieved with ET electrodes, although they are "far-field" recordings and require more averaging to obtain a reasonably reliable response. Studies have been performed comparing various ET electrodes (e.g., Ferraro, Murphy, and Ruth, 1986; Ruth, Lambert, and Ferraro, 1988; Stypulkowski and Staller, 1987). Ruth and Lambert (1989) compared TT electrode tracings with TM electrode tracings and found them to compare favorably. Ferraro and Durrant (2006) described the more recent developments of ET electrodes, including a modified version of the TM electrode first described by Stypulkowski and Staller (1987) and commercially available ET electrodes. In general, each of the different ET electrodes can provide useful ECochG data. The type of ET electrode used and the

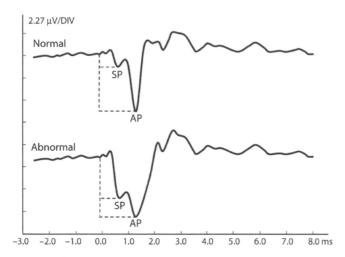

2.27 µV/DIV

Normal

SP

AP

Abnormal

SP

AP

−3.0   −2.0   −1.0   0.0   1.0   2.0   3.0   4.0   5.0   6.0   7.0   8.0 ms

Fig. 12.1 Illustration of normal versus abnormal click electrocochleography (ECochG). Note an enlarged summating potential (SP) for the abnormal ECochG. AP, action potential.

skill of the examiner placing the electrode often dictates the quality of the test results. ET electrodes have advantages clinically in that they are noninvasive and can be placed in the clinic by an audiologist. A disadvantage of ET electrodes is that the amplitudes are comparatively smaller than TT electrodes and may be less reliable depending on ET electrode placement and the overall amplitude of the desired ECochG components. Although many different ET electrodes have been described in the literature, a discussion of the two electrodes commonly used by clinicians, TIPtrodes and TM electrodes, will follow.

TIPtrodes

TIPtrodes are commercially available foam insert earphone tips covered in gold foil. The design of the tiptrode allows for simultaneous use of the electrode as a transducer. The amplitude of the ECochG recording with the TIPtrodes is generally less than with an electrode placed on the TM and thus may provide less robust and less reliable results. The technique and skill on preparing and placing this type of electrode can be a factor in good test results (Hall, 2007).

Tympanic Membrane Electrode

As the name implies, TM electrode is placed directly on the TM and can easily be made in the clinic with the proper supplies. It is also commercially available for purchase. The TM

electrode will generally give the largest amplitude of the ET electrodes. **Table 12.1** lists the materials used in our clinic to make a custom TM electrode.

Making a custom TM electrode is not difficult, even for the novice clinician. However, patience is required, and the specific materials listed in **Table 12.1** are needed. The steps for making a custom TM electrode are as follows:

1. The components of a TM electrode are shown in **Fig. 12.2A**.

2. Cut a 3-inch section of very small, Teflon-coated wire. Remove the coating from each end of the wire to expose bare wire. The exposed wire will connect with the alligator clip electrode on one end and will be embedded within the spongy foam on the other end (**Fig. 12.2B**). Cut a 1½- to 2-inch section of the very flexible tubing noted in the materials list in **Table 12.1**. Cut a small, triangular-shaped wedge from the foam sponge. Cotton can be used in place of the foam sponge, as described by Ferraro and Durrant (2006).

3. Thread the wire through the tubing and pull until the foam sponge is snug.

4. Snip around the foam sponge until it forms a ball at the end of the tubing. Pull some of the foam sponge snugly into the tubing. Do not allow the foam sponge to be pulled all the way into the tubing.

Table 12.1 Materials to Make a Custom Tympanic Membrane Electrode

Silastic tubing (size: 0.58-inch inner diameter, 0.077-inch outer diameter), which may be ordered from Helix Medical, Inc. at http://www.helixmedical.com
Silver wire (Teflon-coated, 0.008-inch bare diameter, 0.011-inch insulated diameter), which can be ordered from A-M Systems, Inc. at http://www.a-msystems.com
Foam sponge material (very fine upholstery foam works well)
Needle syringe
Electrode gel, such as ultrasonic gel
Alligator clip electrode

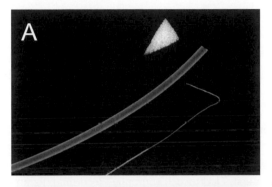

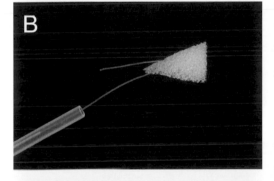

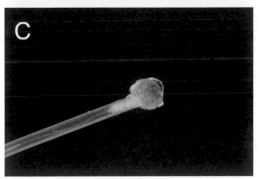

Fig. 12.2 (A–C) Construction of a TM electrode. (A) Components of a TM electrode, (B) assembly of a TM electrode, and (C) completed TM electrode, injected with gel. See text for further details.

5. Holding the electrode, carefully inject the foam sponge with electrode gel that has been placed in a syringe. The gel should fill the foam sponge completely and go slightly into the tubing (**Fig. 12.2C**).

6. Connect the other end of the exposed wire to the alligator electrode, twisting the exposed wire around the end of the clip.

Pearl

The tubing and wire must be very small and flexible, and the type of foam sponge used can make a big difference. If the tubing and wire are not small enough, or the foam sponge is not fine enough, the result could be uncomfortable to the patient.

Pearl

Custom TM electrodes are probably best made fresh prior to each session. It would be advisable to make more than one to prevent cross-contamination and for a backup.

◆ Getting Ready to Test

Equipment and patient preparation includes choosing an electrode type, setting up the stimulus and recording parameters, having an analysis plan, and having a well thought out clinical protocol with patient instructions. Having these preparations in place will improve the likelihood of a successful ECochG recording session.

Table 12.2 Click-Evoked ECochG Recording Parameters

Parameter	Suggested Setting
Low-frequency filter cutoff	5 to 10 Hz
High-frequency filter cutoff	1500 to 3000 Hz
Time window	10 msec (can use 5–7 msec)
Time delay	–1 ms (creates "zeroed out" artificial baseline)
Notch filter	Off
Artifact reject	On
Sensitivity	+/– 50 µV
Gain	50,000x (TM electrode); 75,000x (TIPtrode)
Sweeps	1000 to 2000
Transducer	Insert earphones
Stimulus	100 µs (0.1 msec) click
Rate	5.1–7.1/s
Polarity	Alternating
Level	85 to 95 dB nHL

Abbreviations: nHL, normal hearing level; TM, tympanic membrane.

Equipment setup should include labels for a baseline, SP, AP, and duration for a click ECochG. Set the protocol so that the computer calculates the SP/AP ratio, if possible. Labels for a tone-burst ECochG should include frequencies from 500 to 8000 Hz (including 1500 Hz), as well as a baseline, SP, and AP. The SP and the AP will be calculated from the baseline in amplitude (microvolts) in both the click and tone-burst ECochG. The duration is calculated as latency (in milliseconds) from the baseline to the point determined to be the end of the SP-AP complex.

Recording Parameters

The recording parameters for ECochG will differ depending on the desired information one wants to acquire. It will also differ depending on the type of stimulus used. **Tables 12.2** and **12.3** are typical recording parameters for click-evoked ECochGs, with **Table 12.3** listing additional modifications specific to tone burst-evoked ECochGs. The main differences in the recording parameters, other than stimulus types, are different time windows, gain settings, and stimulation rates. The time window is extended for tone bursts to follow the SP through the duration of the stimulus. Gain settings are higher for TIPtrodes because of their more distal placement in the ear canal compared with TM electrodes. Stimulation rates are higher for tone bursts because the SP

Table 12.3 Additional Modifications for Tone-Burst Electrocochleography Recording Parameters

Parameter	Suggested Setting
Time window	20 msec
Stimulus	Tone burst
Frequencies	1, 2, 4, 8 kHz 1.5 kHz may also be useful
Rise/fall	1–2 msec
Plateau	10–12 msec
Rate	33.1/s
Polarity	Alternating
Level	80–95 dB nHL

is the desired stimulus and not the AP. The SP thrives under higher rates, whereas the AP will diminish with increased rate. If one is interested in looking at click ECochG information in relation to the ABR, the time window should be set on a 10-msec window.

Other general recording considerations are The number of sweeps needed may vary depending on the clarity of the recording. Patient and electrical artifact, as well as placement of the TM electrode, can determine how easily the ECochG can be read and thus the number of sweeps needed. The type of electrode used may influence the number of sweeps needed, as the TM electrode will generally give a larger, more consistent tracing than other ET electrodes, requiring fewer sweeps on average.

A tone-burst ECochG can be an additional diagnostic tool for endolymphatic hydrops. Ferraro and Durrant (2006) recommended a 2-msec rise/fall and 10-msec plateau, and Gibson and Arenberg (1991) recommended a rise/fall of 1 msec and a plateau of 12 msec for tone-burst ECochG. The actual stimulus frequency can vary from 1000 to 8000 Hz. Gibson and Arenberg (1991) reported that 1000 Hz was the best diagnostic frequency for endolymphatic hydrops. After adding 750 and 1500 Hz to the protocol in our clinic, we found 1500 Hz to be a useful diagnostic frequency. The intensity of the tone may need to be varied from 80 to 95 dB nHL depending on the clarity of the response.

Electrode Montage

Several electrode montages are available for clinicians to choose from when placing the noninverting (+) and inverting (−) electrodes. Each montage will produce different waveform displays depending on how they are plugged into the electrode headbox. The headbox itself and its labeling convention may vary from manufacturer to manufacturer. For example, some older systems may have headboxes where the noninverting (+) electrode is plugged into the Cz jack. Although this may not be intuitive, this scenario demonstrates the significance of becoming familiar with your equipment. The

most common way of displaying the ECochG is using an AP-down configuration; that is, APs (as well as the SP) are oriented down (negative voltages) rather than up (positive voltages) like the ABR. **Figure 12.3** and **Table 12.4** describe the electrode connections necessary to produce an AP-down configuration with the AP in the negative voltage range. To achieve an AP-up configuration, all the clinician needs to do is manually swap the noninverting and inverting connections on the headbox or continue to use the AP-down montage and simply flip the waveform using the AEP software. The former technique will yield AP voltage values as positive, whereas the latter technique will simply reverse the voltage scale. The ground electrode is typically placed midline on the forehead.

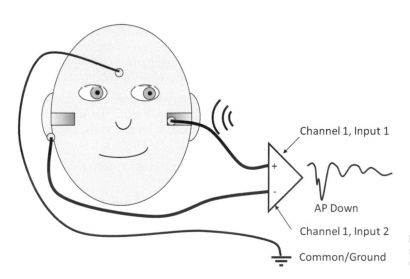

Channel 1, Input 1

AP Down

Channel 1, Input 2

Common/Ground

Fig. 12.3 Electrode placement for action potential (AP) down waveform.

Table 12.4 Electrode Montage for Electrocochleography AP–Down Configuration

Test electrode	Input 1	Noninverting (+)
Nontest electrode	Input 2	Inverting (–)
Ground electrode (Fpz)	Common/ground	Common/ground

When using a TM electrode, one ear is tested, with the desired electrode montage selected. After testing one ear, the TM electrode is removed, and a second TM electrode is then placed in the other ear to be tested. TM electrode should be placed in each ear at separate times, manually changing where the test ear and nontest ear are plugged into the electrode headbox. TIPtrodes may be placed in both ears prior to recording, with each serving as test and nontest ear electrodes for each ear of stimulation. Like the TM electrode, the test and nontest ear electrodes will need to be swapped on the headbox for each ear of stimulation. The Bio-logic Navigator Pro (Natus Medical Inc., Mundelein, IL) has a useful "electrode switching" feature that allows clinicians to connect the electrodes in a predetermined manner and specify in the software which ear is the test ear. This feature can be used with TIPtrodes but should not be selected when using a TM electrode.

Placement of the TM Electrode

Although the TM electrode is not considered invasive, the fact that an object is placed deep within the ear canal either on or next to the TM can cause some discomfort or a feeling of fullness. It is critical for the clinician to talk the patient through each step of the procedure to minimize anxiety and discomfort. The clinician should have all supplies ready to go and well within reach. Prior to inserting the TM electrode, an otoscopic examination is necessary to get a view of the ear canal shape and the location of the TM. If there is significant cerumen or debris, it should be removed prior to insertion of the TM electrode. If cerumen removal is not in the scope of practice of the clinician performing the ECochG, the appointment should be rescheduled until after the cerumen can be removed. If the TM appears abnormal or exhibits a perforation, it is not advisable to perform the ECochG test. The remaining steps are as follows:

- Place surface electrodes on the nontest ear lobe and the forehead. Plug in all electrodes (including the alligator clip electrode) to the electrode headbox. Bring up the impedance check window/screen.

- Prepare strips of surgical tape for securing the TM electrode, alligator clip, and transducer for the earphones.

- Instruct the patient. Example: "I will be placing this small, flexible tubing and sponge into the ear and easing it down the ear canal. The soft sponge will eventually rest on the eardrum. It should not hurt, although you may feel a little discomfort or pressure. Let me know when you have a feeling of pressure or your ear feels full. If you feel any pain, we will bring the electrode out and start again." It can be helpful to show the patient the electrode and how flexible it is. Most patients will have heard that they are not supposed to put anything "smaller than an elbow" in the ear and will be worried about the process.

- With one hand, straighten the ear canal in a manner similar to otoscopic examination. Holding the TM electrode between the thumb and forefinger of the other hand, gently insert the TM electrode. A very slight twisting motion sometimes assists in easing it safely down the ear canal. An occasional light tap with the thumb of the hand holding the ear can help ease the tubing in as well.

- The patient may feel some discomfort as the electrode is going around the second bend. Ask the patient to let you know of any pain or discomfort.

- Monitor the impedance reading while placing the TM electrode.

- When the electrode is on the eardrum, the patient will feel some pressure. If pain is felt, draw the electrode back and ease it in again. A slightly different angle can make a lot of difference in comfort.

- It is not uncommon to need to bring the electrode partially out and place it again. As the patient becomes acclimated to the procedure, he or she will often relax, and placement will be easier. Additional electrode gel (not electrode paste) may need to be added to the sponge foam tip if electrode reinsertion is required.

- The feeling of fullness is often an indication that the electrode is in the proper place.

- The impedance reading will likely be very high (>40 µV). We have seen reliable ECochG tracings in our clinic with very high impedance readings. A good impedance reading and a poor tracing can coexist, and vice versa. Some equipment will not allow an ultra-high impedance reading. If no reading can be obtained with the impedance check, try testing anyway, as it may be possible to get a tracing. Hall (2007) indicated that electrode impedance is not consistently correlated with ECochG AP amplitude. This is in agreement with the author's clinical experience.

- To prevent the TM electrode from moving, it is helpful to secure the tubing of the TM electrode to the ear with a piece of tape, taking care to not push the tubing farther into the ear canal.

- Gently and carefully place the insert earphone foam plug into the ear canal while continuing to hold the electrode with the free hand. The tan pediatric insert ear foam tip works well, as it allows room for the tubing and the insert earphone (**Fig. 12.4**). Secure the transducer to keep it from slipping.

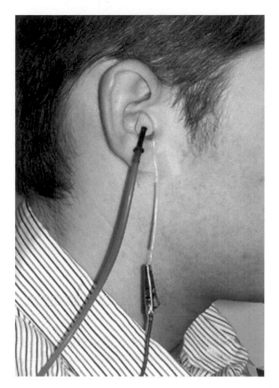

Fig. 12.4 Tympanic membrane (TM) electrode with insert earphone setup on a patient. Ideally, the insert earphone tip would be pushed in farther if space allows to accommodate both the TM electrode tubing and the insert earphone tip. Superficial placement of the insert earphone tip may result in decreased intensity at the level of the TM.

> **Pearl**
>
> Sometimes the ECochG waveform is either too large or too small. Adjusting the scale (not the gain) of the analysis window within the software may help.

> **Pearl**
>
> If the tracings are not good or are not large enough to get a reliable tracing, withdraw the electrode and reinsert it. It may take several attempts, but it will be worth the effort. Electrode placement, especially of the TM electrode, can make the difference between a good recording and a poor one. The experience and patience of the clinician, with good instructions to the patient, are key.

◆ The Patient's Role in Getting a Good Recording

Aside from getting a good TM electrode placement, the way that the patient is positioned is an important part of getting a good tracing. The patient should be in a reclining or supine position. If the patient is sitting up too much, there will likely be too much artifact rejection as a result of high myogenic (muscle) activity. ECochG testing is even more sensitive to this artifact than ABR testing. Relaxation of the neck, arms, and hands is important, as well as good support to the head. The patient's eyes should remain closed during the test procedure. Before starting the recording, instructions to the patient might be: "You are going to hear some loud clicking sounds. Close your eyes and keep them closed. Imagine the tension in your neck and arms flowing from your fingertips. You may take a nap if you like." If the tracings are not good after certainty that the patient is relaxed, the TM electrode should be reinserted. This will be time well spent in the long run.

◆ Interpretation of Test Results

With endoymphatic hydrops, an enlarged SP is the most common characteristic of the abnormal waveform of both the click- (**Fig. 12.1**) and tone burst-evoked ECochG (**Fig. 12.5**). There is no standard for the outside limits of the normal ECochG response for clicks or for tone bursts. An ET electrode will give a smaller response than will a TT electrode. In our clinic, we have used a 0.50 SP/AP ratio (the SP at 50% of the AP, measured from the same baseline) or better, as within the normal range, using the TM electrode (Henderson, Pultro, Montague, and Yarbrough, 1991). The measurement of the duration of the SP-AP complex may prove to be valuable in the diagnosis of endolymphatic hydrops. Ferraro (2010) described the use of an SP/AP area ratio as useful, although the software for this measurement is not commercially available as of this writing.

Tone-burst waveforms can give valuable diagnostic information with the appearance of an enlarged SP. In a tone-burst ECochG, the AP is seen at the onset of the response, whereas SP persists as long as the stimulus (Ferraro and Durrant, 2006). It has been suggested that measuring the amplitude of the SP from a baseline to the midpoint of the SP be considered (Ferraro and Durrant, 2006; Gibson and Arenberg, 1991). No standard has been established for the amplitude that would fall outside the normal range. In a normal ear, the tone-burst SP

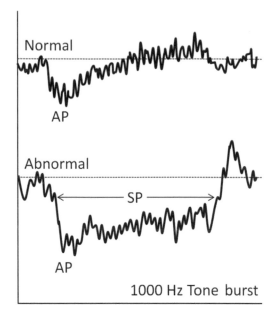

Fig. 12.5 Illustration of a normal versus abnormal tone-burst electrocochleography (ECochG) at 1000 Hz. Note the enlarged summating potential (SP) and lack of recovery to the baseline for the abnormal tone burst ECochG. Even though alternating polarity is used, the cochlear microphonic (CM) may not be completely canceled out. Thus, a small CM can appear to be "riding" on top of the waveform. This small CM appears to be more prominent with lower-frequency tone bursts. AP, action potential.

is very small, so there is little change from the baseline to the midpoint of the SP. In an abnormal ear, however, the SP may be enlarged and may not recover to the baseline by the midpoint latency (**Fig. 12.5**). It has been suggested that measuring the amplitude of the SP from a baseline to the midpoint of the SP be considered (Ferraro and Durrant, 2006; Gibson and Arenberg, 1991). No standard has been established for the amplitude that would fall outside the normal range. Although no measurement standards exist for tone-burst ECochG, an enlarged tone-burst SP may be evident with endolymphatic hydrops. Ferraro, Thedinger, Medianvilla, and Blackwell (1994) found that, although amplitudes were smaller on TM electrode recordings than on TT recordings, the response patterns were the same with patients suspected of having Meniere disease, with most patients tested displaying enlarged SP amplitudes to tone bursts and to clicks.

The strongest ECochG diagnostic finding for endolymphatic hydrops would be an enlarged SP for both clicks and tone bursts. However, it is possible to have a normal click ECochG and an enlarged SP for tone bursts or an abnormal click ECochG and normal tone-burst tracings. Either condition would be suggestive of endolymphatic hydrops. ECochG can be diagnostically useful in determining which ear is involved when a patient is complaining of vertigo.

Labeling ECochG Components

Labeling of the SP and the AP for clicks is the peak amplitude relative to the baseline. The duration between the baseline and the point at which the AP recovers (the "width" of the SP-AP complex) is the duration latency. With endolymphatic hydrops, the duration of the SP-AP complex may have a longer latency than in the ECochG tracing of a normal ear. The following are tips to consider when analyzing and labeling ECochG components:

- The relationship of the SP to the AP, or the SP/AP ratio, is measured in microvolts as amplitude. Both the SP and the AP are measured relative to the baseline.

- The SP will occur as a hump or smaller downward slope between the baseline and the AP. The AP will occur between 1 and 2 msec (if the computer program is set to take into account the insert earphone delay and subtracts it out) and will appear as a large downward slope. If the computer does not subtract the insert earphone delay of sound (~0.8 msec later than when testing with standard earphones), the AP should correspond to the known latency of wave I of the ABR on that computer (2–3 msec).

- A slow rate (5.1 to 7.1 clicks/s) should give the best tracing possible. A slight increase in rate may help determine the SP. With a rapid rate, the AP will get smaller and less distinct, and the SP sometimes will become more defined. This may help determine the

location of the SP. The goal is to have the largest AP possible and still be able to see an SP.

- The duration or the latency from the baseline to the end of the SP-AP complex can also be labeled. This duration would be the time in milliseconds from the beginning to the end of the SP-AP complex (Hall, 2007). In our clinic, we measure duration from the baseline to the point where the AP recovers back to the baseline.

- Calculate the SP/AP ratio by dividing the SP by the AP amplitude readings in microvolts. Most AEP software packages will calculate this if set up properly.

- Although there is no true standard, an SP/AP ratio of 0.50 or greater (an SP that is ≤ 50% of the AP) has been used in our clinic and shown to be within the normal range for ET electrodes. Gibson and Arenberg (1991) suggested a 0.33 (33%) ratio for TT electrodes. An SP/AP ratio greater than 0.50 (SP > 50% of the AP) may be considered outside the normal range.

- There are several ways described in the literature to measure the SP and the AP. Ruth and colleagues (1988) described the method of determining a prestimulus baseline and then measuring the SP and AP at the most negative deflection of each component. This is the method used in our clinic. Another method is to measure the SP and AP from separate single points (Ferraro and Durrant, 2006).

- Test–retest reliability of the TM electrode was found to be very high when testing both normal patients and patients with a complaint of symptoms of endolymphatic hydrops. When the TM electrode was removed and then reinserted, the results were within 0.5% of the original tracing (Henderson et al, 1991).

Labeling for a tone-burst ECochG should include the baseline and SP midpoint, as well as the AP. These points may not always need to be marked, depending on the results obtained. In a normal tone-burst ECochG recording, it may not be relevant to measure the SP or the AP. These components may not even be visible. If the SP is enlarged, it would be useful to measure the amplitude from the baseline to the midpoint of the SP. There is no standard for the degree of enlargement of the SP that is outside the normal range using an ET electrode.

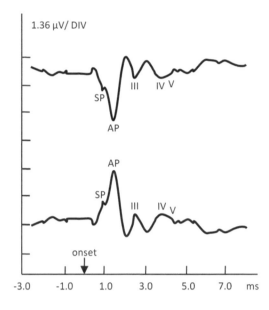

Fig. 12.6 Illustration of an auditory brainstem response (ABR) waveform using an extratympanic electrode for electrocochleography. Note the enhanced wave I and diminished waves III and V. The inverted tracing shows a more typical ABR configuration.

◆ Enhancement of Wave I of the Auditory Brainstem Response

One use of the click ECochG is the enhancement of wave I of the ABR. At times it may be difficult to clearly identify the wave. Because the AP of the ECochG tracing is the same as the wave I of an ABR tracing, a test using an ECochG electrode may be useful in helping to identify the wave. It would be wise to remember that if the ECochG testing is done with the AP down, the waveform will need to be inverted to see the ABR in the more common, wave-up mode. If the major objective is to enhance the wave I for an ABR, it may be useful to use a TIPtrode rather than a TM or TT electrode. The AP of the ECochG (wave I of the ABR) will be larger, yet the other waveforms of the ABR may still be fairly easy to read with a TIPtrode. With the very robust ECochG measurements obtained with a TT and TM electrode, the later ABR waveforms are often diminished (**Fig. 12.6**).

Troubleshooting

ECochG testing can be challenging. Electrical interference can be unpredictable and inconsistent in a busy clinic. It may be a matter of moving cords around, turning off other equipment and lamps, unplugging everything in the room, and more. I have been known to get the patient settled in a dental chair, reclining at just

the right height, unplug the chair, unplug everything in the room except the testing equipment, and even go into the next clinic room to unplug equipment and lamps. Sometimes it may be as simple as moving to a different area of the room and plugging into a different electrical outlet. Electrical interference from outside the equipment, "noise" from patient tension and movement, and electrode setup and placement all can interfere with testing. **Table 12.5** is a list of steps that may help solve the problem of either electrical interference or a very poor tracing.

◆ Intraoperative Monitoring

ECochG has been useful in preoperative and intraoperative evaluation of patients with endolymphatic hydrops. TT ECochG is used for intraoperative monitoring and provides robust responses. The ECochG can provide rapid information concerning cochlear status, especially disruption of the blood

Table 12.5 Troubleshooting Tips

1. Check all electrodes to be sure that they are correctly positioned.
2. Check electrode impedance. Remember that the TM electrode impedance will be high. If the impedance has significantly changed from the original reading, remove and reinsert the TM electrode.
3. Move the electrode wires so that they are not touching each other, the transducer, or the transducer cord.
4. Retape or reposition the TM electrode so that it is hanging farther from any of the other electrodes or the transducer.
5. Move the transducer box away from the patient's test ear.
6. Move the patient farther from the equipment.
7. Turn off all other equipment in the room, or in some cases, unplug all the equipment not being used.
8. Unplug any nearby lamps. Metal floor lamps used in examining rooms can be especially suspect, even when just plugged into the wall and not turned on.
9. Reinsert the TM electrode, especially if there is no appearance of the action potential (AP) of the ECochG.
10. Check the parameters.
11. Change the stimulus rate. Slower rates usually produce a better overall tracing and a larger AP. Faster rates can help bring out the summating potential (SP). If the overall tracing is good and there is a good AP but no apparent or readable SP, increasing the rate may help bring out the SP. The AP amplitude will decrease as the rate is increased, so increase the rate only enough to bring out the SP.
12. Change the stimulus intensity. Sometimes a louder intensity will give a better result.
13. Decrease the low pass filter cut-off (do not go below 1500 Hz).
14. Test in a sound booth, if a recliner is available.
15. If using a TIPtrode or another extratympanic (ET) electrode, replace it with a TM electrode. A TT placement by a physician can be used in a medical setting if no other electrode gives a readable tracing.

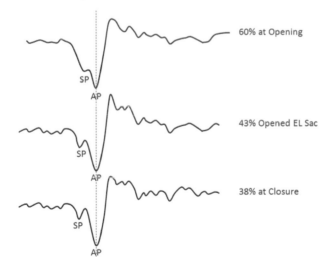

60% at Opening

43% Opened EL Sac

38% at Closure

Fig. 12.7 Intraoperative tracings during endolymphatic shunt removal. Tracings shown are of baseline, opening of the endolymphatic sac, and at closing.

supply (Ruth et al, 1988). This has made ECochG useful in the operating room (OR). Interested readers are referred to Chapter 18 for more information about the ECochG in the OR. The following is a case study of a 24-year-old woman diagnosed with Meniere disease (**Fig. 12.7**). The patient had a history of hearing loss, vertigo, tinnitus, and ear fullness. Endolymphatic shunt surgery had been performed. Her symptoms returned after surgery, and the decision was made to remove the shunt. Intraoperative monitoring was done during endolymphatic shunt removal (**Fig. 12.7**). Clear, reliable results were apparent after 100 to 250 sweeps using a TT electrode and a click stimulus. A baseline recording showed robust, repeatable results. Changes were noted in the SP/AP ratio at baseline of 0.60 at opening to 0.38 at closure. An improved ECochG was seen when the endolymphatic sac was opened (Henderson, Pultro, and Waner, 1992).

◆ Pediatric Applications

Hall (2007) suggested that ECochG measurement was essential for the diagnosis of ANSD and that the classic finding is a clear and often very robust cochlear microphonic (CM) for single-polarity stimuli, with no AP and no ABR. Ferraro (2010) cautioned that strict grounding and shielding must be

applied to identify the CM from stimulus artifact. More information on ANSD is available in Chapter 16.

◆ Summary

ECochG can be a useful tool in diagnosing and monitoring Meniere disease, the enhancement of wave I of the ABR, and intraoperative monitoring. It may also be useful in helping to determine the diagnosis of ANSD. It can be challenging to get a robust, reliable test result with an ET electrode. Clinical application for the audiologist usually involves using an ET electrode that can be placed in a nonmedical setting.

References

Ferraro, J. A. (1997). *Laboratory exercises in auditory evoked potentials.* San Diego: Singular Publishing Group.

Ferraro, J. A. (2000). Electrocochleography. In R. J. Roesser, M. Valente, & H. Hosford-Dunn (Eds.), *Audiology diagnosis* (2nd ed., pp. 400–425). New York: Thieme.

Ferraro, J. A. (2010). Electrocochleography: A review of recording approaches, clinical applications, and new findings in adults and children. *Journal of the American Academy of Audiology, 21*(3), 145–152. PubMed

Ferraro, J. A., & Durrant, J. D. (2006). Electrocochleography in the evaluation of patients with Ménière's disease/endolymphatic hydrops. *Journal of the American Academy of Audiology, 17*(1), 45–68. PubMed

Ferraro, J. A., Murphy, G. B., & Ruth, R. A. (1986, August). A comparative study of primary electrodes used in extratympanic electrocochleography. *Seminars in Hearing, 7,* 279–286.

Ferraro, J. A., Thedinger, B., Medianvilla, S. J., & Blackwell, W. (1994). Human summating potential to tonebursts: observations on TM verses promontory recordings in the same patient. *Journal of the American Academy of Audiology, 5*(1), 217–224.

Gibson, W. P. R., & Arenberg, I. R. (1991, February). *A manual of transtympanic electrocochleography.* Paper presented at the Fourth International ECoG Seminar and Workshop, Denver, CO.

Hall, J. W., III. (2007). *New handbook of auditory evoked responses.* Boston: Pearson.

Henderson, C., Pultro, J., Montague, D., & Yarbrough, S. (1991, October). *Electrocochleography, test/retest reliability of re-insertion of the TM electrode.* Paper presented to Arkansas Speech and Hearing Association meeting, Hot Springs, AR.

Henderson, C., Pultro, J., & Waner, M. (1992, April). *Electrocochleography intraoperative monitoring, a case study.* Paper presented at the annual convention of the American Academy of Audiology, Nashville, TN.

Ruth, R. A. (1989, April). *Trends in clinical electrocochleography.* Paper presented at the annual meeting of the American Academy of Audiology, Kiawah Island, SC.

Ruth, R. A., & Lambert, P. R. (1989). Comparison of tympanic membrane to promontory electrode recordings of electrocochleographic responses in patients with Ménière's disease. *Otolaryngology—Head and Neck Surgery, 100*(6), 546–552. PubMed

Ruth, R. A., Lambert, P. R., & Ferraro, J. A. (1988). Electrocochleography: Methods and clinical applications. *American Journal of Otology, 9*(Suppl), 1–11. PubMed

Stypulkowski, P. H., & Staller, S. J. (1987). Clinical evaluation of a new ECoG recording electrode. *Ear and Hearing, 8*(5), 304–310. PubMed

Chapter 13

Automated Hearing Screening

Nannette Nicholson and Patti F. Martin

The success of universal newborn hearing screening (UNHS) can be attributed in part to advances in hearing technology and the automation of screening tests. Automated hearing screening equipment helps meet the public health criteria for screening (**Table 13.1**). Originally proposed by Wilson and Jungner (1968) and published by the World Health Organization (WHO), these criteria have been modified over time to incorporate aspects of evidence-based practice. Currently, two types of technology are used for newborn hearing screening (NHS): otoacoustic emissions (OAEs) and automated auditory brainstem response (AABR).

> ### Pearl
>
> Screening tests can be conducted in the clinic with diagnostic equipment using protocol modifications; however, many NHS programs use automated digital equipment because of its simplicity. The need for limited training contributes to its cost-effectiveness.

Automated hearing screening tools typically have predetermined algorithms governing stimulus characteristics or conditions, data acquisition and analysis features, and decision rules regarding characteristics of the response. The recorded response elicited from the infant is automatically compared with the default criteria or decision rules programmed into the system. If the response meets the preset criteria or decision rules, the response is considered a "pass." If the response does not meet the criteria, it is considered a "refer" or "fail." For example, some manufacturers use a template-matching decision rule. If the response matches the template, it is considered a pass (**Fig. 13.1**). If the response fails to match the template, it is considered a fail. Regardless of the type of technology used, the result of the hearing screening simply indicates one of the following options: (1) the baby passed the screening and does not need follow-up, (2) the baby did not pass the screening or failed the screening and will be referred for additional testing, or (3) the baby will be monitored over time (in cases where high-risk factors have been identified). The purpose of screening, by definition, is to separate individuals who do not have a disease or problem from those who cannot be readily excluded.

> ### Pitfall
>
> Calibration of acoustic transient stimuli remains an issue and is likely to cause slightly different pass/fail rates across auditory brainstem response (ABR) or OAE screening techniques and across manufacturers.

Table 13.1 Criteria for Public Health Screening Programs

Condition of interest	• Important condition • Untreated natural history understood • Recognizable latent or early stage
Treatment options	• Acceptable treatment • Diagnostic and treatment facilities available • Early treatment should lead to better outcomes than late treatment
Test selection and choice	• Test should be sensitive, specific, reproducible, validated, and safe • Distribution and cutoff points for the test should be known • Acceptable to patients • Inexpensive
Screening program components	• Target population agreed • Continuous screening (interval agreed) • Adequate resources • Supporting randomized controlled trials in favor of screening

Source: Adapted from Wilson and Jungner (1968).

The predetermined aspects of automated equipment vary by test procedure and are chosen by the manufacturer based on evidence in the research literature and independent in-house research. Engineers, biologists, and physicists, as well as researchers from other professions, have contributed to this body of literature over many years. Manufacturers typically have research and development departments responsible for sifting through the research evidence and making decisions about the aspects of hardware and software design that impact clinical results. Each generation of equipment incorporates new data as well as new technology. It is important to know how the equipment works and what criteria are used to determine a pass or fail so that educated decisions can be made about which equipment might work best in the NHS program.

There are four main sections in this chapter. The first section is a general overview of NHS program components and logistics. The second provides information about automated hearing screening technology: OAEs and AABR. The third addresses protocol considerations for well-baby nurseries and neonatal intensive care units (NICUs). The last section in this chapter provides case studies for problem-based

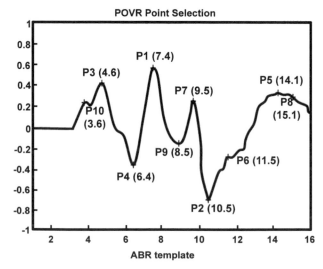

Fig. 13.1 An example of a template-matching paradigm using a statistical algorithm called point-optimized variance ratio (POVR). POVR is similar to Fsp, but uses a known, expected waveform derived from babies with normal hearing. A number of points are selected on the target waveform to which the incoming screening auditory brainstem response is compared. (Reprinted from Sininger, Y., Hyde, M., & Don, M. (2001). U.S. Patent No. 6,196,977 B. Washington, DC: U.S. Patent and Trademark Office., with permission of Yvonne Sininger, PhD.)

learning exercises. OAE and AABR protocols are provided in the appendices. A large body of research regarding newborn hearing screening has accumulated over the past 20 years and is summarized in guidelines, position statements, and other documents. Throughout this chapter, the reader is referred to these seminal publications.

◆ Newborn Hearing Screening Program Components and Logistics

The components of the Early Hearing Detection and Intervention (EHDI) program are defined by the National Center for Hearing Assessment and Management (NCHAM, 2010a) in partnership with the Maternal and Child Health Bureau (MCHB) and the Centers for Disease Control and Prevention (CDC) (**Table 13.2**). Despite the success of the EHDI initiative, continued challenges include competency-based screener training and expertise, identification of and access to competent pediatric diagnostic centers, education of pediatricians and family practice physicians, full disclosure by manufacturers regarding propriety algorithms, and automated hearing screening calibration standards (see Chapter 22).

Pearl

The components of an NHS program work together as a system, with each component critical to the success of EHDI efforts. NHS components are consistent across all applications and are independent of site, facility, or choice of equipment.

Spivak (1998) provided an in-depth presentation of the theoretical and practical aspects of setting up a newborn hearing screening program. The 2007 Position Statement developed by the Joint Committee on Infant Hearing (JCIH) is the most comprehensive current clinical practice guideline and is regarded as the standard of

Table 13.2 Early Hearing Detection and Intervention Components

- Newborn hearing screening
- Early childhood hearing screening
- Diagnostic audiology
- Early intervention
- Family support
- Medical home
- Data management
- Financing and reimbursements
- Program evaluation

Source : National Center for Hearing Assessment and Management (NCHAM, 2010a).

care. The EHDI process is viewed in three distinct phases: (1) hearing screening before 1 month, (2) pediatric diagnostic evaluation before 3 months, and (3) intervention before 6 months. This is known as the 1-3-6 plan. The national EHDI goals developed by the CDC and state representatives illustrate the comprehensive nature of the EHDI initiative, setting benchmarks for goal performance (CDC, 2001, 2003).

The American Academy of Pediatrics (AAP) devoted an entire supplementary issue of their journal to "Pursuing Excellence in EHDI Initiatives" (Koop, 2010). In this issue, Shulman and colleagues (Shulman, Besculides, Saltzman, Ireys, White, and Forsman, 2010) identified five key areas for future program improvements: improving data systems to support surveillance and follow-up activities, ensuring that all infants have a medical home, building capacity beyond identified providers, developing family support services, and promoting the importance of early detection.

Most NHS programs are designed for hospital-based well-baby nurseries or screening programs conducted in NICUs. Program logistics to consider include the target population, personnel, communication, referrals, and data management (**Table 13.3**). Although the hearing screening team is multidisciplinary in nature, an audiologist should be involved in each component of the hearing screening program and can give guidance in the development of a business plan, providing administrators with the information needed to support and advocate for the program.

Table 13.3 Newborn Hearing Screening Program Logistics

Target Population
• Personnel
○ Staff
○ Training
• Communication
○ Parents
○ Physicians
• Referrals
• Data management

Source: National Center for Hearing Assessment and Management (NCHAM, 2010b).

This involvement should occur at the hospital level if possible or minimally in a consultative role at the state program level.

> **Pearl**
>
> The target population is an important consideration. JCIH (2007) recommends different screening protocols for NICU and well-baby nurseries.

It is important to have clearly defined roles and responsibilities. Ideally, a physician would be designated to oversee the medical aspects of the screening program in hospitals and/or agencies at the local level. Staff selection influences selection of equipment, rescreening procedures, and other processes within the program. Regardless of who conducts the hearing screening, it is critical that all service providers complete training in hearing screening procedures, communicating results to the parents, referrals for rescreening, and reporting requirements to the primary care physician (PCP) and state EHDI program. Training is one of the most important roles of the team audiologist.

NCHAM's competency-based curriculum addresses topics such as preparing to screen, screening with OAEs, screening with AABR, communicating with parents and medical providers, completing the screening process, screening babies with risk indicators, and outpatient screening/rescreening. Parents should be informed in a culturally sensitive and understandable manner that their infant did not pass the hearing screening and urged to seek prompt follow-up (JCIH, 2007). A rescreening appointment should be scheduled before discharge, which increases the chances for successful follow-up. If the hospital does not provide rescreening, an appointment with an appropriate professional referral source at the community or state level should be made. In addition to recording the results in the hospital chart, results should be communicated directly to the PCP when screening results are a refer (JCIH, 2007). The NCHAM Newborn Hearing Screening Training Curriculum (NCHAM, 2010b) provides samples of how information could be communicated to parents and physicians.

> **Pearl**
>
> The manner in which screening results are communicated to the parents is very important because it may influence the parents' choice regarding follow-up.

Accurate and timely reports to the state EHDI program help facilitate follow-up. When the child returns for a follow-up screening, these results must be promptly reported to the PCP and the state EHDI office. If the state EHDI program does not receive follow-up information, the case is eventually listed as loss to follow-up/loss to documentation (LTF/D). The national average for loss to follow-up is ~50% but varies widely by state (American Speech-Language-Hearing Association, 2008). State and national efforts have focused on evaluating system issues as well as potential family factors contributing to LTF/D to bridge the gap between screening and follow-up.

> **Pitfall**
>
> One of the biggest EHDI challenges is that of LTF/D. Barriers to successful follow-up include inadequate skill level or expertise of screeners, lack of service-system capacity, lack of provider knowledge, challenges to families in obtaining services, and information gaps (Shulman et al, 2010).

Each NHS program manager/administrator should be familiar with local and state resources. Data provide information related to patient care, personnel needs (e.g., staff, training, and responsibilities), and program logistics (e.g., equipment, procedures, protocols, communication, referrals, and community resources). It is critical for data-driven decision making. Program evaluation includes a comparison of hospital screening program results to state reports and aggregate state data to national EHDI goal benchmarks.

◆ Newborn Hearing Screening Equipment

Technological advances have led manufacturers to develop equipment dedicated to NHS applications. Current hearing screening choices include AABR and OAEs. Research evidence supporting the use of these instruments for NHS applications has been steadily accumulating since the late 1980s. Today these procedures are generally accepted as the standard of care because of the wealth of research studies demonstrating their overall test efficiency (i.e., reliability, validity, sensitivity, and specificity) and cost-effectiveness (**Table 13.4**); however, several factors must be taken into consideration when making choices about the purchase of new equipment. These include test performance, type of technology, digital signal processing (DSP) strategies used to determine pass/refer criteria, and equipment features. Readers are referred to the EHDI e-book (Appendix A) for a myriad of questions that one might consider when choosing equipment (NCHAM, 2010c).

Test Performance

Clinical decision analysis is nothing more than a formal method of decision making, a task done automatically dozens of times a day without giving it much thought. For this process, information is gathered, options are considered, the potential consequences are evaluated, and the decision is made. Outcomes are monitored to determine progress. Numerous variables such as time, reimbursement, inherent risks (Gorga and Neely, 2003), and test results affect NHS program costs. The goal is to choose an automated technology that is efficient (i.e., has diagnostic accuracy) as well as cost-effective.

Test efficiency is a measure of diagnostic accuracy, or the ability to correctly classify individuals according to their true condition (Zweig and Campbell, 1993). For example, test selection is focused on choosing one that does a good job of classifying individuals who may have a hearing loss or who need monitoring into a refer category and those who do not have a hearing loss into a pass category. Descriptive statistical measures are used to help quantify test performance.

Table 13.4 Definitions of Terms Used to Describe Test Performance

Test efficiency	Overall diagnostic accuracy of a screening test
Reliability	Extent to which the test or procedure yields the same results during independent repeated trials
Validity	Degree to which a test procedure accurately measures what it was designed to measure
Sensitivity	Ability of a test to accurately identify those individuals who have a hearing loss
Specificity	Ability of a test to accurately identify those individuals who do not have a hearing loss
Cost-effectiveness	Economical in terms of the impact of services and programs, their costs, and the consequences of choosing one option over another

> **Pearl**
>
> Although there is no screening test that is 100% accurate, a technology must be chosen that does a good job of correctly separating individuals in a population into one of two categories: individuals for whom there is no concern and individuals requiring follow-up.

A test with high sensitivity has few false negatives. A false negative is a case in which an individual with a hearing loss is classified as normal, or "pass" (type I error). Conversely, a test with high specificity has few false positives. False positives refer to those individuals who are identified as having hearing loss for further testing when in fact they do not (type II error). The consequences of this error (type II) are not as severe as the consequences of misclassifying a patient with hearing loss and not recommending future follow-up (type I). When a type II error is made, a child is referred for a rescreen and/or follow-up, and there is another opportunity to find the truth. The goal is to choose the test with the highest sensitivity and reasonable specificity.

> **Pitfall**
>
> A false positive is a case in which an individual with normal hearing is classified as potential hearing loss, or refer (type II error). Inordinate numbers of false positives add a burden of increased expense to the cost of the screening program.

Technology Options

Diagnostic ABR and OAE are not tests of hearing sensitivity. Behavioral assessment is the only true measure of hearing sensitivity; however, because newborn infants are unable to indicate the softest level that can be heard because of the lack of cognitive and motor development, another means of assessment must be used. ABR and OAE are tools that assess the physiologic function and integrity of the auditory system and are used as indicators of hearing sensitivity. They rely on the observation of an expected response pattern occurring in reaction to various stimuli presented at varying intensities. ABR assesses the integrity of the auditory system from the external auditory canal to the level of the inferior colliculus. The presence of these objective electrophysiologic responses indicates synchronous neural activity and may be used to estimate hearing thresholds; a normal pattern indicates integrity of the sensory and neural systems. For OAEs, the electrophysiologic response is an indication of outer hair cell function; a normal response pattern at specific suprathreshold levels is characteristic of normal sensory function. Diagnostic assessment relies on the decision-making skills of the clinician in the interpretation of the response pattern.

With automated techniques, the responsibility of clinical decision making by screening personnel is alleviated and assigned to the intelligent DSP algorithms developed based on a collection of knowledge and evidence about the behavior and performance of the auditory system. Algorithms coupled with statistical theory can be used to separate infants who have normal hearing from those who may be in need of additional testing.

Automated Auditory Evoked Response

Today, diagnostic ABR assessment is recognized as the gold standard for the diagnosis of hearing loss in infants. The idea of using AABR for NHS was proposed in 1979 by Schulman-Galambos and Galambos (1979). By the late 1980s, researchers had focused their efforts on the evaluation of AABR instruments for NHS purposes. Since that time, numerous studies have demonstrated the efficacy of using AABR for NHS. More details about the technical aspects of AABR screening systems can be found in Sininger, Hyde, and Don (2001).

Otoacoustic Emissions

Two types of otoacoustic emissions are used clinically: transient evoked otoacoustic emissions (TEOAEs) and distortion-product otoacoustic emissions (DPOAEs). These are named for the type of stimulus used to elicit the response from the auditory system. There are numerous descriptions of these technologies and their application to NHS. Kemp (2003) provided an account of the discovery and development of OAE technology. The first TEOAE equipment became commercially available in 1988. Commercial DPOAE equipment was introduced in 1992. Since that time, numerous research endeavors have focused on the efficacy of OAE screening in well-baby and NICU nurseries, as well as outpatient clinics.

OAEs are low-level signals caused by the motion of the tympanic membrane in response to vibrations from deep within the cochlea. Healthy ears produce this motion when an acoustic stimulus is presented to the ear, whereas unhealthy cochleas do not. Signals are recorded from the ear canal via a miniature microphone following the delivery of stimulus. Both the speaker and the microphone are secured in a small probe assembly that is positioned in the ear canal. The middle ear has to be working efficiently to allow the vibration from the cochlea to be transmitted to the tympanic membrane. The presence of fluid in the middle ear prevents recording of the response if present. Given a healthy middle ear, the most important aspect of recording an OAE is the probe fitting. Because OAEs are so dependent on middle ear status, some NHS programs find the use of high-frequency tympanometry (HFT) a critical addition to their protocol.

> **Pearl**
>
> A good-fitting probe ensures closure of the ear canal, excluding unwanted external sounds and increasing the sound pressure in the ear canal.

Digital Signal Processing Strategies

Statistical analysis is often used to differentiate between random and meaningful events. In NHS, statistics can be used to help make clinical decisions. Several statistical techniques have been employed to develop DSP algorithms to automatically detect the presence or absence of a response at a specified intensity. Some of the techniques used to predict this dichotomous choice are the use of cross-correlation, binomial statistics, signal-to-noise and spectral analysis, and template matching. In all cases, the goal is to automate the process in such a way that the solution to the algorithm is accurately predicted as either a pass or refer. Analysis techniques vary by manufacturers even though the goal is the same. Many dedicated NHS devices use a combination of statistical approaches. Contact the manufacturer for more information about specific equipment.

Cross-Correlation

Cross-correlation compares two (or more) sets of data stored in separate buffers with each other and attempts to identify the presence or absence of a replicated response, which is assumed to be the ABR or OAE, depending on the technology employed. Care must be used when employing this strategy in isolation, as this technique cannot differentiate between a response and noise. This leads to an increased probability of a false positive or false negative and results in reduced sensitivity and specificity.

Binomial Distribution

The term *binomial distribution* applies to events that have two possible outcomes. Some algorithms are weighted to make the assumption that the results will be a refer until enough responses have been acquired and averaged to conclude with a very high probability level (99%) that the baby has typical auditory neural function (ABR) or hair cell function (OAEs). Because the conditions of a refer can be precisely controlled, the sensitivity of this algorithm can be set a priori.

Signal-to-Noise and Spectral Analysis

Signal-to-noise analysis involves an examination of the amount of noise remaining in the response after averaging or accumulating a given number of samples, with a comparison to the averaged response. For ABR, the random electroencephalogram (EEG) activity is assumed to average to zero. In the case of OAEs, the residual response following cross-correlation is considered noise. There are several variations on this technique depending on the technology; however, as with the cross-correlation method, differentiation between the response and noise is mathematical. Spectral analysis looks at the response in the frequency domain.

Template Matching

Template matching evaluates the latency and amplitude of the response in the time domain. Expectations regarding frequency and latency characteristics are derived from empirical data. Age is a critical input variable for instruments relying on this technique because frequency, amplitude, and latency characteristics are widely variable by age. Responses matching the expected pattern are considered a pass. Normative data are based on expected waveforms or responses of thousands of neonates. An example of an AABR template-matching paradigm is provided in **Fig. 13.1**.

It is important to know and understand what is occurring inside the equipment being used. Although the equipment is automated, the audiologist is ultimately responsible for choosing or making recommendations about the technology and equipment that best meet the needs of an individual facility in a precise geographic location serving a specific population. Some equipment offers flexibility so that the audiologist can change the pass/fail criteria depending on choices regarding test sensitivity and specificity (i.e., false-positive and false-negative rates).

Special Consideration

For most dedicated screening equipment, clinicians (or technicians) are no longer viewing waveforms or responses but relying on DSP decision rules built into the equipment software.

◆ Newborn Hearing Screening Protocols

The purpose of NHS is to identify infants with permanent congenital, conductive, sensory, and neural (auditory neuropathy spectrum disorder, ANSD) hearing loss. JCIH (2007) stated that hearing screening should identify infants with specifically defined hearing loss on the basis of investigations of long-term developmental consequences of hearing loss, currently available physiologic screening

techniques, and availability of effective intervention in concert with established public health screening principles (**Table 13.1**). Separate hearing screening protocols are recommended for well-baby nurseries and NICUs (JCIH, 2007). Choices for well-baby nurseries include OAE and AABR. Choices for NICU settings are AABR or both AABR and OAE. The protocol for outpatient rescreening will vary in some aspects from newborn screening protocols.

Hearing screening protocols include information about staff responsible for conducting the test, required competency training, what equipment will be used, stimulus parameters for the test signal, decision criteria to rule the response as pass or refer, number of times the test can be repeated before the patient is discharged, parental consent if needed, how the results will be communicated to the parents and physician, state reporting requirements, process for rescreening, appointments for referrals, follow-up, and data management (**Table 13.3**). The screening form should have a place to indicate high-risk factors associated with permanent congenital, delayed onset, or progressive hearing loss in childhood (**Table 13.5**), demographic data for infant and parents, emergency contact information, screening and rescreening test results, recommendations, and follow-up appointment.

In some well-baby nursery screening programs, a two-stage sequential or parallel approach may be taken in which the infant is first screened with OAEs, and if the baby fails, an AABR is conducted. In a two-stage sequential approach, the second test (AABR) is completed only if the baby does not pass the first test (OAE). In many NICUs, a two-stage parallel approach is used. Both tests are given, and the baby must pass both, or the child will be referred for outpatient rescreening or for pediatric diagnostic testing. The addition of HFT to the screening protocol may help in determining the next steps if the baby does not pass.

A screening test is completed one time. If the baby refers, the protocol typically suggests that the screener troubleshoot by cleaning the probe tip, repositioning the earphone or electrodes, and so on. The screening test may be repeated, or another screener may repeat the screening, but this is not considered a rescreen. If the test still results in a refer, the baby should be rescreened after several hours by another

Table 13.5 High-Risk Indicators Associated with Permanent Congenital, Delayed Onset, or Progressive Hearing Loss in Childhood

1	Caregiver concern regarding hearing, speech, language, or developmental delay
2	Family history of permanent childhood hearing loss
3	Neonatal intensive care of more than 5 days for any of the following, regardless of length of stay: ECMO, assisted ventilation, exposure to ototoxic medications (gentamycin and tobramycin) or loop diuretics (furosemide/Lasix), and hyperbilirubinemia that requires exchange transfusion
4	In utero infections, such as CMV, herpes, rubella, syphilis, and toxoplasmosis
5	Craniofacial anomalies, including those that involve the pinna, ear canal, ear tags, ear pits, and temporal bone anomalies
6	Physical findings, such as white forelock, that are associated with a syndrome known to include a sensorineural or permanent conductive hearing loss
7	Syndromes associated with hearing loss or progressive or late-onset hearing loss, such as neurofibromatosis, osteopetrosis, and Usher syndrome; other frequently identified syndromes include Waardenburg, Alport, Pendred, and Jervell and Lange-Nielson
8	Neurodegenerative disorders, such as Hunter syndrome, or sensory motor neuropathies, such as Friedreich ataxia and Charcot-Marie syndrome
9	Culture-positive postnatal infections associated with sensorineural hearing loss, including confirmed bacterial and viral (especially herpes viruses and varicella) meningitis
10	Head trauma, especially basal skull/temporal bone fracture, that requires hospitalization
11	Chemotherapy

Abbreviations: CMV, cytomegalovirus; ECMO, extracorporeal membrane oxygenation.

Source: Joint Committee on Infant Hearing. (2007).

screener. If this test results in a refer, the hospital or screening center may make one of two recommendations: return to the hospital or local outpatient center for rescreening or participate in a rescreening/diagnostic evaluation at a pediatric diagnostic center. A follow-up appointment should be scheduled for the family at this time.

> **Pitfall**
>
> Repeated excessive screening increases the likelihood of inadvertently calling a hearing screen a pass, when in fact the infant has a hearing loss (type I error).

Well-Baby Nurseries

The prevalence for hearing loss in the well-baby population is ~3 per 1000. The JCIH guidelines (2007) endorse either OAE or AABR screening for well-baby nurseries. In many well-baby programs, an OAE is completed as the initial screening measure and repeated prior to discharge if necessary. When OAEs are used as the screening tool, conductive and sensory hearing loss of 25 or 40 dB or greater will be identified depending on the stimulus intensity, DSP algorithm, and decision rules. If the baby fails the initial screening and the rescreening, the infant should either participate in an outpatient screening at the hospital or at a general outpatient clinic within 2 weeks or be referred to a pediatric diagnostic center for follow-up (see Appendix B for sample OAE protocol). Other well-baby nurseries employ AABR technology as the screening procedure. AABR technology identifies conductive and sensory hearing loss of 30 to 40 dB or greater, as well as neural pathologies. If a baby fails the initial AABR and rescreening prior to discharge, the infant should be referred to a pediatric diagnostic center (see Appendix C for sample AABR protocol). Several research studies suggest that two-step protocols decrease the false-positive rate at discharge—thus, decreasing the need for outpatient follow-up. In a two-step sequential process, infants who do not pass the OAE screening but pass an AABR prior to discharge are considered a pass. In cases where AABR is the initial procedure, and the baby fails (i.e., NICU), the baby should not be rescreened with an OAE and considered a pass, as the child is at risk for ANSD.

Neonatal Intensive Care Units

Infants in the NICU have ~10 times the risk of hearing impairment because of the fragility of their health condition. The prevalence of hearing loss in the NICU population is ~3 per 100. NICU infants are at greater risk as a result of immature development for premature infants, the presence of conditions (e.g., hyperbilirubinemia) or disease (e.g., cytomegalovirus), and treatment effects (e.g., ototoxic medication, ventilation, extracorporeal membrane oxygenation [ECMO], and chemotherapy). The JCIH guidelines recognize AABR as the only appropriate screening technology for use in the NICU. Some NICUs use a two-stage parallel approach where both OAE and AABR are used together in the screening protocol. For infants who do not pass the initial and/or the rescreen prior to discharge, referral should be made directly to a qualified pediatric audiologist at a pediatric diagnostic center as opposed to a general outpatient clinic. When indicated, a comprehensive diagnostic ABR will be conducted to diagnose type, degree, and configuration of hearing loss.

♦ Case Studies

The following case studies are some real-life scenarios extracted from parent interviews (Nicholson and Vanbiervliet, 2007; National Institutes of Health Office of the Director, 1993) and used with parental consent. Read each case and identify aspects from this chapter regarding the processes and procedures that could have improved each parent's experience of universal newborn hearing screening.

Case 1 (Mom): Referred Newborn Hearing Screening/Risk Factors

As we were being released from the hospital, the nurse who was discharging us just randomly said, "Your daughter hasn't passed the newborn hearing screening. We gave it to her yesterday, and she didn't pass, so we gave it to her today, and she isn't responding." She said it as if she were saying something off her grocery list. It was just, like, "Okay, when you go home, do this and this and this and this, and by the way, your daughter failed her newborn hearing screening." When I left the hospital, I was just shocked. I mean, we had no idea that that was coming. I had the feeling that something was wrong, and she [daughter] had a lot more wrong than just that, but the initial feeling was just disbelief. . . . I immediately scheduled the follow-up testing, . . . One of the pediatricians said when we went for our follow-up, "Oh, it is not unusual; a lot of times they are born with fluid in their ears." He made it seem like it wasn't a big deal. We did not have information on [her] hearing loss for 3 months. . . . The nurse and the audiologist were very, very sympathetic to the problems we were having. We did get [her] admitted to the hospital, and we had a long list of things that were wrong with her. When we got all of that straightened out, after neurosurgery and cardiology, after all of that we came back to the hearing loss. We had her tested in conjunction with another surgery, and they just did a fantastic job breaking the news. It was something that we knew, but, you know, she had failed it. We knew that there was some hearing loss; we just didn't know how much. They said that it was severe hearing loss, that she wasn't completely deaf, but that she would require hearing aids, and did we want to go ahead and order them? We left with a packet of information. We left with a video, which I took back. [She] was still at the hospital, so I was living there for 4 months. So I took the video back to the room and watched it. . . . That information really helped a lot because it had parents talking. It had real people who were going through the same thing. All of the information in the world doesn't change the fact that she has a hearing loss. Just knowing that other people have gone through the same thing . . . it helps.

Discussion Points: Competency-based screener training and expertise, personnel, communication, referral, well-baby and NICU protocols, risk factors

Case 2 (Dad): Referred Newborn Hearing Screening/Classified as LTF/D

We found out about his hearing loss when he was 3 years old, actually. . . . We had been going to an audiologist, and she had been telling us that he was fine, and he did not need amplification; that he was just was just taking a little longer to learn his speech because if you would get down on his level, he would communicate with you, but across the room he could not. As we started noticing this, and we ran a little test, it was like a gym class with a bunch of little kids, and my son was talking to one of these lady's daughters, and she noticed that he was reading her lips, and she was an audiologist and she said, "I think you need to get a second opinion," and so we did. . . . I had been to those other appointments with the previous audiologist, but we were going every 6 months and getting the hearing screenings, and he [son] would fail one, and she would say, "Oh, he is fine." We always felt like we were rushed with that lady, and I don't think she specialized in children. You know, I hate to say it that way, but I really think he was just pushed through like an adult, and he was sort of tricking her, and you could tell. She was pressing the button, and he was, like, "I hear it." . . . Once, though, my wife went along, thinking it was just a normal hearing screening, and so she finds out that day that my son can't hear at all out of his right ear and that in his left ear he only has, like, 50%, 60%. Since then he has lost another 10 to 15%.

Discussion Points: Identification of and access to competent pediatric diagnostic centers, personnel, referrals, community resources, data management, well-baby screening protocols, LTF/D.

Case 3 (Mom and Dad): Passed Newborn Hearing Screening/No Risk Factors

Dad: [Our daughter] passed her newborn hearing screens. When we left the hospital, we did not find out that she had hearing loss until she was almost 3 years old. My wife started suspecting that she was not hearing right because her speech wasn't quite up to the level of her cousin, who is the same age, and friends she was around and stuff. She could still speak just fine, but she wasn't developing the language as fast as they were. Just little clues like that. So [my wife] took her to have her hearing checked and found out at that point that she did in fact have a mild hearing loss, which, especially for dads, you go immediately into denial, start testing her at home, making loud noises to get her to turn her head: "Oh, she can hear fine; she just doesn't pay attention" and that sort of thing.

Mom: I have three daughters; my oldest daughter is 8, and she was diagnosed with hearing loss at age 3. My second daughter is 4, and she was diagnosed at 1, and my third daughter is 18 months, and so far her hearing is normal. . . . Our oldest daughter . . . her speech was slightly behind my nephew's, who is the same age. . . . So we let it go for a little while because we thought you are not supposed to compare kids, and then I just kept being concerned. I was noticing she was ignoring us, and people would say that is just how kids are, they just ignore you. Since this was our first, I listened to what people said for a while, and we finally got her ear infections cleared up. We took her to an audiologist, and she did have hearing loss, and that was our initial, official diagnosis that she had hearing loss. We have no family history, no one in our family, unless they are senior adults, who have any hearing issues. So we did not know what to do with that information. . . .

Dad: Our second child passed her newborn hearing screen. When she was diagnosed at a year, we were just religious in testing her from birth on because we knew this was a possibility. So far we have done the same thing with our third child as well, and her results have all been normal hearing. Genetic testing showed it was a dominant nonsyndromic progressive hearing loss with both of the older girls.

Discussion Points: EHDI components, referrals, well-baby nursery, risk factors

◆ Appendix A Suggested Online Resources

1. The EHDI e-book is available for free download from the NCHAM website (http://infanthearing.org/ehdi-ebook/index.html). This is an excellent resource guide for new and not-so-new EHDI programs.

2. EHDI Patient Checklist for Medical Home Providers developed by the AAP can be downloaded from http://www.medicalhomeinfo.org/downloads/pdfs/Checklist_2010.pdf (American Academy of Pediatrics Task Force, 2010).

3. NCHAM has recently developed a Newborn Hearing Screening Training Curriculum (NCHAM, 2010b) that is available via a set of two DVDs, streaming video from the Web, or free downloadable slides available from http://www.infanthearing.org/nhstc_dvd/index.html.

4. Annual CDC EHDI Hearing Screening and Follow-Up Survey (Centers for Disease Control and Prevention, 2010) statistics are available at http://www.cdc.gov/ncbddd/ehdi/data.html.

5. The *Hearing Review* technology guide from July/August 2010 provides an extensive side-by-side matrix showcasing a variety of AABR and OAE screening devices from the industry's leading manufacturers (Hearing Review, 2010). This guide can help answer questions regarding critical equipment selection prior to purchase. Download the pdf document at http://www.hearingreview.com/issues/pdf/TechGuideScreening2010.pdf.

Note: Although each of the above URLs and Web links are current at the time of publication, they are subject to change and/or updates.

◆ Appendix B: Sample OAE Protocol

1. **Personnel and competency training:** All screening personnel will complete the competency-based Newborn Hearing Screening Training Curriculum developed by the National Center for Hearing Assessment and Management under the supervision of an audiologist (http://www.infanthearing.org/nhstc_dvd/index.html).

2. **Screening procedure:** Otoacoustic emissions (DPOAE or TEOAE).

3. **Equipment:** EchoCheck (http://www.otodynamics.com).

4. **Stimulus parameters for the test dignal:** DPOAE = stimulus frequencies (f_2 = sine waves of 6, 4, 3, and 2 kHz), frequency ratio (f_2 = 1.22 f_1), stimulus intensities (65/55 dB SPL [sound pressure level]); TEOAE = 84 dB pe [peak equivalent] SPL $+/-1$ transient click, 260 sweeps of 16 stimulus presentations.

5. **Decision rule criteria for pass/fail:** DPOAE default pass criteria = SNR (sound-to-noise ratio) of 6 dB and minimum signal greater than -5 dB SPL in at least 1.28 s of data collected using three frequency bands; TEOAE default pass criteria = SNR of 6 dB and a minimum signal greater than -5 dB SPL in at least two frequency bands.

6. **Parental consent:** Explain screening test process to parents, answer questions, and obtain consent if required (varies by state). Provide parents a copy of consent form and contact information of state EHDI program.

7. **Screening procedure and number of times for repeat testing prior to discharge:** Position the probe in the sleeping baby's ear and calibrate the stimulus. Conduct the test if probe fit is okay. If the baby does not pass, reposition the probe and repeat. If the baby does not pass, do not repeat the test until immediately prior to discharge. Immediately prior to discharge, repeat the process. If the baby does not pass the screening test, complete the screening form and report screening as a fail. Schedule the baby for a rescreen appointment and counsel parents.

8. **Communication of results to parents/physician:** Complete state EHDI form and give a copy to the parents; forward a copy to the primary care physician. Stress the importance of completing the rescreen for babies who did not pass the initial screen.

9. **State form and reporting requirements:** Complete all sections of the state EHDI screening form. The screening form should have a place to indicate high-risk factors associated with permanent congenital, delayed onset, or progressive hearing loss in childhood, demographic data for infant and parents, emergency contact information, screening and rescreening test results, recommendations, and follow-up appointment.

10. **Process and appointments for rescreening:** Schedule an appointment within 2 weeks for rescreening for families whose infant failed the initial birth screen. The rescreen appointment can be scheduled as an outpatient at this hospital or at a local rescreening site convenient to the family. The baby will receive an OAE rescreen followed by an AABR if the OAE rescreen does not result in a pass.

11. **Appointments for referrals:** If the baby fails the OAE rescreen and AABR screen, make an appointment for the baby at the nearest pediatric diagnostic facility at the earliest convenience. Diagnostic ABRs are much easier to conduct on babies younger than 3 months. Babies older than 3 months often require sedation.

12. **Follow-up and data management:** Enter data in the hospital database; send state EHDI form to the state EHDI program.

◆ Appendix C: Sample Automated Auditory Brainstem Response Protocol

1. **Personnel and competency training:** All screening personnel will complete the competency-based Newborn Hearing Screening Training Curriculum developed by the National Center for Hearing Assessment and Management under the supervision of an audiologist (http://www.infanthearing.org/nhstc_dvd/index.html).

2. **Screening procedure:** AABR.

3. **Equipment:** EchoScreen (http://www.natus.com/documents/051611C.pdf).

4. **Stimulus parameters for the test signal:** AABR stimulus intensity = 35 dB nHL (normal hearing level); Stimulus polarity = alternating clicks.

5. **Decision rule criteria for pass/fail:** Template-matching method.

6. **Parental consent:** Explain the screening test process to the parents, answer questions, and obtain consent if required (varies by state). Provide parents with a copy of the consent form and contact information of state EHDI program.

7. **Screening procedure and number of times for repeat testing prior to discharge:** Attach electrodes to the baby as indicated (refer to equipment manual). Fit the probe to the baby's ear canal, ensuring a secure fit. Apply echo couplers to the ears and attach using the Y probe cable. If the baby does not pass, reposition the probe and repeat. If the baby does not pass, do not repeat the test until immediately prior to discharge. Immediately prior to discharge, repeat the process. If the baby does not pass the screening test, complete the screening form and report screening as a fail. Schedule the baby for rescreen appointment and counsel parents; call physician.

8. **Communication of results to parents/physician:** Complete state EHDI form and give a copy to the parents; forward a copy to the primary care physician. Stress the importance of completing the rescreen for babies who did not pass the initial screen.

9. **State form and reporting requirements:** Complete all sections of the state EHDI screening form. The screening form should have a place to indicate high-risk factors associated with permanent congenital, delayed onset, or progressive hearing loss in childhood, demographic data for infant and parents, emergency contact information, screening and rescreening test results, recommendations, and follow-up appointment.

10. **Process and appointments for rescreening:** Schedule an appointment within 2 weeks for rescreening for families whose infant did not pass the initial birth screen.

The rescreen appointment can be scheduled as an outpatient at this hospital or at a local rescreening site convenient to the family. The baby will receive repeat AABR followed by a diagnostic ABR if the baby does not pass the rescreen.

11. **Appointments for referrals:** If the baby fails the AABR rescreen, and a diagnostic ABR cannot be conducted, make an appointment for the baby at the nearest pediatric diagnostic facility at the earliest convenience. Diagnostic ABRs are much easier to conduct on babies younger than 3 months. Babies older than 3 months often require sedation.

12. **Follow-up and data management:** Enter data in the hospital database; send state EHDI form to the state EHDI program.

References

American Academy of Pediatrics Task Force. (2010). *Early hearing detection and intervention guidelines for pediatric medical home providers*. Retrieved from http://www.medicalhomeinfo.org/downloads/pdfs/Algorithm1_2010.pdf.

American Speech-Language-Hearing Association (2008). *Loss to follow-up in early hearing detection and intervention* (technical report). Retrieved from www.asha.org/policy.

Centers for Disease Control and Prevention. (2003). *National EHDI goals*. Retrieved from http://www.cdc.gov/ncbddd/hearingloss/documents/goals.pdf.

Centers for Disease Control and Prevention. (2010). *The annual CDC EHDI hearing screening and follow-up survey*. Retrieved from http://www.cdc.gov/ncbddd/ehdi/data.htm.

Gorga, M.P. & Neely, S.T. (2003). Cost-effectiveness and test-performance factors in relation to universal newborn hearing screening. Mental Retardation and Developmental Disabilities Research Reviews 9, 103-108. PubMed

Hearing Review. (2010). *Technology guide*. Retrieved from http://www.hearingreview.com/issues/pdf/TechGuideScreening2010.pdf.

Joint Committee on Infant Hearing. (2007). Year 2007 position statement: Principles and guidelines for early hearing detection and intervention programs. *Pediatrics, 120*(4), 898–921. PubMed

Kemp, D. T. (2003). *The OAE story*. Retrieved from http://www.oaeilo.co.uk/downloads/advisories/the%20oae%20story.pdf.

Koop, C. E. (2010). Foreword: Pursuing excellence in early hearing detection and intervention programs. *Pediatrics, 126*(Suppl 1), S1–S2. PubMed

National Center for Hearing Assessment and Management. (2010a). *Early hearing detection and intervention components*. Retrieved from http://www.infanthearing.org/components/.

National Center for Hearing Assessment and Management. (2010b). *Newborn hearing screening training curriculum*. Retrieved from http://www.infanthearing.org/nhstc_dvd/index.html.

National Center for Hearing Assessment and Management. (2010c). *The EHDI e-book*. Retrieved from http://www.infanthearing.org/ehdi-ebook/index.html.

National Institutes of Health Office of the Director. (1993). *NIH consensus ztatement: Early identification of hearing impairment in infants and young children*. Bethesda, MD: Author.

Nicholson, N., & Vanbiervliet, A. (2007). *Making EHDI decisions: A DVD tool for EHDI programs* (1R41DC008232-01A2). Bethesda, MD: National Institute on Deafness and Other Communication Disorders (NIDCD).

Schulman-Galambos, C., & Galambos, R. (1979). Brain stem evoked response audiometry in newborn hearing screening. *Archives of Otolaryngology—Head and Neck Surgery, 105*(2), 86–90. PubMed

Shulman, S., Besculides, M., Saltzman, A., Ireys, H., White, K. R., & Forsman, I. (2010). Evaluation of the universal newborn hearing screening and intervention program. *Pediatrics, 126*(Suppl 1), S19–S27. PubMed

Sininger, Y., Hyde, M., & Don, M. (2001). U.S. Patent No. 6,196,977 B. Washington, DC: U.S. Patent and Trademark Office.

Spivak, L. (1998). *Newborn hearing screening*. New York: Thieme.

Wilson, J., & Jungner, G. (1968). Principles and practice of screening for disease. *WHO Chronicle, 22*(11), 1–493. Retrieved from http://whqlibdoc.who.int/php/WHO_PHP_34.pdf.

Zweig, M. H., & Campbell, G. (1993). Receiver-operating characteristic (ROC) plots: A fundamental evaluation tool in clinical medicine. *Clinical Chemistry, 39*(4), 561–577. PubMed

Chapter 14

Threshold Estimation Using the Auditory Brainstem Response

Paul M. Brueggeman and Samuel R. Atcherson

Although there are several different techniques for assessing hearing sensitivity, the auditory brainstem response (ABR) test is currently the gold standard for estimating puretone thresholds in infants (as well as other difficult-to-test patients). Wave V is generally the largest of the ABR waves and is the last to disappear with progressive decrease in stimulus intensity level. When the patient is under sedation or anesthesia, or resting quietly, and the test conditions are optimal, the lowest intensity level that produces an identifiable and repeatable wave V can be within 5 to 15 dB of an infant's or adult's behavioral audiometric threshold (Stapells, 2000). The lowest level at which wave V is actually obtained may vary depending on the frequency of the stimulus tone burst used, the envelope function imposed on the tone burst, how well the system has been calibrated, the number of stimulus repetitions used, the amount of residual noise in the averaging process, the impedances achieved, the electrode montage chosen, and the individual anatomy and physiology of the patient.

The estimation of behavioral thresholds using ABR requires not only technical skills but also a degree of patience and discernment. Because time is usually not on the clinician's side during assessment of thresholds, the clinician must possess the skill to know when to wait, when to stop, when to troubleshoot, and when to move on to the next intensity level, another stimulus frequency, or the other ear. Moreover, the clinician must command confidence in the interpretation and be able to recognize and be willing to report any limitations on the part of the test results. This is all particularly true when determining ABR thresholds in awake children. An astute clinician will have multiple distractors at their disposal to help in keeping the child engaged with a preferred activity. Think of your time as limited from the moment the child enters the room with the parent. With this mindset, you will find yourself using precious time collecting threshold data, rather than pursuing lengthy case history and setting up the equipment. The time for such things can be found either before the child arrives at the appointment or after the testing is completed.

In addition to mastering certain skills, clinicians today have some choices to make, not only with recommended recording and stimulus parameters, but also with different commercial systems, each of which may have proprietary or unique features. For example, the Bio-Logic Navigator Pro (Natus Medical Inc., Mundelein, IL) uses Fsp as an additional confidence measure to enhance objective detection of ABRs (refer to Chapter 3), whereas the Vivosonic Integrity system (Vivosonic Inc., Toronto, Canada) uses Kalman filtering to allow ABRs to be recorded without sedation and anesthesia (Li, Sokolov, and Kunov, 2002). Without these

Table 14.1 Pretest Form Items

- Building and office location where the auditory brainstem response evaluation will take place
- Date and time of the evaluation, as well as the recommended arrival time
- Audiologist who will be conducting the evaluation
- Simple explanation of the procedure (e.g., what the test measures, use of electrodes, and the method of sound delivery)
- If sedation or anesthesia will be given, basic information about what is to be expected
- General rules about eating or drinking prior to, during, and after the evaluation
- Approximate length of time the evaluation will take
- Items to bring (favorite sleeping toys, blankets, pillow, etc.)
- Simple explanation about what is to be expected after the evaluation
- Estimated date when the results will be available

proprietary features, most commercial ABR systems will suffice for threshold estimation testing. Thus, clinicians will need to familiarize themselves with their equipment by consulting with the user manuals and performing as many practice recordings as possible in advance of the first patient. This chapter is not intended to be exhaustive, but it should help guide new or returning clinicians with skill and protocol development in this exciting yet challenging area of auditory evoked potential recording.

♦ Family Preparation and Pre–Auditory Brainstem Response Evaluation Information

Infants and young children who do not pass their hearing screenings may have parents who are experiencing feelings of sadness, confusion, anger, fear, or frustration (Abdala de Uzzcategui and Yoshinaga-Itano, 1997). If a hearing disorder is diagnosed using ABR, parents are very likely going to experience shock and upset (Gilbey, 2010). With this in mind, it is extremely important to prepare the family and the child well for the ABR evaluation experience. This will be true whether or not the ABR evaluation involves sedation or anesthesia. The moments prior to the ABR evaluation are just as important as the time after the evaluation is completed and results are ready. When parents are calm and adequately prepared at the outset, the child to be tested will also very likely be calm. To prepare families, a letter or handout explaining the procedures and any

materials that they should bring are extremely beneficial. **Table 14.1** lists items that would be helpful in such a letter or handout.

♦ Patient Preparation and Orientation

Preparing a child or adult for an ABR consists of several steps that ensure a valid test will be performed. The very first step is to ensure a comfortable environment for the ABR assessment to take place. This is an often overlooked detail that can end up impacting evaluations negatively. If the clinic room is too hot or cold, too bright, or just too small, a pediatric ABR evaluation may be unsuccessful because the child may become uncomfortable and agitated. If there is a paging system installed, be sure to turn down the volume. If there is a phone in the room, turn off the ringer. Always ask the front desk staff to disrupt an ABR evaluation only in cases of emergency, as it is very frustrating to parents to have to reschedule an evaluation because a staff member woke up the baby being evaluated. For ABR assessments under sedation or anesthesia, the setting is not nearly as important, as the patient will be unaware of the environment for a period of time.

Once the details of the evaluation have been explained to the patient or the patient's parents, the next step is to prepare the skin areas where the electrodes will be placed. There are multiple products available to prepare the skin for electrode placement, but they generally all achieve the same result.

Skin preparation is done to remove dead skin, makeup, skin oils, and dirt/debris to allow for a clean surface for the electrodes so as to obtain the lowest impedances possible. Commercially available electrode prep pads have been used for years to help clear the skin of residue when preparing for electrophysiologic testing. These prepackaged pads generally contain isopropyl alcohol and pumice. There are also commercially available abrasive gels that can be used to clear the skin of debris. It is much easier to prepare the electrode sites once using moderate pressure than going back over the sites several times with little to no pressure after one finds the electrode impedances too high. It also is costly when using disposable surface electrodes, as reprepping an electrode site often requires a fresh disposable electrode. Suggested electrode sites are discussed later in this chapter.

Once the electrode sites are prepared, the electrodes are ready to be placed. Single-use disposable electrodes or permanent reusable electrodes (disk or cup electrodes) are both reasonable options to use for different purposes. If you are primarily performing adult ABR evaluations, where the electrodes are very likely not going to be pulled at or removed by the patient, it makes clinical and financial sense to continue using reusable electrodes. During pediatric evaluations, when more movement and electrode pulling are likely, single-use, pre-gelled surface electrodes tend to be a better option. The adherent properties of today's single-use electrodes allow for moderate tugging without becoming dislodged. Most pediatric clinicians who have made the switch to single-use electrodes will attest that they would not go back to the reusable electrodes because of the increased testing efficiency and easier clean-up. If you are using disposable pregelled electrodes, be sure to employ light pressure around the the gel to adhere them. Failure to do so will cause the gel to be pushed outward onto the adhering part of the electrode. The end result is having an electrode that does not adhere well to the skin. When using reusable electrodes, be sure to fill each electrode cup with a slightly rounded amount of electrode contact paste. When placing each electrode, use gentle, steady pressure. Having multiple 1- to 2-inch lengths of tape already cut and

nearby before starting to place the electrodes will help reduce preparation time. Once the electrodes are in position, place the electrode wires up and over the ear as appropriate so that the wires are not in the patient's field of vision. You are now ready to check the impedance of the electrodes and begin testing.

◆ Testing Methods

Obtaining clear, reliable ABRs to estimate thresholds can be a challenge when working with infants, young children, and other patients who are difficult to test. They must be physiologically quiet either by sleeping or undergoing sedation or anesthesia; for some specialized ABR equipment, they can be awake but not excessively active. These methods of obtaining clear, reliable responses are discussed as follows.

Natural Sleep

Children under the age of 3 years often have a natural naptime that is part of their everyday routine. This is particularly true of children under the age of 1 year. In the first 3 months of life, most children will take midmorning or afternoon naps, which supplement the sleep they get at night. Even some children as old as 4 years still routinely take naps. An audiologist should consider timing an ABR evaluation during one of these regular sleeping-interval times to get reliable data on hearing function.

Scheduling an ABR at a particular time of day for a particular child may be difficult to do if a clinician, like most, has a very busy schedule. It may also be difficult for the parent to know when exactly the child will fall asleep during the day. A common practice among clinicians is to ask the parent to withhold sleep from a child the morning and/or early afternoon of the ABR evaluation. This presents its own challenges for the parent. There have been many times when a parent has said, "I tried everything in my power to keep him awake on the drive here. I had the radio up, I tickled his feet while I drove," and so on. Clearly, there are times when you cannot expect a parent to entirely deprive a child of a nap before an evaluation. When a child has already taken a nap on the way to the appointment, it is usually best to move forward with a nonsedated ABR instead of trying to make a child sleep. That usually is just a waste of time, as the need for a nap is a natural sleep cycle for the child that cannot be "doubled up." The caveat moving forward with a nonsedated ABR is that one needs appropriate equipment to do a nonsedated ABR in very young children, such as that described in the following section. The other options are attempting the natural sleep ABR on a different day or completing a sedated ABR, if applicable.

If a child is sleepy and is clearly ready to take a nap, it is recommended that patient preparation be completed before he or she is already in a restful state. Patient preparation is almost always going to wake children. As such, it is highly recommended at a minimum, that the electrode skin sites are prepared and the electrodes placed before anything else is done.

Sedation and Anesthesia

When ABRs cannot be recorded during natural sleep, or when it is anticipated that an infant or young child will not be able to cooperate, sedation or anesthesia may be recommended to reduce physiologic noise and collect information as quickly as possible. Sedatives are drugs that depress the central nervous system and are used to calm patients or put them to sleep. Anesthetics, in contrast, cause partial or complete loss of sensation to local parts of the body or the whole body. The administration of both types of drugs requires qualified medical personnel. The most popular sedative used with ABR is chloral hydrate. It is administered orally in liquid or capsule form or rectally with a suppository. However, there can be gastrointenstinal and respiratory side effects (Keengwe, Hegde, Dearlove, Wilson, Yates, and Sharples, 1999; Ronchera-Oms et al, 1994; Vade, Sukhani, Dolenga, and Habisohn-Schuck, 1995). Propofol is another drug for use with young children undergoing ABR recordings. It is a popular choice for short procedures because ABR amplitudes are relatively unaffected (Purdie and Cullen, 1993), and recovery is rapid and complete without troublesome side effects (McLeod and Boheimer, 1985; Sanderson and Blades, 1988). However, some clinicians have reported rare or previously unknown adverse reactions, or medical contraindications, to propofol. Regardless of the drug used, the clinician will benefit from a physiologically quiet child but still needs to work quickly to gain the most information possible before the child is brought back to consciousness.

Because of the potential risks involved with sedatives and anesthetics, clinicians need to work closely with their sedation/ anesthesia teams and observe strict protocols. There may be feeding or fasting requirements, such that food and liquids are generally restricted a few hours before the procedure. It will be up to the sedation/ anesthesia team to decide whether fasting is necessary (e.g., Keidan, Gozal, Minuskin, Weinberg, Barkaly, and Augarten, 2004). The sedation/anesthesia team may conduct multiple reviews of the child's medical history in advance of any scheduled ABR as well as the day before or prior to the scheduled ABR. The audiology clinician who will be conducting the ABR can be instrumental by identifying conditions, syndromes, and craniofacial anomalies that may present complications and require additional equipment and personnel. In some cases, ABRs may be recorded while the infant or child is already under anesthesia for another procedure.

Special Consideration

ABR threshold estimation in infants and young children who must be sedated or undergo anesthesia require medical personnel (usually a physician or nurse) who are qualified to administer the drugs and provide airway and respiratory support in the event of an adverse reaction. Although sedation or anesthesia can offer a distinct advantage in the recording of ABRs, even at very soft intensity levels, there may be times when the medical risks outweigh the potential benefit in obtaining information about hearing sensitivity.

Nonsedation

ABRs recorded during natural sleep, deprived sleep, or restful cooperation are a few examples of nonsedation options. There are multiple reasons why it makes intuitive sense not to require a young child to undergo sedation to have his or her hearing evaluated. There is an increased cost resulting from the need for physician oversight, nursing consult, the actual sedative itself, and the increased time away from work for the parents because of the need for medical surveillance after the procedure is over. That said, many of the current ABR systems on the market do not reject myogenic and other artifacts in an effective manner as to allow unsedated ABR assessments to be completed while very young children are fully awake. However, the introduction of the Vivosonic Integrity system has recently presented another interesting nonsedation option. The Integrity system allows for some amount of physical movement by the child without affecting the ABR waveform as a result of the use of Kalman filtering. As described in the previous section, there are certainly advantages to having a child sleep through an ABR evaluation, but as any parent knows, children sometimes fight going to sleep only to become increasingly agitated and overtired in the process. What might have been scheduled as a sleep-deprived appointment can lead to a nonsedated awake appointment if a child will not sleep. An astute clinician will realize that the child will not sleep and will quickly move to engage the child with play to keep the appointment moving. Allow a child 15 minutes to settle into sleep after the disposable electrodes are placed. If the child will not settle in that time, move quickly to a nonsedated ABR routine using distractors/toys/DVD movies to engage the child.

Children are amazing. They have the ability to stay engaged with sensory experiences that allow for growth and development. One method to keep children engaged during an ABR evaluation is to allow them to explore sensory and animated toys. The issue is that sometimes we, as professionals, do not know what sensory preferences a very young toddler has. Because of this, when scheduling a nonsedated ABR assessment with young children, you need to have multiple toys ready that offer different types of sensory experiences. Some examples that have worked well are pop-up toys, baby rattles, sensory balls, bubbles, switch-activated toys, and light boxes. Small fans, animated toys, lights, and buzzers all create different sensory experiences for children as well. If you use a switch, even a very young child can activate it while you change toys throughout the evaluation.

Another method that has proven very effective is to use media as distractors. The use of a personal computing tablets (e.g., Apple iPad; Cupertino, CA), TV/DVD combination system, or even your work laptop can serve as a means to distract young children with their favorite movie or TV show. The parents should be contacted before the day of the ABR appointment to find out what types of toys are most appropriate and also to request that the parents bring one or two of the child's favorite movies along with them to the evaluation. If the program selected is short, be sure to select the DVD to repeat continuously during the evaluation. Think of distraction techniques this way. As a child, if the circus came to town and you saw the trucks coming down the street with all of the sights, colors, and animals present, it would be very hard to distract yourself away from that. Consider yourself as the circus to the child you are testing during a nonsedated ABR. The child will follow your every move and be overly engaged in the sensations that occur during patient preparation if you do not keep him or her engaged in other sensory experiences. Because of this, be sure to stay out of the child's visual field if he or she is engaged in a movie and when it is clear that your presence is somewhat disconcerting to the child.

To an infant, there is nothing more naturally important than the touch, smell, and sound of their mother, father, or other caregiver. As a clinician, remember that the very best comforters, distractors, and playmates are the parents. The child will likely be most comfortable sitting on a parent's lap or lying on a parent's shoulder. For children who can sit upright, having them sit on the floor near a parent can allow for a comfortable place to play and engage with the parent. Asking the parent to help keep the child's hands off the electrode wires is useful and necessary during the evaluation. Let parents know that if a child under 2 years of age manages to get one of the electrodes off once, there is a likelihood that it will become a new challenge for the child to do it again. When parents ask how they can help, simply ask them to play and talk with their child like they do at home. If the child needs a bottle, let him or her have it. If the child needs to be burped, so be it. Larger rooms with comfortable furniture may help the parent and child become comfortable and feel safe just being themselves.

Because the Vivosonic Integrity system is fully wireless, a small stimulus box can be placed on a parent's shoulder/arm near a child younger than 2 years. For children over the age of 2, the use of a backpack containing this box allows full freedom of movement around the room, and building if need be. There have been many ABR assessments with the Integrity system that this author has completed while playing kickball with a child in a gym or letting a child explore a sensory room. Playing on a swing, walking the hallways, and simply eating a snack have occurred, all while reliable ABR threshold data were being collected.

♦ Instrumentation and Setup

Stimuli

Two types of stimuli are used for threshold estimation: clicks and tone bursts. Because of the virtually instantaneous onset of a click, the energy introduced to the cochlea has the effect of synchronizing a broad range of auditory nerve fibers. Broadly stimulating the cochlea certainly has its advantages in producing a clearly defined ABR with most, if not all, complementary waves present. However, the click is considered a broadband stimulus and therefore is not frequency specific. Pure tones are highly frequency specific, but they must be shaped in a particular manner so that they do not have instantaneous onsets like a click and their rise times are not too slow. Because neural synchrony remains a requirement to produce an ABR, tone-burst stimuli must be short (usually 4 or 5 cycles long) with relatively fast rise/fall times. Tone bursts are typically ramped using a linear or Blackman envelope function with rise/fall times encompassing 2 cycles and a plateau of either 0 or 1 cycle. **Table 14.2** provides an example of

some published ABR stimuli and their specific parameters. Readers are encouraged to consult with these published sources to guide their own clinical stimulus and testing protocols.

For clicks and higher-frequency tone bursts, use of a single stimulus polarity (rarefaction or condensation) is sufficient. For lower-frequency tone bursts, a highly periodic stimulus artifact can appear to be a single stimulus polarity that may obscure the ABR waveform, although not in all cases. An alternating stimulus polarity may reduce, if not eliminate, the periodic stimulus artifact. **Figure 14.1** shows an example of a 500-Hz ABR recorded to rarefaction, condensation, and alternating polarities. Notice how the stimulus artifact was removed with the alternating polarity. Care must be taken, however, not to miss a possible diagnosis of auditory neuropathy spectrum disorder (ANSD), which requires a single stimulus polarity (see Chapter 16). In addition, for patients with ANSD, threshold estimation will likely not be possible.

Stimulation rate for threshold estimation is generally set higher than would be expected for an ABR neurodiagnostic protocol. Rates no more than ~40/s (e.g., 37.7 or 41.1/s) will still produce strong wave V responses, especially in infants, while allowing test time to be relatively quicker.

As would be expected, stimulus intensity will need to be changed during the recording session in order for thresholds to be estimated. Although there is no firm consensus about starting intensity levels, what intensity step sizes to use, or even which stimulus frequencies to begin testing, the goal of any threshold estimation protocol is to obtain the most useful and reliable information, all within the finite period of time that you have with the infant or child. Most ABR threshold estimation protocols include stimuli that will estimate low-, mid-, and high-frequency hearing sensitivity. Published protocols often include tone-burst frequencies of 500, 1000, 2000, and 4000 Hz, although some substitute specially constructed 250-Hz tone bursts for 500-Hz tone bursts and clicks for 4000-Hz tone bursts. Some protocols begin with a high-intensity click (~70 dB nHL [normal hearing level]) in each ear to initially rule out ANSD. If there is no suspicion of ANSD, click stimulation continues until threshold is obtained. Some authors view the click as a valid estimate of high-frequency

Table 14.2 Examples of Published Auditory Brainstem Response Stimulus Parameters

Source	Stimulus Types and Frequencies	TB Duration	TB Envelope Function	Rise/Fall Times	Polarity	Stimula-tion Rate	Ipsilateral Noise
Gorga et al (2006)	Clicks* and TB (0.25, 1, 2, or 4 kHz)	4 msec (0.25 and 1 kHz); 3 msec (2 kHz); 2 msec (4 kHz)	Blackman	2 msec (0.25 and 1 kHz); 1.5 msec (2 kHz); 1 msec (4 kHz)	Rarefaction clicks and 0.25 kHz TB; condensation for others	17/s or 27/s for clicks; 37/s for TBs	N/A
British Columbia Early Hearing Program (2008); Stapells, 2005/2006	TB (0.5, 1, 2, and 4 kHz) and clicks if necessary	6 msec (0.5 kHz), 5 msec (1 kHz), 2 msec (2 kHz), 1 msec (4 kHz)	2-1-2 linearly gated or 5-cycle Blackman	4 msec (0.5 kHz), 2 msec (1 kHz), 1 msec (2 kHz), 0.5 msec (4 kHz)	Alternating polarity	39.1/s	1-octave narrow-band noise centered on stimulus frequency
Karzon and Lieu (2006)	*Clicks and TB (0.5, 1, and 4 kHz), 2 kHz if asymmetric	Same as above	2-1-2 or 5-cycle Blackman	Same as above	Rarefaction for all stimuli	33.3/s for AC, 11.1/s for BC	N/A
Ontario Infant Hearing Program (2008)	TB (0.5, 1, 2, and 4 kHz) and *clicks if necessary	6 msec (0.5 kHz), 5 msec (1 kHz), 2 msec (2 kHz), 1 msec (4 kHz)	2-1-2 linearly gated	Same as above	Alternating polarity	39.1/s	N/A for ipsi, discretionary for BC

Abbreviations: AC, air conduction; BC, bone conduction; TB, tone burst.

*Clicks are 100 μsec in duration.

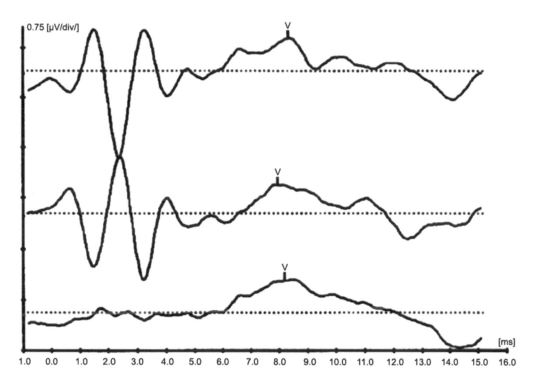

Fig. 14.1 Case example of an air-conduction 500-Hz auditory brainstem response (ABR) recording requiring alternating polarity. The top waveform was produced using a rarefaction polarity, the middle waveform was produced using a condensation polarity, and the bottom waveform was produced using alternating polarities. Notice that the stimulus artifact was eliminated in the bottom waveform.

hearing sensitivity (Gorga, Johnson, Kaminski, Beauchaine, Garner, and Neely, 2006). However, if a protocol includes clicks and high-frequency tone bursts (e.g., 2000 and/or 4000 Hz), beginning with high-frequency clicks at the outset could be viewed as redundant and wasteful (Sauter, 2007). Regardless of the stimuli used, most protocols attempt to optimize time efficiency. Examples of optimizing time efficiency include the following:

- Using an ascending approach

- Using 20- to 40-dB step sizes at suprathreshold levels with a descending approach

- Not testing below some minimum required intensity level (cf. British Columbia Early Hearing Program, 2008; Gorga et al, 2006; Ontario Infant Hearing Program, 2008)

- Not using step sizes < 10 dB (5-dB step sizes > 70 dB nHL are recommended)

- Not repeating runs at suprathreshold levels

- Testing at a higher frequency first, followed by the lowest frequency, and filling in the rest

- Testing the assumed better ear first

A final important consideration for stimuli is calibration. The issues relevant to calibration are discussed in depth in Chapter 22; however, some information bears repeating here. Although there are two published international standards, there is currently no American National Standards Institute (ANSI) standard for the calibration of short-duration stimuli, such as clicks and tone bursts. Because of this, it is entirely possible for different commercial ABR systems, both diagnostic and screening, to yield different results. Thus, it is strongly encouraged that clinicians "know their equipment by checking each stimulus they intend to use to see whether 0 dB nHL on the monitor screen or dial corresponds with the behavioral threshold in a group of ototologically and audiometrically normal individuals. This means that the ABR system is used like an audiometer with each stimulus, and the average softest intensity level is recorded. This assessment should be performed in a sound booth and well in advance of the first patient. If any average behavioral threshold does not equal 0 dB nHL, then a correction factor may need to be applied. Experienced clinicians may be comfortable enough to change the ABR system's calibration settings. In the absence of an ANSI standard, readers are encouraged to consult with their manufacturer, calibration expert, and the ISO 389–6 (International Organization for Standardization, 2007) standard on calibration information and concerns.

> **Pitfall**
>
> It is commonly thought that a click stimulus can best estimate the audiogram between 2 and 4 kHz. There are two reasons for this assumption. First, the spectrum of a click recorded through an artificial ear coupler on average demonstrates maximal energy between 2 and 4 kHz. Second, high-frequency sensorineural hearing losses can degrade the ABR morphology, whereas low-frequency sensorineural hearing losses may show intact ABR morphologies. The fact remains that the click is a broadband stimulus, and any surviving neural elements in the cochlea can respond to the click. Thus, a patient with significant cochlear damage beyond 2 kHz can still produce an ABR to a click when neural elements below 2 kHz respond (e.g., Oates and Stapells, 1998; Sauter, 2007; Sininger, 2007).

Electrode Montage

Gorga et al (2006) and Stapells (2005; 2006) use high forehead (Fz) as the noninverting electrode site, with the ipsilateral mastoid (M1/M2) as the inverting electrode site and the contralateral mastoid (M1/M2) as the ground, whereas Hall (2007) uses earlobe ipsilateral to the stimulus (Ai) as the noninverting electrode site, with either low forehead (Fpz) or contralateral earlobe (Ac) as the ground. Each of these electrode montages is suitable for one-channel recordings. If both ipsilateral and contralateral

recordings are desired (as is recommended for bone-conduction ABRs), both mastoids (or earlobes) will be inverting electrodes, and the ground is typically placed at Fpz. To further enhance wave V in infants, a nape of the neck reference (C7) can also be used. **Figure 14.2** illustrates the three 1-channel electrode montages described here.

> **Pitfall**
>
> In infants, the anterior fontanelle (or soft spot) is the largest region of cartilage on top of the head between several cranial bones that is not replaced by bone until the second year of life (**Fig. 14.3**). Although it is possible to place the noninverting electrode at Cz (vertex) in infants for both ABR and auditory state-state response (ASSR), caution is strongly urged.

In contrast to conventional ABR systems, the Vivosonic Integrity is a unique one-channel electrode system where the preamplifier, called the Amplitrode, is placed on the head at the ground electrode site (Fpz). The noninverting electrode (reference) is then placed at Fz, while the inverting electrode is placed on the mastoids, earlobes, or nape of the neck (around

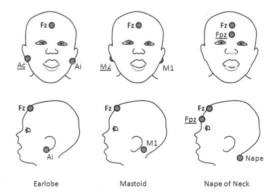

Fig. 14.2 Three commonly used electrode montages for one-channel auditory brainstem response (ABR) recordings with earlobe, mastoid, or nape of the neck as reference (inverting). For illustrative purposes, the left ear is the stimulation ear. Fz is the noninverting electrode. Ai, M1, and nape (usually C7 or Oz) is the inverting or reference electrode. Ac, M2, and Fpz serve as the ground.

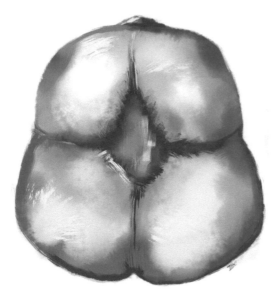

Fig. 14.3 Anterior fontanelle of an infant (anterior is up). (Figure drawn by Timothy Lim, AuD.)

Oz or C7), with a manufacturer preference for the earlobe placement. Once all electrodes are placed, the clinician can then drape the electrode wires over and behind the child's ear and the top of the child's ear out of the visual field. If earlobe references are used, the clinician will need to ensure that the inverting electrode is always on the ear of stimulation.

Controversial Point

Although an electrode placed at the nape of the neck (Oz or C7) may yield slightly larger wave V responses as a result of its more parallel (vertical) arrangement with the auditory brainstem dipole (e.g., Sininger, Abdala, and Cone-Wesson, 1997), one group argues that there could be increased noise that offsets this benefit (British Columbia Early Hearing Program, 2008). Furthermore, although several investigators have chosen to use the ipsilateral mastoid as the inverting electrode site (e.g., Gorga et al, 2006; Stapells, 2005/2006), others (Hall, 2007) have recommended the inverting site on the ipsilateral earlobe to minimize the stimulus artifact that can be seen in some ABR recordings.

Amplifier Gain

Most commercial ABR systems set the amplifier gain at 100,000 times by default. However, some published protocols recommend an amplifier gain of 150,000 times. Any amplifier gain below 100,000 times is not recommended.

Filter Settings

The typical filter settings for threshold ABR in children are 30 to 3000 Hz or 30 to 1500 Hz when compared with the typical 100- to 3000- Hz filter setting used in a high-intensity neurodiagnostic application. One or both cutoff frequencies are lowered for at least two reasons: First, the infant ABR has been shown to be lower in spectra content when compared with adults (Sininger, et al, 1997). Second, the ABR waveform morphology inherently becomes lower in spectral content with decreases in intensity (Malinoff and Spivak, 1990). For tone-burst frequencies 1000 Hz or greater, a filter setting of 100 to 3000 Hz may be sufficient (Gorga et al, 2006). In addition, it is recommended that the filter skirts not be excessive (no more than 6 or 12 dB per octave) to avoid distorting the waveform.

Averaging

The general rule of thumb is to use as many stimulus presentations (or sweeps) as needed to obtain a clear and repeatable wave V. At higher intensity levels, fewer sweeps may be allowable (e.g., ~1500), although the British Columbia Early Hearing Program (2008) and Ontario Infant Hearing Program (2008) recommend a minimum of 2000 sweeps. However, as many as 3000 to 6000 sweeps may be necessary at intensity levels near the ABR threshold (British Columbia Early Hearing Program, 2008; Sininger et al, 1997). Using an objective online detection statistic, such as Fsp, can help with averaging, especially when signal-to-noise ratio can vary in a signal recording session. As described in Chapter 3, the computer may stop averaging when a particular Fsp criterion is met. Conversely, if the Fsp criterion is not met, the computer will continue to average until all sweeps have been completed. Again, at higher intensity levels, Fsp may stop with as few as 1000 sweeps but require 3000 to 6000 sweeps at lower intensity levels.

Analysis Time

Regardless of the type of stimulus used, wave V latency will prolong with decreases in stimulus intensity level. Thus, it is recommended that the analysis time window extend the standard 10 msec. An analysis window of 15 msec should be sufficient for higher-frequency tone bursts and clicks, whereas an analysis window of 20 to 25 msec may be necessary for lower-frequency tone burst stimuli.

◆ Estimating and Plotting Behavioral Thresholds

One of the goals of using ABR for behavioral threshold estimation is to have the ability to paint an audiometric picture, especially for infants, young children, and other patients for whom conventional pure-tone audiometry is inappropriate or cannot be completed. Here, the ABR is recorded using a variety of acoustic stimuli (e.g., 500, 1000, 2000, and 4000 Hz tone bursts and 100 clicks) and at various intensity levels to identify the margin between which a wave V response is present and when it is absent. It is good practice, near threshold, to repeat ABR to ensure that the observed wave V response is reliable and valid. To repeat ABR at all suprathreshold intensity levels could be considered wasteful in terms of clinical time and efficiency. (Recall in the Stimulus section of this chapter that step sizes of 20 to 40 dB are used at suprathreshold levels and a step size of 10 dB is used near threshold.) It is also considered good practice to repeat the ABR when there is no wave V response. These two practices help promote clinician confidence in defining the margin between present or absent response.

Once the margin between present and absent wave V is identified, the clinician has a number of issues to resolve to estimate behavioral thresholds and for transferring the information to an audiogram. First, the clinician needs to make a decision about how he or she defines threshold. For example, if a clinician uses a final step size of 10 dB and the margin for the wave V response is 35 dB nHL (absent) and 45 dB nHL (present), is the ABR threshold at 45 dB nHL or is it somewhere in between such as 40 dB nHL? Second, thresholds obtained using ABR often overestimate (i.e., elevated or poorer) behavioral thresholds between 10 and 20 dB in individuals with normal hearing and 5 and 15 dB in individuals with sensorineural hearing loss (Stapells, 2000). Third, it may not be necessary to continue to track wave V if it is present at some minimum intensity level thought to be consistent with normal hearing (e.g., 20 dB nHL; Gorga et al., 2006).

If we define ABR threshold only on the basis of the final intensity level at which a wave V is present, it is likely not going to be useful for clinical interventions such as hearing aid selection and fitting because of overestimation. It is for this reason that we recommend one of two methods for estimating behavioral threshold and plotting them onto an audiogram. One method advocated by Hall (2007) is to plot ABR thresholds on the audiogram with standard audiometric symbols and then to add a vertical line topped off with a horizontal marker indicating the estimated behavioral threshold. Hall (2007) uses a 10 dB correction factor at all ABR test frequencies. One value of this method is that allows for a rapid comparison of the ABR threshold and the estimated behavioral threshold on the same audiogram. This method probably provides a reasonably good, "middle of the road" estimate given that adults and children have known ear canal differences and individuals with and without hearing loss can have ABR to behavioral threshold overestimation between 5 and 20 dB.

The other method, developed by Bagatto and her colleagues (2005) and recommended for routine clinical practice by Beck, Samsson, and Moodie (2009), is to plot ABR thresholds in dB nHL as behavioral, estimated hearing loss (EHL) thresholds using the following correction factors: subtract 20 dB at 500 Hz, 15 dB at 1000 Hz, 10 dB at 2000 Hz, and 5 dB at 4000 Hz. Again, the clinician would use standard audiometric symbols and would clearly indicate on the audiogram form that ABR thresholds were converted to EHL thresholds. One major benefit to this method is its application for infants, taking into account known physical differences in ear canal acoustics, and making the EHL thresholds readily transferred to the Desired Sensation Level hearing aid fitting algorithm (DSLi/o v5; National Centre for Audiology, University of Western Ontario, London, Ontario, Canada).

◆ Case Studies

Case 1: Infant with Normal Hearing (Natural Sleep)

A 4-month-old female infant passed her otoacoustic emission newborn hearing screening (NHS); however, both of her parents had histories of sensorineural hearing loss: one caused by ototoxicity (stable moderate to moderate-severe sensorineural hearing loss) and one caused by large vestibular aqueduct syndrome (progressive sensorineural hearing loss presently at profound levels). An ABR was requested by the parents during the first few months of their daughter's life. ABR results were judged to be within normal limits not only for clicks, but also for 500-Hz tone-burst stimulation. The left ear results are shown in **Fig. 14.4**.

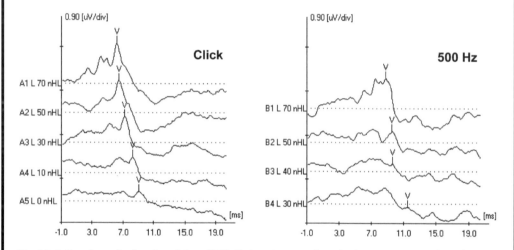

Fig. 14.4 Case 1 results showing click and 500-Hz tone burst auditory brainstem responses (ABRs) at normal levels. Only the left ear results are displayed in this example. Notice that step sizes ranged from 10 to 20 dB, depending on the intensity level. Equipment: Bio-Logic NavPro system with nape of neck reference.

Case 2: Preadolescent with Sensorineural Hearing Loss (Relaxed with Eyes Closed)

A preadolescent male patient with a sensorineural hearing loss of unknown etiology was referred for ABR threshold estimation to determine whether hearing sensitivity had changed prior to the purchase and fitting of new hearing aids. The patient had little in the way of communication abilities and was very low functioning. He was enrolled in a special education program in the county school district. In years past, visual reinforcement audiometry and play audiometry were successful in obtaining reasonable estimates of audiometric thresholds, but never with a great deal of confidence. The latest attempt at obtaining audiometric information proved unreliable. Other than enjoying playing video games and basketball, the patient would lose interest even while doing mundane tasks and would choose not to participate. To the clinician's delight, however, he would sit cooperatively without protest for relatively long durations without interruption. We made an unusual attempt to collect ABR thresholds initially with clicks and then with 500-, 1000-, and 2000-Hz tone bursts in each ear. ABR thresholds converted to dB estimated HL (EHL) showed what appeared to be a bilateral moderately severe sensorineural hearing loss. The left ear results for click and 500-Hz tone burst stimuli (1000 and 2000 Hz are not shown) are presented in **Fig. 14.5**.

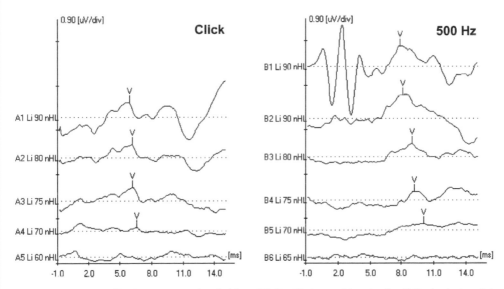

Fig. 14.5 Case 2 results showing ABR thresholds at 70 dB nHL (normal hearing level) for both the click and 500 Hz tone burst stimuli. Using a dB EHL (estimated hearing level) correction factor would put these results in the moderate-to-severe hearing loss range. Notice the stimulus artifact for the 500-Hz tone burst stimulation at 90 dB nHL. This came about when using rarefaction polarity. Switching to an alternating polarity effectively diminished the stimulus artifact. Equipment: Bio-Logic NavPro system with stimulation earlobe reference.

Case 3: Child with Conductive Hearing Loss (Unsedated)

A 4-month-old female infant presented with a previous diagnosis of sensorineural hearing loss. The purpose of the evaluation was to provide a second opinion as to the degree of sensorineural hearing loss the child had before she was to be fitted with hearing aids at another audiology private practice. The previous evaluation, which was performed at another clinic, involved the use of 226-Hz tympanometry and ABR testing. The 226-Hz tympanograms were interpreted as normal in each ear, and the ABR evaluation was consistent with a mild to moderate hearing loss with a reverse-slope configuration.

On the day of the testing, the patient was found to have flat 1000-Hz tympanogram tracings in each ear. The ABR testing verified a bilateral mild to moderate conductive hearing loss in each ear (**Fig. 14.6**). The results of masked bone-conduction ABR testing revealed normal ABR responses down to a level of 5 dB nHL bilaterally. There was no indication that this child had any form of inner ear hearing loss. Two months later, the patient had surgery for pressure equalization (PE) tube placement in each ear. The physician again referred the child to our facility for testing to ensure that there was no residual conductive hearing loss that was unrelated to the fluid/effusion in her ears. The results of this subsequent air-conduction ABR were consistent with normal hearing sensitivity to click and tone-burst stimuli. The parents were elated to learn that their child had normal hearing. They had previously been told by the first facility's audiologist that their daughter had a bilateral permanent hearing loss that would likely become worse. This case points out the necessity of using other test measures to help verify the nature of each patient's hearing loss. It also illuminates how important accurate waveform analysis is.

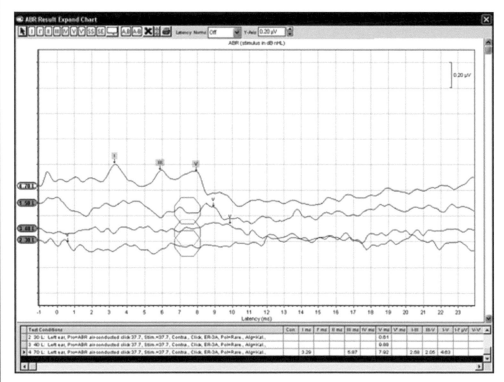

Fig. 14.6 This screen shot shows that the wave V waveforms were delayed in latency in this 4-month-old child with conductive hearing loss. The waveforms were obtained using a Vivosonic Integrity ABR system.

Case 4: Autistic Adolescent with Normal Hearing Sensitivity

A 13-year-old male patient had been previously diagnosed with autism. He was nonverbal but did communicate through a picture-exchange system. His verbal and nonverbal IQs were estimated to be somewhere between 50 and 55. Previous hearing evaluations at other facilities had involved behavioral evaluations, including visual reinforcement audiometry (VRA) and speech detection testing in the sound field. The earlier test results indicated a mild hearing loss in at least one ear. Ear-specific tests of hearing were not attempted in the past because of the patient's level of tactile defensiveness; he would become physically agitated if his ears were touched or manipulated.

On the day of the ABR evaluation, one of the first questions asked of his mother was what reinforced this boy to complete tasks. It was found that a type of fruit candy was very reinforcing to him, as well as deep pressure on his head and upper back. It was quickly found that the boy would not allow the audiologist to place any sort of probe tip in his ears. The reinforcement strategies were attempted but were unsuccessful. The boy was then asked to place the probe in his own ear for tympanometry after it was modeled for him. It was found that he would copy placing the probe and insert the earphone. Essentially, this boy placed the headphones and electrodes himself with hand-over-hand assistance from the audiologist. Because this evaluation was completed using a Vivosonic Integrity wireless ABR system, the actual waveforms were collected while the boy and the audiologist walked around the clinic hallways and into a gym area that had a basketball hoop. As the waveforms were collected on the laptop, the audiologist and the patient played basketball (**Fig. 14.7**). The boy was estimated to have normal hearing in each ear, as recorded via air-conduction ABR testing. The point of this case study is to provide a sample of what strategies can be employed to assist in successfully completing ABR assessment in difficult-to-test populations.

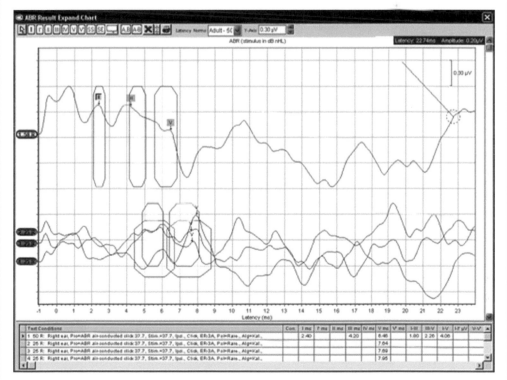

Fig. 14.7 Sample air-conduction waveforms from an 13-year-old boy with autism for whom previous testing was unable to be completed because of behavioral issues. Using a Vivosonic Inegrity System, these waveforms were collected while the audiologist played basketball with the patient. The patient placed the electrodes and insert earphones himself with the aid of a mirror. The Vivosonic unit was placed in a backpack and worn by the boy during the testing procedure.

◆ Summary

Threshold estimation using ABR remains the test of choice for infants and young children before they are able to complete behavioral testing. With experience, preparedness, patience, effective protocols, and proper instrumentation, fairly accurate threshold estimations can be obtained using conventional evoked potential systems either with natural sleep or sedation. Although not yet in widespread clinical use, newer technologies, such as the Vivosonic Integrity system, may offer a more patient-friendly option for obtaining ABR thresholds without sleep or sedation. Clinicians would do well to stay current with published guidelines, research, calibration method issues, and developing technologies. Regardless of the technology, the popularity of the ABR as a diagnostic, threshold estimation, and screening tool will likely continue to grow.

References

Abdala de Uzzcategui, C., & Yoshinaga-Itano, C. (1997). Parents' reactions to newborn hearing screening. *Audiology Today, 9*(1), 24–25.

Bagatto, M., Moodie, S., Scollie, S., Seewald, R., Moodie, S., Pumford, J., & Liu, K.P.R. (2005). Clinical protocols for hearing instrument fitting in the desired sensation level method. *Trends in Amplification, 9*(4), 199–226.

Beck, D. L., Samsson, M. L., & Moodie, S. (2009). Facilitating a smooth transfer from ABR to hearing aid fittings. *The Hearing Journal, 62*(12), 20–28.

British Columbia Early Hearing Program (2008). *Diagnostic audiology protocol.* Retrieved from http://www.phsa.ca/NR/rdonlyres/06D79FEB-D187-43E9-91E4-8C09959F38D8/40115/aDAAGProtocols1.pdf

Gilbey, P. (2010). Qualitative analysis of parents' experience with receiving the news of the detection of their child's hearing loss. *International Journal of Pediatric Otorhinolaryngology, 74*(3), 265–270. PubMed

Gorga, M. P., Johnson, T. A., Kaminski, J. R., Beauchaine, K. L., Garner, C. A., & Neely, S. T. (2006). Using a combination of click- and tone burst-evoked auditory brain stem response measurements to estimate pure-tone thresholds. *Ear and Hearing, 27*(1), 60–74. PubMed

Hall, J. W. (2007). *New handbook of auditory evoked responses.* Boston: Allyn & Bacon.

International Organization for Standardization. (2007). *Acoustics—reference zero for the calibration of audiometric equipment:6. Reference threshold of hearing for test signals of short duration* (ISO 389–6). Geneva: Author.

Karzon, R. K., & Lieu, J. E. (2006). Initial audiologic assessment of infants referred from well baby, special care, and neonatal intensive care unit nurseries. *American Journal of Audiology, 15*(1), 14–24. PubMed

Keengwe, I. N., Hegde, S., Dearlove, O., Wilson, B., Yates, R. W., & Sharples, A. (1999). Structured sedation programme for magnetic resonance imaging examination in children. *Anaesthesia, 54*(11), 1069–1072. PubMed

Keidan, I., Gozal, D., Minuskin, T., Weinberg, M., Barkaly, H., & Augarten, A. (2004). The effect of fasting practice on sedation with chloral hydrate. *Pediatric Emergency Care, 20*(12), 805–807. PubMed

Li, X., Sokolov, Y., & Kunov, H., (2002). inventors; Vivosonic Inc., assignee. (2002, October 8). System and method for processing low signal-to-noise ratio signals. U.S. Patent No. 6,463,411.

Malinoff, R. L., & Spivak, L. G. (1990). Effect of stimulus parameters on auditory brainstem response spectral analysis. *Audiology, 29*(1), 21–28. PubMed

McLeod, B., & Boheimer, N. (1985). Propofol ("Diprivan") infusion as main agent for day case surgery. *Postgraduate Medical Journal, 61*(Suppl 3), 105–107. PubMed

Oates, P., & Stapells, D. R. (1998). Auditory brainstem response estimates of the pure-tone audiogram: Current status. *Seminars in Hearing, 19*(1), 61–85.

Ontario Infant Hearing Program. (2008). *Audiologic assessment protocol.* Retrieved from http://www.mountsinai.on.ca/care/infant-hearing-program/documents/IHPAudiologicAssessmentProtocol3.1FinalJan2008.pdf

Purdie, J. A. M., & Cullen, P. M. (1993, Mar). Brainstem auditory evoked response during propofol anaesthesia in children. *Anaesthesia, 48*(3), 192–195. PubMed

Ronchera-Oms, C. L., Casillas, C., Martí-Bonmatí, L., Poyatos, C., Tomás, J., Sobejano, A., et al. (1994). Oral chloral hydrate provides effective and safe sedation in paediatric magnetic resonance imaging. *Journal of Clinical Pharmacy and Therapeutics, 19*(4), 239–243. PubMed

Sanderson, J. H., & Blades, J. F. (1988). Multicentre study of propofol in day case surgery. *Anaesthesia, 43*(Suppl), 70–73. PubMed

Sauter, T. B. (2007). Initial audiologic assessment of infants: Comments on Karzon and Lieu (2006). *American Journal of Audiology, 16*(1), 75–76, author reply 77–78. PubMed

Sininger, Y. S. (2007). The use of the auditory brainstem response in screening for hearing loss and audiometric threshold prediction. In: R. F. Burkard, M. Don, & J. J. Eggermont (Eds.), *Auditory evoked potentials: Basic principles and clinical application* (pp. 254–274). Philadelphia: Lippincott Williams & Wilkins.

Sininger, Y. S., Abdala, C., & Cone-Wesson, B. (1997). Auditory threshold sensitivity of the human neonate as measured by the auditory brainstem response. *Hearing Research, 104*(1–2), 27–38. PubMed

Stapells, D. R. (2000). Threshold estimation by the tone-evoked auditory brainstem response: A literature meta-analysis. *Journal of Speech-Language Pathology and Audiology, 24*(2), 74–83.

Stapells, D. R. (2005/2006). *Recommended recording parameters and stimulus parameters for clinical tone evoked ABR in infants.* Retrieved March 22, 2010, from http://www.courses.audiospeech.ubc.ca/haplab/TONE-ABR_PARAMETERS.html

Vade, A., Sukhani, R., Dolenga, M., & Habisohn-Schuck, C. (1995). Chloral hydrate sedation of children undergoing CT and MR imaging: Safety as judged by American Academy of Pediatrics guidelines. *AJR American Journal of Roentgenology, 165*(4), 905–909. PubMed

Chapter 15

Auditory Steady-State Responses: Clinical Applications

Julie Strickland and Alyssa Needleman

Auditory steady-state response (ASSR) is an electrophysiologic method for assessing frequency-specific hearing thresholds. It is used following a conventional auditory brainstem response (ABR) test when more specific information is needed. The ASSR can be clinically useful in an audiological setting when accurate thresholds cannot be obtained voluntarily or behaviorally. Typically, this application is useful for pediatric patients, but it can also be used when adults attempt to malinger or feign elevated thresholds. Young children and teenagers occasionally need an electrophysiologic assessment of hearing thresholds when attempts to test them behaviorally yield inconclusive or suspicious results. The ASSR can estimate the degree and the configuration of the hearing loss.

The ASSR is a frequency-specific electrophysiologic measurement that differs from ABR in that it is analyzed in the frequency rather than in the time domain. It uses modulated pure-tone stimuli and a statistical computer algorithm to determine whether a response is present. It takes most of the subjectivity away from the conventional methods of reading waveforms either via broad-spectrum click stimuli or tone-burst stimuli. Instead, clinicians rely on the computer to give a statistically significant indicator to determine whether a response is present at specific frequencies and intensity levels. For a more in-depth discussion of ASSR, including its history, comparison with other auditory evoked potentials (AEPs), instrumentation, and stimuli, interested readers are directed to Chapter 8.

> **Pearl**
>
> The beauty of the ASSR test is that there is no additional patient equipment or hardware needed other than what you would typically use for the ABR. Most manufacturers have designed equipment and computers with multipurpose software that includes both conventional ABR and ASSR. The patient does not have to change locations or positions or have electrodes added for the ASSR test following an ABR.

◆ Description of Typical Test Protocol

There are three important criteria to obtain before attempting the ASSR. First, it is best to establish normal middle ear function. A normal tympanogram and a normal otologic examination will save time in the long run. There is no sense testing a patient with middle ear dysfunction, as you will just have to repeat the test once the pathology has been treated or has resolved on its own. Second, establish that a patient has normal neural transmission through the auditory brainstem pathways by completing an ABR (Chapter 14). You will do that by stimulating the patient with a fairly high-intensity click, such as 70 to 80 dB nHL (normal hearing level). You need to establish the presence of the most important neural generators and ensure that interpeak latencies (IPLs) and amplitude ratios are normal. Assess waves I–III, III–V, and I–V IPLs. The waveform should have normal morphology, repeatability, and symmetry between sides. Third, you will want to establish a threshold for the click. To establish a threshold, decrease the intensity until you no longer see a reliable, repeatable wave V. Repeat each tracing at least twice to ensure repeatability and reliability. This will help you to determine an approximate intensity level to start in the ASSR program. If you start at too high an intensity level, you might disturb the patient's sleep or relaxation state and waste time.

Once you have finished the ABR and tympanogram, you will probably need to change to the software for the ASSR program. You should not have to change transducers, electrode configurations, or patient position. Select the ear you wish to start with; select the frequency or frequencies to test, then set the intensity based on the previously established click ABR.

Pearl

It will be important to have at least two transducer types for most settings. Most clinicians use insert earphones. However, for babies with microtia/atresia or stenotic ear canals, you should have a pair of circumaural headphones available. These can be taken out of the metal headband and propped up against the ear with a cloth or blanket. Avoid having a parent hold the earphone on the ear, as it will slide or move easily without notice. This may lead to erroneous testing of the baby's cheek instead of the ear. Caution should also be taken to avoid holding an earphone on an infant's ear by putting firm pressure, as you may collapse the canals and cause additional hearing loss.

Bone-conduction ASSR is not yet in widespread use because of the uncertainty of stimulus levels with this type of transducer (Small and Stapells, 2006, 2008; Swanepoel, Ebrahim, Friedland, Swanepoel, and Pottas, 2008). Further research is recommended before a bone-conduction stimulus is used. Likewise, obtaining ASSR thresholds with amplification has had limited study (Damarla and Manjula, 2007). However, this information will likely be very useful to the pediatric practitioner in the near future.

Standard electrodes are used for ASSR testing just as for ABR testing. Some clinicians use the standard skin prep/electrode cream/tape method. Others use disposable electrodes. Either is acceptable provided you get low, matched impedances. As recommended for standard electrophysiologic assessment, impedances should be less than 5 kΩ (kiloohms), ideally less than 1 to 3 kΩ, and matched within 2 kΩ (Hall, 1992). Attempts to do any electrophysiologic testing with unmatched electrodes and high impedances will result in a poor test session with unreliable data.

The electrode montage required for ASSR is also a standard montage for ABR. No changes are required for ASSR. We typically test vertex (Cz, noninverting) to the ipsilateral mastoid or earlobe (inverting), with the contralateral ear serving as the ground. When the soft spot (or fontanel) in infants is a concern, the noninverting electrode could also be placed on the high forehead (Fz). Other montages frequently used are dual vertex to mastoid and vertex to nape with a ground on the shoulder.

Most ASSR systems offer the ability to test four frequencies. Typically, the selection includes 500, 1000, 2000, and 4000 Hz. At least one system we are aware of offers a wider range of test frequencies (e.g., 250–8000 Hz). Additional frequencies can be very beneficial, depending on your clinical caseload. Those involved with pediatric testing will find the flexibility of more frequencies helpful. Interoctave testing may be required for patients who have hearing loss with unusual configurations. Likewise, patients receiving chemotherapy or other ototoxic drug therapy may need additional frequencies tested to determine the extent of the hearing loss. Some manufacturers offer the ability to test multiple frequencies simultaneously, whereas others require you to test only one frequency at a time. You will have to determine the needs of your caseload in your particular setting. Although testing multiple frequencies in both ears sounds attractive, we have found the correlation of the ASSR to subsequent behavioral thresholds to be superior when testing only one frequency in one ear at a time (see also Swanepoel, Hugo, and Roode, 2004). Some equipment will require you to lower the modulation rate when testing only one frequency at a time. It is not known whether or not this lower modulation rate is the reason for superior clinical correlations.

If you are testing a patient who had a normal click threshold (e.g., 20 dB nHL), testing all four frequencies simultaneously in one ear at threshold (if you have that option) will help provide information about the audiometric configuration. If you are unable to get results in the normal range from 500 to 4000 Hz, then you will want to establish thresholds at individual frequencies. In our clinic we start at 500 Hz, then move to 1000, 2000, and finally 4000 Hz. Remember, in most cases your click stimulus will generally reflect activity from 1500 to 4000 Hz, with most of the energy centered on 2000 to 4000 Hz.

In patients with a higher threshold, test each frequency starting at an intensity level around the click threshold and increase or decrease your intensity as needed. For patients who have no click response at 90 dB nHL, test each frequency separately starting at 100 dB. Try not to exceed 100 or 110 dB, as you may get a response that is artifactual in nature. If you do not get a response at this high-intensity level, move on to another frequency. Make sure to mask, when appropriate, per regular electrophysiologic rules for masking.

Patients who do not have normal neural transmission, including those with auditory neuropathy spectrum disorder (ANSD), those with significant neurologic diagnoses, and those with an asynchronous brainstem response, are not likely to be candidates for ASSR testing. Test results for these individuals will not necessarily correlate with subsequent behavioral test results. This may be due to the differences in filter settings between the ABR and ASSR (Cone, 2008). There are certain instances when it is inappropriate to follow up ABR testing with ASSR testing. Some examples include when a click response at a high intensity appears to be a reversing cochlear microphonic (CM), when a click response at a high intensity does not yield any response from the rostral brainstem generators (i.e., no wave V), when a click response at a high intensity has repeatable but uninterpretable waveforms, and when a click response at a high intensity yields poorly formed, asynchronous waveforms. In these situations, the ASSR rarely correlates well with behavioral thresholds.

◆ Instrumentation, Setup, and Patient Preparation

Several manufacturers have commercially available ASSR systems and they are typically paired with ABR systems. When looking for equipment, you will want to "test drive" a system for several weeks. Ask the manufacturer's representative to provide enough training to get you started, then use the system on your patients. If you are in a hospital setting, you will need to have the biomedical department safety check the system before using it on a patient. This is a simple procedure that takes about 2 minutes. The technician plugs the system into a unit that checks for electrical leakage. If the system passes, the technician will place an approved sticker on the system. Every piece of patient-related equipment goes through this process.

When making the decision to purchase equipment, you will want to consider ease of use, appropriate features for your setting, size, portability, cost, warranty, service, and technical support. The more intuitive a software program is, the easier it will be to use. As mentioned, look for flexibility in the software. That is, you will want to determine whether you can make changes to the protocol without going into a programming mode. Can you make impromptu changes during a test session? Is there a pause button? You will want to be able to pause when a patient is moving or changing sleep stages. Find out whether the system has the ability to switch electrode montages internally. This is called electrode switching. Some systems will require you to reposition the test ear electrode in another jack on your patient connection box if you do not have automatic electrode switching. Stopping to change electrodes when switching between test ears wastes time. This is something you can easily forget and will end up testing the contralateral ear, yielding inaccurate information.

Some software programs provide the clinician with the ability to print an estimated electrophysiologic audiogram. Some have a default setting that automatically adjusts the threshold. Others provide a larger range for threshold possibilities. Still others allow for an adjustment but have the flexibility to leave the threshold just where it was obtained. These features will have to be explored with your particular system.

Your test environment should be designed the same as for an ABR test. The environment should be peaceful and conducive to relaxation and sleep. Consider a calming color on the walls with minimal or no artwork so as not to stimulate a patient of any age. Light switches should be on a rheostat so they can be dimmed during the test while still allowing adequate lighting for the clinician. A reclining chair for adults and older children works very well and does not take up as much room as a full-size bed or exam table. A recliner that is also a rocking chair will double for parents who will hold their babies in their arms during the testing. For those babies who will not sleep well in their parent's arms, a crib is necessary. The crib will double as a diaper-changing table. A room with a sink is also helpful when your patient population includes infants.

The ASSR is much smaller than the ABR (Hall, 2004). That is, ABR amplitudes are measured in microvolts (μV), whereas the ASSR is measured in nanovolts (nV). Therefore, the patient's state and test environment are critical to the success of the test session and results. Physiologic as well as ambient environmental and electrical noise must be kept to a minimum. We also recommend that the patient be in a natural sleep state or sedated to obtain the most reliable results.

The natural sleep state for infants requires the parents to follow specific pretest instructions. First, the parents must try to keep the baby awake during the trip to the test facility. Frequently a second adult in the car is necessary to help the parent. It is best if the test is scheduled close to a feeding time so the baby comes to the appointment both hungry and tired. Most babies will fall asleep after a feeding. The baby should be burped, have a clean diaper, swaddled, and made as comfortable as possible. Adjust the lighting per the parents' request. They will know what works best for their child. Sometimes a pacifier is required to get the baby to sleep, but remember that the sucking may interfere with the recording session by producing too much myogenic (muscle) noise. To get the parents to follow these directions, reminder phone calls and written information sent to the home in advance of the appointment are helpful.

For pediatric patients too old to fall asleep naturally, sedation may be necessary. Many institutions have the ability to develop a protocol for sedation that involves additional medical professionals. Sedated testing can be labor intensive; it must be done in a controlled environment with adequate emergency backup equipment and support personnel in the event of a serious reaction to the medication. In our facility, we use conscious sedation for patients 12 months and older. The parents must follow rigorous presedation instructions, including sleep deprivation and no eating or drinking several hours prior to testing. As with the nonsedated patients, specific instructions are given by telephone and in writing before the appointment. These patients are examined by a pediatric nurse practitioner, who will complete a history and physical. The patient must be healthy and have clear lungs/normal airway, normal ear exam, and no contraindications to the medication. The patient may not have fever, otorrhea, and/or congestion. If the parents deviated from the instructions in any way (e.g., the patient had a sip of water within the past 2 hours before the test), the testing is rescheduled. Unfortunately, despite our best efforts, some parents fail to follow instructions and are sent home without results. Although this seems harsh, it is best not to take any chances with the safety of our patients. Once the pre-sedation questionnaire is completed and the patient is examined, the nurse will determine whether the presedation criteria were met. The patient is weighed and given 50 mg/kg of chloral hydrate sedation by mouth. If the patient has not fallen asleep in 20 minutes, an additional 20 mg/kg is given (Rady Children's Hospital San Diego, 2008). Patients fall asleep on a bed and are placed on their back whenever possible to have equal access to both ears.

Some facilities can offer anesthesia for testing. This requires the services of an anesthesiologist or a nurse anesthetist and either an inhalation agent or intravenous access for delivery of a drug to sedate. Each facility exploring either option would have to evaluate the availability of personnel, reimbursement possibilities, location, space availability, emergency backup equipment, and emergency code team response time in the event of a serious complication.

Older pediatric patients can be sleep-deprived and scheduled for an appointment after the end of the school day. Most older children and teenagers are ready for a nap at that time. Attempt to test adults in a natural state of relaxation the first time. If you cannot get adequate information and threshold information, which is critical for a legal or workers' compensation case, consider requesting a mild sedative, such as Valium. The patient must have someone available to drive him or her home before leaving the facility.

◆ Measurement Techniques

The ASSR uses broadband amplitude- and frequency-modulated pure tones to elicit a response. Consider an amplitude-modulated pure tone (**Fig. 15.1**). In **Fig. 15.1**, the carrier frequency is a pure tone (i.e., 1000 Hz), and the carrier tone is amplitude modulated at 85 Hz. This means the carrier tone's envelope ramps up and down 85 times per second.

Consider a system that allows you to use four carrier tone frequencies at once. Each pure tone is modulated at a different rate. If we add all these waveforms together, we have created a complex amplitude- and frequency-modulated signal. When this modulated signal is presented to the ear, it will have the effect of stimulating the cochlea at four different regions along the basilar membrane (relative to the 500-, 1000-, 2000-, and 4000-Hz tones in the example). As the cochlea is stimulated, the brain "hears" the different modulation rates, which can be extracted from the electroencephalographic (EEG) activity (**Fig. 15.2**). The reason we can simultaneously present four frequencies is because each carrier tone is modulated at a different frequency, and the modulation frequencies are what is measured in the EEG. If the same modulation frequencies were used, you would not be able to identify the carrier frequency to which it was related. It is knowing which modulation rate is used with each of the carrier frequencies that allows us to examine the responses to multiple frequencies simultaneously.

Some systems now use "chirp" stimuli to elicit the ASSR. Chirps incorporate higher harmonics in the detection algorithms. For example, if the frequency is 90 Hz, the ASSR will occur at 90, 180, 270, 360, and so on. The theory behind this is that it enables more hair cells to be stimulated at lower intensity levels while producing response amplitudes twice as large as previous stimuli (Elberling, Don, Cebulla, and Stürzebecher, 2007). It is thought that chirp stimuli allow for faster data collection,

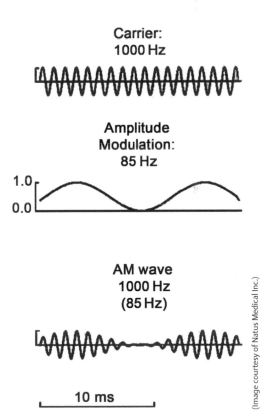

Fig. 15.1 Amplitude-modulated (AM) waveform with 85-Hz modulation frequency and 1000-Hz carrier frequency.

(Image courtesy of Natus Medical Inc.)

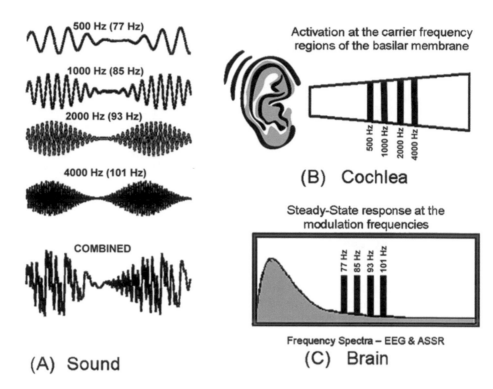

(Image courtesy of Natus Medical Inc.)

Fig. 15.2 **(A)** Auditory steady-state response (ASSR) stimulus: four amplitude- and frequency–modulated waveforms, with carrier frequencies ranging from 500 to 4000 Hz and modulation frequencies ranging from 77 to 101 Hz. **(B)** The carrier frequencies stimulate four distinct regions of the basilar membrane. **(C)** The modulation frequencies can be seen as spikes in the electroencephalogram (EEG) activity.

approaching half the traditional ASSR data collection time.

Another important consideration when selecting the modulation frequencies is where the response is generated. At modulation rates lower than 60 Hz, the auditory midbrain, thalamus, and primary auditory cortex are thought to be stimulated, similar to middle and late evoked potentials, and can be affected by sleep state (Kuwada, Anderson, Batra, Fitzpatrick, Teissier, and D'Angelo, 2002). At higher modulation rates (>60 Hz), the neural generators are similar to that of the ABR. Modulation rates commonly default to >60 Hz in commercially available software for the purposes of threshold estimation.

If you have experience with ABR and/or other AEPs, you are probably accustomed to looking at EEG activity in the time domain. To interpret the signal for an ASSR, a fast Fourier transform (FFT) calculation transforms the signal from the time domain, converts it to the frequency domain, and determines the frequencies within that response and the amplitude of the response at each of the frequencies (**Fig. 15.3**). The spikes are the frequencies of the modulation; these are the ones that are most important to us because this is where we are looking for the response to stimuli.

The technology and interpretation will depend on the manufacturer you choose. Two primary methods are used by manufacturers to determine the ASSR response. The first uses FFT calculations on each sweep of data to convert it to the frequency domain, and an F ratio is used to statistically evaluate the energy at each modulation frequency compared with the energy in surrounding frequency bins. An algorithm in the system then compares the amplitude of the modulation frequency with the amplitude of the noise around it (John, Dimitrijevic, van Roon, and Picton, 2001).

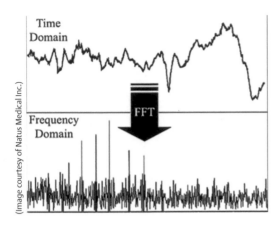

(Image courtesy of Natus Medical Inc.)

Time
Domain

FFT

Frequency
Domain

Fig. 15.3 Fast Fourier transform (FFT) analysis of the electroencephalographic activity from the time domain (*top*) to the frequency domain (*bottom*). The modulation frequencies can be seen as spikes in the frequency spectrum, indicating the auditory steady-state response response above the EEG noise.

The good news is you do not have to make all these calculations; you just need to look at the statistical significance. On the Biologic Multiple Auditory Steady-State Evoked Response (MASTER, Natus Medical Inc.,

Mundelein, IL), a *p* value is used. A statistical calculation determines the probability of the response being present; it is also color-coded on the screen. A *p* statistic greater than .10 suggests the response is not present; the response will show up in red on the screen. A p statistic between .051 and .10 suggests a 90% probability the response is present, and this will show up as yellow on the computer screen. A *p* statistic .05 suggests a 95% probability the response is present; this will show up as green on the computer. You want to accept those responses that are green, or having 95% likelihood of being a response at that intensity level (**Fig. 15.4**).

The second method used for determining the ASSR response incorporates polar plots to evaluate phase coherence (Cone-Wesson, Rickards, Poulis, Parker, Tan, and Pollard, 2002). This method uses an FFT spectral analysis of the EEG signal and looks at the phase of the EEG relative to the modulation frequency. When a response is present, EEG samples are in phase; this is called "phase locking" or phase coherence (**Fig. 15.5**). Any phase lag between the stimulus and the response can be seen on the circular plot. The phase latency of

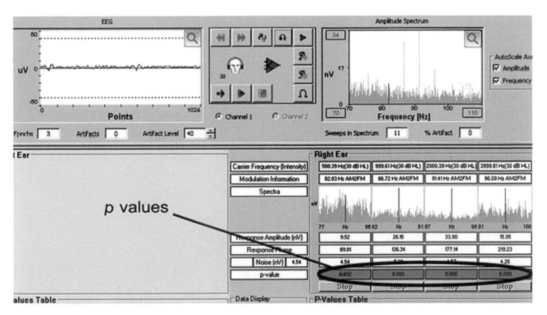

Fig. 15.4 Bio-logic MASTER collection screen of actual patient data indicating probability (*p* values) <.05 (circled). The large spikes on the frequency spectra show the auditory steady-state response above the electroencephalographic noise for each frequency.

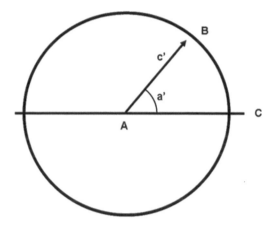

Fig. 15.5 Polar plot depicting phase latency information to detect the auditory steady-state response response. Vectors around the plot indicate phase lag between the modulation frequency and electroencephalogram (a'), as well as the magnitude of that response (c').

each response is plotted as a vector along the circular plot. The vector angle (a') represents the phase lag of the modulation frequency response relative to the EEG at the modulation frequency. The vector length (c') represents the magnitude of the response.

Random EEG activity shows up as noise; resulting in the random distribution in the phase angles (**Fig. 15.6A**). When a response is present, you will see phase coherence on the circular plot. The phase of the vectors of the EEG at the modulation frequencies cluster along the plot; this cluster is a visual representation of phase coherence (**Fig. 15.6B**). The system determines the probability of the phase coherence values being statistically significant or different from the random EEG

noise. Some systems also uses color coding. When EEG activity is detected that is less than the noise threshold, the vector plot in the vector view window is colored black. When the signal strength exceeds the noise threshold, the plot changes to purple. Similarly, the progressive plot displayed in the probability view window is colored black when it has not reached statistical significance and purple once it reaches statistical significance. **Figure 15.7** shows both the vector plot and the probability view (VIASYS Healthcare Inc., 2007).

Whichever method is used to determine the ASSR response, the final result is plotted on an estimated audiogram. **Figure 15.8** shows an example of estimated audiogram using ASSR thresholds, with thresholds at 20 dB or less with an up-arrow symbol. Most ASSR systems provide correction tables to convert the ASSR responses to estimated HL (hearing level) audiograms (Bio-logic, 2008; Interacoustics A/S, 2007; VIASYS Healthcare Inc., 2007). It is always best to collect your own normative data.

◆ Reporting Findings

There will be many pediatric cases where the electrophysiologic assessment will be the only information you have before the time comes when you can obtain a reliable behavioral audiological test result. Some more involved patients will never be successfully tested in a sound booth. It is important to remember that the ABR is not a test of hearing abilities; it is a test of peripheral auditory sensitivity. It can provide an estimate of auditory thresholds

(A)

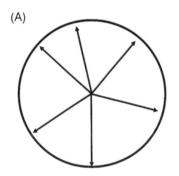

(B)

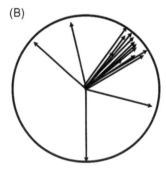

Fig. 15.6 (**A**) Random encephalography; vectors are randomly distributed around the plot. (**B**) Phase coherence; vectors cluster at the modulation frequency.

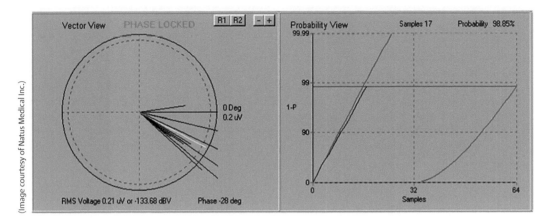

Fig. 15.7 GSI Audera collection screen of actual patient data indicating phase coherence (vectors clustered in the lower right quadrant) and high probability (98.85%) of a response.

Estimated Physiologic Audiogram

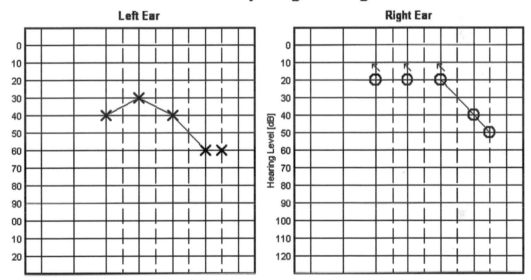

Fig. 15.8 Estimated physiologic audiogram. Arrows indicate responses < 20 dB nHL.

in some cases. The same holds true for ASSR. Although ASSR can provide an estimate of auditory sensitivity at more specific and discrete frequencies, the behavioral threshold audiogram is still the gold standard.

When reporting ASSR findings, be sure to include verbiage that indicates the results are an approximation. Such verbiage might be "ASSR predicted estimated behavioral thresholds in the moderate to severe range for the frequencies 500 to 4000 Hz."

♦ Case Studies

The ASSR can provide a wealth of information that will allow you to more accurately estimate the degree and configuration of hearing loss, as well as more confidently program hearing aids for very young children. By following some of the guidelines set forth in this chapter, we have found that there is a strong correlation between the ASSR and the audiogram once we are able to verify behavioral thresholds.

Case 1

A 14-month-old female patient had a normal birth history and was born without complication, but she did not pass the newborn hearing screening (NHS) for her right ear. There was a family history of right-sided hearing loss, with one sibling exhibiting a draining cyst on the right ear and another relative with stenosis of the right ear canal. ABR testing indicated normal peripheral auditory sensitivity on the left and responses down to 65 dB nHL on the right, suggesting a moderately severe peripheral abnormality for the frequency range 1500 to 4000 Hz. The ASSR predicted auditory thresholds in the moderate to severe range for the right ear. Follow-up behavioral testing in the sound booth confirmed the ASSR findings (**Fig. 15.9**).

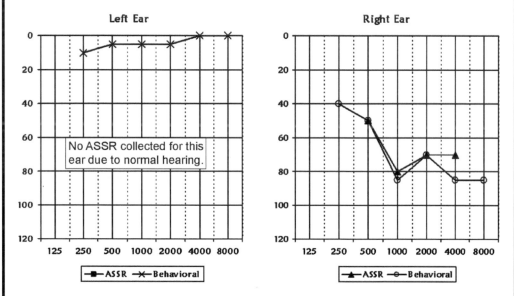

Fig. 15.9 Behavioral audiometric thresholds and auditory steady-state response (ASSR) estimated physiologic thresholds for Case 1.

Case 2

A 6-month-old female patient was the product of a normal pregnancy and born without complication, but she did not pass her NHS. ABR responses were obtained down to 60 dB nHL bilaterally, suggesting a moderate hearing loss for the frequency range 1500 to 4000 Hz. The ASSR predicted thresholds in the normal range at 500 to 1000 Hz, sloping to moderate range at 2000 to 4000 Hz for the left ear, and normal hearing at 500 Hz, sloping to mild to moderate hearing loss at 1000 to 4000 Hz for the right ear. Follow-up audiometric testing in the sound booth confirmed the ASSR findings (**Fig. 15.10**). This case demonstrates why hearing aids should not be fit solely on the click ABR alone. The click ABR suggested a moderate hearing loss, yet hearing sensitivity in the low frequencies was normal.

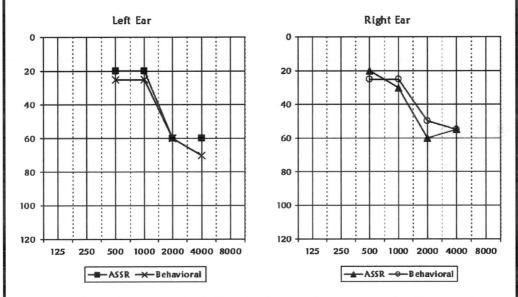

Fig. 15.10 Behavioral audiometric thresholds and auditory steady-state response (ASSR) estimated physiologic thresholds for Case 2.

Case 3

A 15-year-old female patient had a unilateral profound sensorineural hearing loss in the right ear. She reported having this from birth and now wanted a hearing aid. She denied having any communication difficulties at home and very few difficulties at school. Audiometric testing revealed a profound right sensorineural hearing loss, but several inconsistencies were noted. ABR testing indicated normal peripheral auditory sensitivity on the left and responses down to 50 dB nHL on the right, suggesting a moderate peripheral abnormality for the frequency range 1500 to 4000 Hz. The ASSR predicted auditory thresholds in the mild to moderate range for the right ear. On further discussion with the patient, follow-up behavioral audiometric testing in the sound booth revealed greater consistency with the ASSR findings (**Fig. 15.11**). Of note, this ASSR was completed using simultaneous multiple-frequency ASSR. We have found slightly poorer correlation with audiometric thresholds when completing ASSR with this protocol rather than stimulating each frequency separately (e.g., Swanepoel et al, 2004).

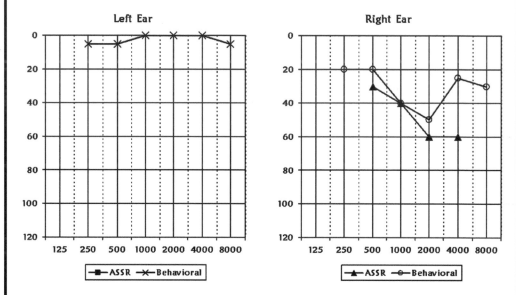

Fig. 15.11 Behavioral audiometric thresholds and auditory steady-state response (ASSR) estimated physiologic thresholds for Case 3.

Case 4

A 4-year-old male patient presented with slight to mild hearing loss bilaterally. There were concerns about auditory processing disorder and hyperactivity, as well as a history of a previous cotton swab injury. ABR testing indicated a slight hearing loss bilaterally for the frequency range 1500 to 4000 Hz. The ASSR predicted thresholds in the normal range at 500 Hz in the left and 500 and 4000 Hz in the right, dropping to a slight loss at 1000 to 4000 Hz in the left and 1000 to 2000 Hz for the right ear. These ASSR findings were consistent with the behavioral results (**Fig. 15.12**). This case demonstrates that the ASSR can be used to accurately assess thresholds for mild hearing losses.

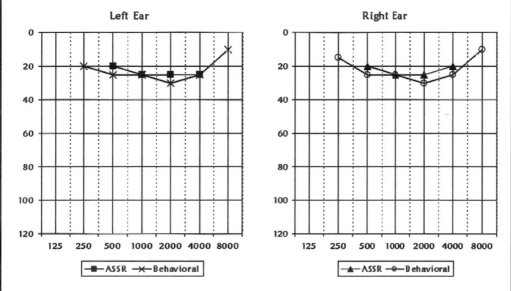

Fig. 15.12 Behavioral audiometric thresholds and auditory steady-state response (ASSR) estimated physiologic thresholds for Case 4.

Case 5

A 6-year-old female patient was born prematurely at 30 weeks' gestational age. The patient remained in the neonatal intensive care unit (NICU) for 6 months following birth, receiving oxygen and ventilator support. There were numerous other complications typical of a premature infant. She reportedly passed the NHS at discharge from the NICU. When seen for electrophysiologic testing, the patient had failed a hearing screening in school, and behavioral test results were judged to be unreliable. Parental concerns regarding the patient's hearing loss began following administration of Viagra for pulmonary hypertension; she had also been treated with loop diuretics. ABR click responses were obtained down to 60 dB nHL bilaterally, suggesting a moderate peripheral hearing loss for the frequency range 1500 to 4000 Hz. The ASSR predicted thresholds in the profound rising to moderate range for the left ear and severe rising to mild range for the right ear. Follow-up behavioral testing in the sound booth confirmed the ASSR findings (**Fig. 15.13**). A conductive component was observed with normal middle ear function and normal computed tomography (CT) scans. Viagra use was discontinued by the cardiologist following the diagnosis of hearing loss; there was no further progression of hearing loss, nor was there any improvement in the conductive component.

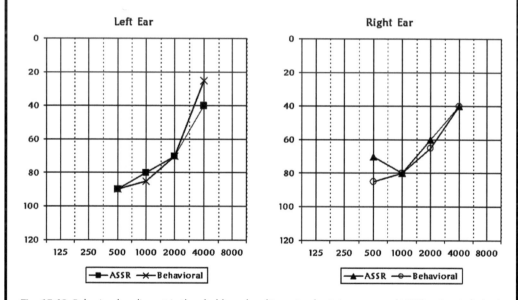

Fig. 15.13 Behavioral audiometric thresholds and auditory steady-state response (ASSR) estimated physiologic thresholds for Case 5.

Case 6

A 5-year-old female patient was the product of a normal pregnancy and delivery. Her history included developmental delays, speech-language delays, attention deficit/ hyperactivity disorder (AD/HD), and prenatal substance abuse. Previous attempts to test her behaviorally were inconsistent. ABR testing indicated normal peripheral auditory sensitivity on the left and responses down to 70 dB nHL on the right, suggesting a severe peripheral hearing loss for the frequency range 1500 to 4000 Hz. The ASSR predicted thresholds in the moderate range at 500 to 2000 Hz, rising to normal at 4000 Hz for the left ear, and in the severe hearing loss range at 500 to 4000 Hz for the right ear. Follow-up audiometric testing in the sound booth confirmed the ASSR findings (**Fig. 15.14**). These test results demonstrate a very unusual configuration and asymmetry between ears. The ASSR in this case can be used to validate the behavioral findings, particularly for a patient who is difficult to test. However, there was a discrepancy between the click ABR and the ASSR/behavioral thresholds. The ABR indicated normal peripheral sensitivity, likely picking up the normal threshold at 4000 Hz. However, relying solely on the click ABR would have missed the significant moderate component in the low frequencies that should be addressed with amplification.

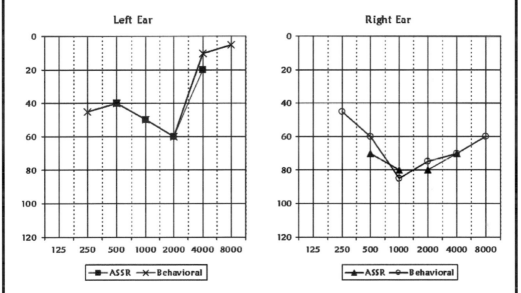

Fig. 15.14 Behavioral audiometric thresholds and auditory steady-state response (ASSR) estimated physiologic thresholds for Case 6.

✦ Summary

This chapter reviews protocols, techniques, and methods used when implementing ASSR testing and incorporating it into the electrophysiologic test battery. The ASSR adds significant value to a pediatric diagnostic test battery and yields additional information that helps to diagnose and treat all degrees of hearing loss in patients of any age.

References

Bio-logic. (2008). *Bio-logic MASTER II: User's and service manual.* Natus Medical Inc, Mundelein, IL: Author.

Cone, B. (2008, June). *The electrophysiology of auditory neuropathy spectrum disorder: Guidelines for identification and management of infants and young children with auditory neuropathy spectrum disorder.* Paper presented at the Guidelines Development Conference at NHS 2008, Como, Italy; 20–29.

Cone-Wesson, B., Rickards, F., Poulis, C., Parker, J., Tan, L., & Pollard, J. (2002). The auditory steady-state response: Clinical observations and applications in infants and children. *Journal of the American Academy of Audiology, 13*(5), 270–282. PubMed

Damarla, V. K. S., & Manjula, P. (2007). Application of the ASSR in the hearing aid selection process. *Australian and New Zealand Journal of Audiology, 29*(2), 89–97.

Elberling, C., Don, M., Cebulla, M., & Stürzebecher, E. (2007). Auditory steady-state responses to chirp stimuli based on cochlear traveling wave delay. *Journal of the Acoustical Society of America, 122*(5), 2772–2785. PubMed

Hall, J. W. (1992). *Handbook of auditory evoked responses.* Needham Heights, MA: Allyn a & Bacon.

Hall, J. W. (2004). ABRs or ASSRs? The application of tone burst ABRs in the era of ASSRs. *Hearing Review, 11*(9), 22–30, 60.

Interacoustics A/S. (2007). *The Eclipse platform: Operation manual.* Eden Prairie, MN: Author.

John, M. S., Dimitrijevic, A., van Roon, P., & Picton, T. W. (2001). Multiple auditory steady-state responses to AM and FM stimuli. *Audiology and Neuro-Otology, 6*(1), 12–27. PubMed

Kuwada, S., Anderson, J. S., Batra, R., Fitzpatrick, D. C., Teissier, N., & D'Angelo, W. R. (2002). Sources of the scalp-recorded amplitude-modulation following response. *Journal of the American Academy of Audiology, 13*(4), 188–204. PubMed

Rady Children's Hospital San Diego. (2008). *Sedation of patients undergoing diagnostic or therapeutic procedures* (CPM 5–09). San Diego: Author.

Small, S. A., & Stapells, D. R. (2006). Multiple auditory steady-state response thresholds to bone-conduction stimuli in young infants with normal hearing. *Ear and Hearing, 27*(3), 219–228. PubMed

Small, S. A., & Stapells, D. R. (2008). Normal ipsilateral/contralateral asymmetries in infant multiple auditory steady-state responses to air- and bone-conduction stimuli. *Ear and Hearing, 29*(2), 185–198. PubMed

Swanepoel, W., Ebrahim, S., Friedland, P. L., Swanepoel, A., & Pottas, L. (2008). Auditory steady-state responses to bone conduction stimuli in children with hearing loss. *International Journal of Pediatric Otorhinolaryngology, 72*(12), 1861–1871. PubMed

Swanepoel, D., Hugo, R., & Roode, R. (2004). Auditory steady-state responses for children with severe to profound hearing loss. *Archives of Otolaryngology—Head and Neck Surgery, 130*(5), 531–535. PubMed

VIASYS Healthcare Inc. (2007). *GSI Audera ASSR software user guide.* Madison, WI.

Chapter 16

Early Latency Auditory Evoked Potentials in Retrocochlear Disease and Auditory Neuropathy Spectrum Disorder

Todd Sauter and Christina L. Runge

This chapter is divided into two sections: the auditory brainstem response (ABR) in retrocochlear disease and the ABR in auditory neuropathy spectrum disorder (ANSD). Although the stimulus and recording parameters are essentially identical, the differences in pathophysiology warrant separate diagnostic approaches and interpretations. Each section features unique recording aspects, as well as sample cases.

◆ The Auditory Brainstem Response in Retrocochlear Disease

Early latency auditory evoked potentials (AEPs), specifically the ABR, have been considered a primary functional measure of retrocochlear ear disease for several decades. Researchers in the 1970s predicted that a major clinical application of the ABR would be in neurodiagnosis. This came to fruition most notably beginning with the work of Selters and Brackmann (1977), who demonstrated the very high sensitivity of the ABR to tumors of the eighth cranial nerve (CN VIII). Throughout the 1980s and 1990s, ABR testing was heavily relied on for diagnosis of lesions in CN VIII and the auditory brainstem, particularly space-occupying lesions and neurodegenerative conditions. Many clinics now bypass ABR testing in favor of imaging techniques in patients suspected to have retrocochlear involvement. This, however, should be considered an incomplete comprehensive evaluation of the auditory nervous system, as tests of structure and function are not 100% sensitive to all forms of disease. One need only look to the second section of this chapter on ANSD to find a form of retrocochlear disease that often yields normal imaging results (Buchman, Roush, Teagle, Brown, Zdanski, and Grose, 2006; Teagle et al, 2010).

◆ Candidacy for Neurodiagnostic ABR Testing

Testing should be considered for any patient with symptoms or test results that suggest retrocochlear disease. Symptoms and test results include unilateral tinnitus, unilateral or asymmetric sensorineural hearing loss, unexplained dizziness, facial nerve symptoms, significant hearing loss with normal otoacoustic emissions, unexplained poor word recognition scores or speech-in-noise scores, head injury, and the onset of auditory processing disorders (APD).

Using the ABR for neurodiagnosis should also be considered in all pediatric patients with the aforementioned symptoms, as well as any children whose ABRs evoked by tonal stimuli for threshold estimation show signs of retrocochlear involvement, such as unexplained prolonged latency compared with age-specific norms (Gorga, Kaminski, Beauchaine, Jesteadt, and Neely, 1989).

◆ Recommended Stimulus and Recording Parameters

The recommendations given here are not intended to be used without flexibility for all neurodiagnostic ABRs. To the contrary, a knowledgeable and effective clinician should be able to make adjustments to parameters when called for by subject or response differences to achieve the best response in an individual patient. The following parameters represent excellent default settings that can be used in most patients.

Recommended Stimulus Parameters

Stimulus Type: 100-μsec Click

The extreme brevity of the click stimulus onset will cause a highly synchronous firing of neurons innervating the basal regions of the cochlea, and the broadband nature of the stimulus will maximize the number of neurons that evoke the response. For patients with severe high-frequency loss or an extreme high-frequency asymmetry, the ABR can be evoked using tone bursts centered at a frequency at which hearing is more symmetric (e.g., 1000 Hz), then compared with the wave V interaural latency difference ILD V.

Rate: 21/s

The goal in setting the stimulus rate is to use the fastest rate that does not significantly alter ABR latency and amplitude. Previous research has demonstrated that, although somewhat variable for individuals, this rate falls between 20 and 30 stimuli/s (Yagi and Kaga, 1979). Maximizing the rate will expedite the overall test time or allow for increased signal averaging that will further improve the signal-to-noise ratio (SNR) and waveform morphology. In cases where wave I identification is difficult, reducing the stimulus rate to 9 or 11/s may improve the amplitude and morphology of this specific peak.

Intensity: 80 dB nHL (Normal Hearing Level) or Greater

A high-intensity stimulus is necessary to ensure identification of all major waveform components. For those with normal or near-normal thresholds, a level of 80 dB nHL (~113 dB pSPL [peak sound pressure level]) is usually sufficient. For those with hearing loss, using a stimulus level of at least 20 dB above the patient's HL thresholds at 2 to 4 kHz should limit latency prolongation resulting from cochlear pathology (Durrant and Fowler, 1996). Because most evoked potential units cannot produce a click stimulus greater than 100 dB nHL (~133 dB pSPL), the audiometric limit of sensorineural hearing loss for which neurodiagnostic ABR should be employed is 80 dB HL. It is recommended that the latencies of all ABRs evoked from ears with thresholds greater than 70 dB HL at 1 to 4 kHz be interpreted with caution. For the purpose of a more equal comparison between ears, the same stimulus intensity used in the worse hearing ear should also be used in the ear with better hearing. Stimulus intensity may also be increased further to increase the amplitude of major waveforms (e.g., wave I) if identification is difficult at a lower intensity.

Masking: Contralateral Wideband Noise 60 dB Below the Stimulus Intensity

Although it can be argued that the use of insert earphones for neurodiagnostic ABR testing negates the need for contralateral masking because of the large interaural attenuation, there is no harm in adding a noise 60 dB below the nHL value of the click to ensure that there is no contribution to the response from the nontest ear.

Polarity: Alternating with the Ability to View Separate Rarefaction and Condensation Traces

Because polarity effects are variable among subjects for click ABR latencies (Don, Vermiglio, Ponton, Eggermont, and Masuda, 1996), it is clinically desirable to have traces to

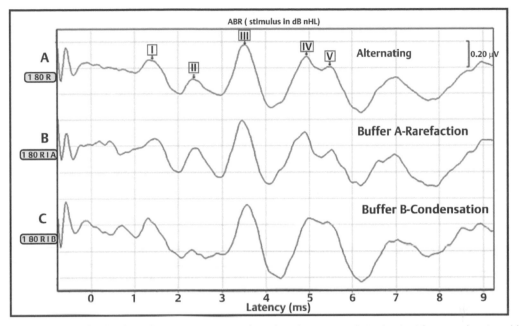

Fig. 16.1 Example of auditory brainstem responses (ABRs) to alternating polarity (top), with traces also viewable in separate buffers according to rarefaction (middle) or condensation (bottom) polarities.

both rarefaction and condensation clicks available for analysis. This can be accomplished via one of two techniques. First, separate traces to rarefaction and condensation clicks can be recorded, then summed digitally to obtain the alternating polarity response. Second, a more efficient technique now available on many systems is to record the response to alternating polarity stimuli while the device places data from every other sweep into separate memories (or "buffers"). The data from the two memories can then be viewed as separate rarefaction and condensation traces, without ever having to record them at different times (**Fig. 16.1**). Even if the alternating polarity trace is ultimately used to mark peak latencies for analysis, viewing the single polarity traces may help in peak identification when alternating polarity morphology is unusual (e.g., bifid waves or fused/downsloping IV–V complex).

Recording Parameters

Electroencephalographic Filtering: 100 to 3000 Hz

The ABR to a high-intensity stimulus includes spectral electroencephalogram (EEG) components mainly between 30 and 1500 Hz. Although it would be desirous to use open

Pitfall

A common assumption by clinicians is that rarefaction clicks produce shorter latencies than condensation clicks in all patients. This assumption is based on an overly simplistic explanation of the upward-downward basilar membrane movement in reference to the inward-outward movement of the tympanic membrane. Indeed, upward movement of the basilar membrane results in excitation of sensory hair cells; however, the traveling wave mechanics along the cochlea may be too complex for such a simple explanation. Rather, clinicians should pick a polarity and use the other one if ABR morphology to the first is deemed poor but not necessarily abnormal.

filtering, which does not eliminate any known spectral ABR energy, the overlap of lower-frequency components with electromagnetic and myogenic interference makes some high-pass filtering necessary, particularly because many patients for this testing are relaxed yet not asleep. The amplitude loss due to high-pass filtering is typically offset by the high-intensity stimulus used. Extending the low-pass filter to 3000 Hz adds a small amount of high-frequency energy, which slightly sharpens the peaks of the waves of interest, assisting in more precise latency analysis. In young children, it is essential that the high-pass filter be lowered to 30 to 50 Hz, as the spectral energy contributing to the response is lower in that population.

Signal Averaging: Variable

Because there is high inter- and intrasubject variability in "noise" while attempting to record the ABR, the amount of signal averaging should vary accordingly. Certainly no device should be set to automatically terminate averaging at the common finite number of 2000 sweeps, as this is not always adequate to resolve a response with an acceptable SNR. The often cited principle of residual noise decreasing by $\sqrt{2}$ for every doubling in the number of sweeps holds true only if the magnitude of the background noise is stable throughout testing. In fact, the magnitude of background noise may change often during testing, especially

when testing relaxed but awake adult subjects. It is recommended that the default ABR protocol allows for maximum averaging, with the audiologist determining averaging based on a combination of the audiologist's clinical judgment of response clarity and available statistical measures of SNR and/or residual noise.

The use of weighted averaging techniques, if available, is highly recommended for neurodiagnostic ABR. Again, in relaxed but awake adults, the magnitude of the background noise may fluctuate significantly over the course of the procedure. Weighted averaging addresses these fluctuations by applying a statistical weighting of less than one for sweeps collected under higher background noise conditions and greater than one for quiet noise conditions. Both Bayesian (Elberling and Wahlgreen, 1985) and Kalman (Kurtz and Steinman, 2005) statistical techniques are used in current devices. The end result is a waveform that is more representative of the quieter periods of recording and allows achievement of a response with an acceptable SNR in a much more efficient fashion. **Figure 16.2** shows an ABR collected in

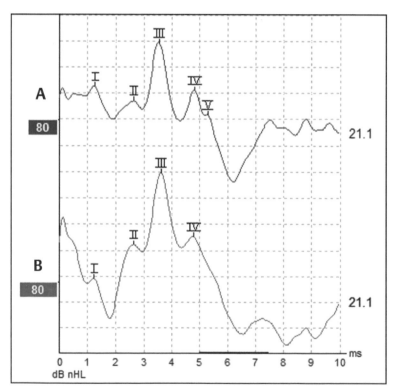

Fig. 16.2 A comparison of weighted (top) versus unweighted (bottom) averaging.

an awake subject with weighted signal averaging after 2000 sweeps are collected, and shows the same subject after 2000 sweeps without weighted averaging.

Artifact Rejection: Approximately ± 25 µV

Artifact rejection will remove any sweeps in which the EEG voltage exceeds a set criterion from the overall average. Too lenient a setting will allow sweeps with extensive noise to contaminate the average, whereas too strict a setting may reject too high a percentage of sweeps to allow testing to proceed. This setting is typically set higher (more lenient) for neurodiagnostic ABR because the amplitude of the response (and SNR) is greater than for threshold ABR applications, where even slight contamination of the response may lead to interpretation errors. Weighted averaging also allows for a more lenient rejection setting without significant response deterioration.

Electrode Montage: Cz/Fz (+) to Ipsilateral Earlobe (−)

Placing the noninverting recording electrode at true vertex is known to maximize brainstem AEP amplitude compared with other locations. For this reason, it is recommended that this electrode be placed as close to Cz as feasible. In some patients with thick scalp hair, preparing the skin and placing and securing the electrode may prove difficult and interfere with the clinical efficiency of the test, especially with the current popularity of the thicker, disposable EEG electrodes. Although some would argue that Cz should always be the noninverting site at any cost, the primary effect of moving to a more frontal (Fz) location is a slight loss of waveform amplitude. This may be critical in threshold estimation applications of the ABR, but in neurodiagnosis amplitude it is not nearly as important for interpretation and not difficult to achieve when using high-intensity click stimuli. Given the significant variety of hairline locations among individual patients, the recommendation is to use a midline location as close to true vertex as possible without requiring time-consuming hair/scalp preparation.

For the inverting (−) electrode, the earlobe location is recommended rather than the mastoid not because of any significant amplitude advantage, for which evidence is underwhelming, but to better avoid contamination of the response with postauricular muscle (PAM) artifact. The PAM sonomotor reflex can be problematic in neurodiagnostic ABR interpretation, as it is easily evoked in awake subjects who have not relaxed adequately when using a high-intensity stimulus. The latency of the PAM response (~12 msec) can overlap with the later ABR waveforms and complicate peak marking and interpretation. Even with an earlobe electrode, PAM artifact is sometimes problematic and the use of a noncephalic (off the scalp) inverting electrode site is necessary, such as the nape of the neck at the seventh cervical vertebra.

An excellent alternative to using the earlobe as the inverting site is to use an ear canal electrode, such as a TIPtrode (Bauch and Olsen, 1990; Brantberg, 1996). This is known to create an amplitude enhancement for wave I, presumably by moving the electrode closer to its anatomical generator (the distal end of CN VIII). The wave I–V interpeak latency (IPL) is known to be one of the most powerful neurodiagnostic ABR measures, though at times the wave I peak is poorly formed or absent, especially in patients with high-frequency sensorineural hearing loss, making the I–V IPL impossible to calculate. The use of an ear canal electrode should make wave I marking easier and more accurate or even allow identification of the wave when it did not exist using an earlobe or mastoid recording site. In fact, a strong argument can be made to routinely use ear canal electrodes for the inverting location if their placement does not significantly prolong testing.

> **Pearl**
>
> Clinicians should consider the use of an ear canal inverting electrode (e.g., TIPtrode) to enhance wave I for neurodiagnostic ABRs.

We do not routinely record from a contralateral channel (Fz to contralateral earlobe) in our clinic for neurodiagnostic purposes, although this is popular in many clinics and laboratories, as we feel the possible clinical advantages are outweighed by the additional waveform overcomplicating interpretation or even perhaps being mistaken for the ipsilateral waveform. The one time we may record a contralateral response is to assist in the identification of the wave V peak when there is a highly fused wave IV–V complex that cannot be resolved by looking at the rarefaction and condensation polarity traces individually (see the discussion of polarity later in this chapter).

◆ ABR Analysis and Interpretation

Peak Picking

Because latency values of the major waveform peaks account for the vast majority of neurodiagnostic ABR interpretive measurements, a discussion of peak-picking skills is warranted. One aspect that makes peak picking even more complicated is that even the normal ABR waveform peaks can be extremely varied. Although waves II, IV, and VI have little known diagnostic value, their variations can complicate the overall judgment of the waveform. One must also be wary of evoked potential devices that offer automated peak-picking functions that are based mainly on voltage maximums and do not account for missing, fused, and bifid peaks.

Consistency in how peaks are marked in a clinic or laboratory is of significant importance.

Most clinicians mark the absolute peak of a wave, but others prefer to mark the "shoulder" of the wave following the true peak. The method must be consistent, and the normative data used by the clinic must have been collected using the same technique. The reader is directed to Chapter 3 for more information on peak picking.

Determining a Normal or Abnormal Neurodiagnostic ABR

A review of the literature indicates that the two most powerful ABR indices are the wave I–V interpeak latency (IPL) and the interaural latency difference of wave V (ILD V) (Bauch, Olsen, and Pool, 1996). Other useful indices with somewhat lesser sensitivity and specificity are the absolute latency of waves III and V, the wave I–III and III–V IPLs, the I–V ILD, and the wave I/V amplitude ratio. Cutoff values for these indices should be based on clinical goals and algorithms within the diagnostic test battery as a whole. If a clinician uses the ABR as a screening tool prior to ordering imaging studies, then it is recommended that strict cutoff values be used that err on the side of sensitivity (i.e., ILD V of 0.2 msec), although this still does not guarantee a positive test in all radiologically detectable auditory lesions (Cueva, 2004). If the ABR is used simply (and correctly, in our opinion) as the functional measure of the auditory nerve and brainstem, and the decision to pursue imaging studies is not entirely dependent on the result, then somewhat more lenient cutoff values are recommended to describe an abnormal study (e.g., ILD V of 0.4 msec).

The effects of high-frequency hearing loss must be considered not only for candidacy for ABR testing, but also in latency interpretation. One common scenario involves a patient with a unilateral high-frequency hearing loss with a prolonged wave I but relatively normal wave V latency, which results in a shortened wave I–V IPL compared with the "normal" ear. The I–V ILD may then be asymmetric and be suggestive of retrocochlear disease on the "normal" side. Clinicians should be aware of the effects of both sensorineural and conductive hearing losses on ABR wave latencies so as not to confuse the expected effects of peripheral hearing loss with neural pathology.

We do not recommend using correction factors in patients with high-frequency sensorineural hearing loss. Selters and Brackmann (1977) recommended accounting for high-frequency hearing loss by subtracting 0.1 msec from the wave V latency for every 10 dB of hearing loss greater than 50 dB HL at 4000 Hz. The main goal of the correction factor was to improve the specificity (i.e., reduce the number of false-positives) of the ABR for tumor detection. Subsequent studies, however, have shown that a universal correction factor may not perform well, as there is high variability in the amount of latency shift caused by cochlear hearing loss from patient to patient. We recommend accounting for hearing loss by using higher intensity levels (80–100 dB nHL) when necessary, recognizing that a clear distinction between sensory and neural effects on the ABR may not be possible in cases of severe high-frequency loss. Our opinion is that, although reducing false-positives is an excellent goal, one should always err on the side of sensitivity, especially in today's health care environment in which clinical liability is heightened. Cashman, Stanton, Sagle, and Barber (1993), in a retrospective study of 1539 ABRs, found that using the Selters and Brackmann correction factor essentially halved the false-positive rate but doubled the false-negative rate.

◆ Discussion

Local or Outside Normative Data?

Locally collected normative data are advantageous in that the exact same equipment, parameters, and techniques are used for collection and comparison (Sininger, 1992). Conversely, it is tempting to take advantage of large, powerful outside databases when collecting data on a similar number of subjects locally is impractical. For example, the database by Joseph, West, Thornton, and Hermann, (1987) comprises 2730 subjects and includes separate norms for patients with normal hearing and sensory loss (**Table 16.1**). To use a vast outside database such as this, a clinic must ensure that the stimulus and recording parameters match those used to collect the norms

as closely as possible. It is also recommended that local normative data are collected on a smaller sample of subjects and compared with the outside database to ensure that the measures are acceptably comparable. Significant latency differences between the local and outside norms would preclude use of the external database, at least for the absolute latencies. IPL and ILD criteria may still be applied with confidence.

Advanced Techniques and Future Directions in Neurodiagnostic ABR

We will review a sample of many advanced techniques that have been suggested to improve ABR performance, particularly in the detection of small CN VIII/cerebellopontine angle (CPA) tumors. A popular theoretical method for improving ABR sensitivity has been using rapid stimulus rates, which has been proposed since the first decade of ABR research. The general theory is that auditory nerve fibers affected by retrocochlear pathology will have longer refractory periods than unaffected fibers, and when stressed by repetitive transient stimuli presented with very small interstimulus intervals, the evoked ABR would break down, specifically in the form of a longer than expected latency shift or a missing wave V. Although this theory is intriguing, most literature is, at best, suggestive, and there are certainly no peer-reviewed, large-scale studies that convince clinicians of its additional value compared with standard-rate ABR, particularly regarding the effects of space-occupying lesions. Perhaps the most applicable study was by Tanaka, Komatsuzaki, and Hentona (1996). In their study of 40 patients with vestibular schwannomas, they found that 90/s ABRs were abnormal in five patients who had normal ABRs using a rate of 9/s. The only measure used for this comparison, however, was the I–V IPL, and the other common indices were not examined. The case for the effectiveness of faster-rate ABR in the detection of neurodegenerative conditions (e.g., multiple sclerosis) is slightly more convincing, although there are conflicting conclusions in the literature. From a physiologic perspective, the relative change in interstimulus interval is quite small when increasing the stimulus rate from, say, 21 to 81/s, when you consider that auditory nerve fibers are capable of firing close to 1000 times per

Table 16.1 Example of a Large Outside Normative Database for Normal Hearing and Sensorineural (Cochlear) Hearing Loss

Normal Hearing (N = 786)

Measure	Mean	SD	99%
Absolute latency			
I	1.65	0.14	1.97
III	3.80	0.18	4.22
V	5.64	0.23	6.18
Interwave latency			
I–III	2.15	0.14	2.49
III–V	1.84	0.14	2.16
I–V	3.99	0.20	4.45
Interaural absolute latency			
I	−0.02	0.08	0.21
III	−0.03	0.10	0.26
V	0.00	0.11	0.29
Interaural interwave latency			
I–III	−0.01	0.10	0.25
III–V	0.00	0.10	0.25
I–V	0.00	0.11	0.28

Cochlear Loss (N = 1944)

Measure	Mean	SD	99%
Absolute latency			
I	1.80	0.23	2.34
III	3.95	0.24	4.54
V	5.82	0.27	6.44
Interwave latency			
I–III	2.17	0.18	2.59
III–V	1.84	0.16	2.21
I–V	4.02	0.24	4.58
Interaural absolute latency			
I	−0.01	0.25	0.65
III	−0.03	0.23	0.59
V	−0.03	0.20	0.52
Interaural interwave latency			
I–III	−0.02	0.16	0.41
III–V	0.01	0.14	0.37
I–V	−0.02	0.18	0.46

*All measurements in milliseconds. Stimulus parameters: 0.1-msec click, 13/s, 75 dB HL.

Abbreviation: SD, standard deviation.

Source: From Joseph, J. M., West, C. A., Thornton, A. R., & Herrmann, B. S. (1987, August). Improved decision criteria for the evaluation of clinical ABRs. Paper presented at the biennial meeting of the International Electric Response Study Group, Charlottesville, VA.

second. Recording ABRs to stimulus rates greater than 100/s is possible using the maximum length sequence (MLS) technique, which employs rapid trains of clicks presented in pseudo-random patterns; however, this algorithm is not known to be available as an option in any currently marketed evoked potential system.

A pilot study by Bush, Jones, and Shinn (2008) showed some promise in improving ABR sensitivity by comparing the physiologic ABR threshold with the behavioral threshold of the same stimulus. All patients with confirmed vestibular schwannomas had physiologic to behavioral threshold differences greater than 30 dB. One can envision an efficient three-step clinical protocol in which the behavioral click threshold is rapidly obtained, followed by two ABR recordings, one at 90 dB and one at an intensity level 30 dB SL (sensation level) relative to the behavioral click threshold. In doing so, an absent waveform at 30 dB SL would be considered a positive finding.

Certainly the mostly widely discussed advanced ABR technique in the past decade has been the stacked derived-band ABR technique developed by Don, Kwong, Tanaka, Brackmann, and Nelson (2005). The problem the stacked ABR is attempting to solve is the relative insensitivity of standard ABR measures (I–V IPL and ILD V) to some small tumors. Theoretically, this occurs not only because of the small size of these tumors, but also because of their location on the CN VII/VIII nerve bundle in the instances when low-frequency fibers alone have been affected by the mass. Because the latency of the click-evoked ABR is affected primarily by the high-frequency fibers arising from the basal end of the cochlea as a result of their high relative synchrony of activation compared with fibers arising from apical regions, a small tumor in this region may not affect conventional ABR latencies at all. Stacked ABR accounts for this weakness by first combining clicks with ipsilateral high-pass masking noise of progressively lower cutoff points, then using a subtraction process of the resulting ABRs to create more frequency-specific, derived-band ABRs. As would be expected, the ABRs resulting from the apical lower-frequency derived bands have significantly longer latencies compared with the basal ABRs, so if one were to simply combine the derived-band ABRs in their original form, much of the low-frequency

ABR would cancel out. The stacked ABR software adjusts for this by realigning the marked wave Vs of all of the derived bands to an equal latency before combining the waveforms into a single (stacked) ABR waveform. The result is a waveform that, to have what is considered a normal wave V amplitude, must have contributions from both basal and more apical regions. A small tumor affecting the fibers responsible for any of the derived-band ABRs, including the lower-frequency apical bands, would affect the stacked ABR overall and be considered a positive finding. Data on using the stacked ABR in patients with small acoustic tumors were excellent. Use of this technique, however, is not widespread. Many clinicians have found that the considerable time necessary (up to 2–3 h) to record quality ABRs for all of the high-pass masking conditions is not feasible for a screening test.

An exciting future possibility for the ABR technique that is based on the stacked ABR theory for tumor detection involves the use of the rising-frequency chirp stimulus (Don, Elberling, and Maloff, 2009). A chirp is a stimulus that rises from low to high frequency over the course of each transient. The rate at which the chirp ascends in frequency is based on one of several models of cochlear traveling wave delay. The goal of the chirp is that the earlier, low-frequency portions of the stimulus will reach and activate apical hair cells at the same time the delayed mid- and high-frequency positions of the stimulus are stimulating their more basal regions. This results in a synchronous neural discharge that is more representative of the entire cochlear partition, rather than being skewed toward basal regions resulting from traveling wave delay. The resulting ABR evoked by this stimulus is a more equivalent representation of nerve fibers from a wider-frequency region than the click and has been shown to have a significantly greater wave V amplitude, especially at lower intensity levels. Elberling and Don (2008) have described the chirp as input compensation for cochlear traveling wave delay in evoking the ABR, as opposed to output compensation, which occurs when derived-band ABRs are temporally realigned following recording, as in the stacked ABR technique. The obvious advantage to the chirp ABR over the stacked ABR is test efficiency. Stacked ABR technique requires six recordings to create the derived bands, whereas a chirp ABR requires only a single recording. Because inefficiency has contributed to the limited clinical use of stacked ABR, the chirp ABR may turn out to be an acceptable alternative if a similar improvement in sensitivity to acoustic tumors can be proven in research.

Practical Factors in the Use of Neurodiagnostic ABRs in the Clinic

We recommend performing ABRs in all cases suspicious for neural involvement, particularly immediately following audiometry testing. There are several clinical and practical advantages to this. Clinically, if you are basing the click intensity level on the audiogram, same-day ABR ensures that thresholds have not shifted. It also allows for immediate analysis of the audiologic test battery as a whole.

The ability to perform ABRs in an efficient manner has been improved by the development of devices with advanced hardware and software, such as the Vivosonic Integrity system (Vivosonic Inc., Toronto, Canada). The hardware of the Integrity (other than a Bluetooth-enabled laptop computer) consists of only the Vivolink module, which is small enough to be worn around the neck of patients. This allows for ABR testing in virtually any testing environment, including the same room/booth used for conventional audiometry. Neurodiagnostic ABR testing can be performed in any reasonable testing space when using stimulus levels of 80 dB nHL or greater and properly seated insert earphones. The device also uses a novel preamplifier that is mounted directly on the ground electrode. This allows for analog filtering and differential amplification to occur prior to electromagnetic artifacts being introduced via the electrode leads. This, combined with weighted averaging, provides a remarkably effective device for the recording of ABRs in awake patients.

ABR Testing in the Era of Magnetic Resonance Imaging

In the 21st century, ABR use has declined significantly because of the increasing popularity and expansion of advanced imaging techniques, mainly magnetic resonance imaging (MRI), as the test of choice to detect and diagnose lesions of the central nervous system. It is a reality that MRI-G (MRI with gadolinium) can detect space-occupying lesions that sometimes are too small or are located in an area of CN VIII or the brainstem that does not significantly affect ABR. Many authors have openly called for the end of ABR as a screening tool for CN VIII tumors (Cueva, 2004). Although the use of ABR as a screening tool certainly can be called into question, its continued use as the most powerful functional measure of the auditory nerve and brainstem cannot. It should also be noted that certain retrocochlear pathologies can be missed by imaging techniques as well. The second section of this chapter describes auditory neuropathy spectrum disorder, a type of pathology that, though not always truly neural, always presents with an abnormal ABR as a test result. In most cases, however, ANSD presents with normal imaging studies.

The wisdom of describing all abnormal ABR tests that are contradicted by negative imaging studies as false-positives should be brought into question. Although a negative MRI-G certainly may rule out most space-occupying lesions of CN VIII and the brainstem or significant degenerative plaques in the same areas, it does not contraindicate retrocochlear disease in all of its forms. An appropriate ABR candidate with a grossly abnormal response, such as a response with a completely absent wave V with a wave I–V IPL greater than 6 msec, should be considered as having a neural contribution to the auditory disorder regardless of the outcome of imaging studies. That is, a normal MRI study does not render an abnormal ABR null and void. MRI is also not immune to false-positive results. Several case studies (e.g., Arriaga, Carrier, and Houston, 1995; House, Bassim, and Schwartz, 2008) have demonstrated MRI results indicative of space-occupying lesions that are not found under surgical exploration. This is not to suggest that an abnormal ABR should be a requirement for surgical treatment, as normal ABRs are possible in the presence of tumors, as discussed previously, but to demonstrate that tests of structure and function are not infallible.

♦ Case Studies

Case 1: Acoustic Neuroma with Abnormal ABR

This represents the classic case of neurodiagnostic ABR in an acoustic tumor (**Fig. 16.3**). The 45-year-old patient complained for several years of a gradual decrease in hearing along with tinnitus in the left ear. Pure-tone audiometry revealed a mild to moderate sloping sensorineural hearing loss in the suspect ear. Immediate neurodiagnostic ABR testing was performed. In **Fig. 16.3**, the wave I latencies are relatively symmetric between the ears, but the later waves are significantly prolonged in the left ear trace. With the exception of waves I and V in the left trace, it is difficult to identify which deflections represent waves II to IV. This is a trivial matter at this point, however, as the marked data are all that are necessary to deem the evaluation positive for retrocochlear involvement in the left ear. MRI clearly indicates enhancement of the left CN VIII.

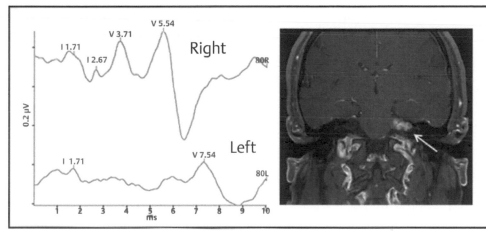

Fig. 16.3 Acoustic neuroma on the left side. Notice the prolonged I–V interpeak latency in the left auditory brainstem response trace.

Case 2: Vestibular Schwannoma with Normal ABR

A 31-year-old woman's primary complain was unilateral tinnitus in the left ear for less than 1 year (**Fig. 16.4**). Her pure-tone audiogram was essentially normal, with no significant asymmetry noted. Word recognition scores, as well as middle ear muscle reflexes, were normal bilaterally. The ABR was immediately recorded and indicated a normal response, with all absolute, interpeak, and interaural latency values within acceptable clinical limits. Despite the normal ABR, an MRI was ordered to investigate the persistent bothersome unilateral tinnitus; this study revealed a 2-mm mass in the left internal auditory canal. This demonstrates that the ABR can be normal in patients with small acoustic tumors but was still of great value in this patient. The normal ABR was monitored regularly as a functional measure of CN VIII function, as well as potentially serving as a baseline measure for intraoperative monitoring if hearing-preservation surgery was elected in the future.

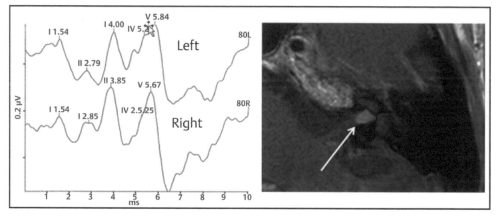

Fig. 16.4 Normal auditory brainstem responses with 2 mm vestibular schwannoma confirmed by magnetic resonance imaging (MRI).

Case 3: Abnormal ABR with Normal MRI

A 45-year-old woman had left-sided tinnitus and dysequilibrium (**Fig. 16.5**). Her audiogram indicated minimal asymmetric loss on the left side, with normal acoustic reflexes and word recognition bilaterally. An immediate ABR was performed that yielded a typical retrocochlear pattern, with symmetric wave I responses from each ear but significantly prolonged waves III and V in the left ear. The wave V ILD was 0.92 msec, well beyond the often used cutoff of 0.4 msec. The wave I–III IPL of 2.63 msec in the left ear was also beyond our clinical tolerance limit. Interestingly, MRI-G was completely normal in this patient. Despite the absence of a radiologically confirmed space-occupying lesion, this patient is still considered to have a neural cause for her auditory and vestibular symptoms, based on the ABR result, and is being closely monitored for other neurologic deficits.

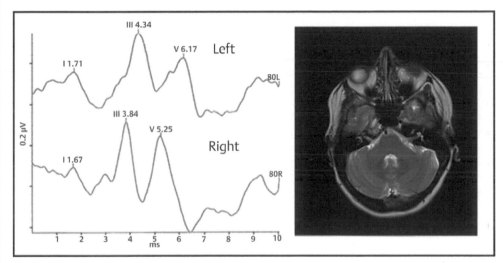

Fig. 16.5 Abnormal auditory brainstem response in the left ear with normal magnetic resonance imaging.

◆ Auditory Neuropathy Spectrum Disorder

ANSD is a relatively newly defined type of auditory impairment. In strict terms, it is a type of sensorineural hearing loss in that the site of the lesion involves the cochlea and/or the auditory nerve; however, ANSD and sensorineural hearing loss are distinct with respect to diagnostic criteria and clinical presentation. ANSD is defined as present outer hair cell (OHC) function accompanied by dyssynchronous auditory neural responses. As such, evoked potential measures are the defining features in the diagnosis of ANSD, specifically, present otoacoustic emissions (OAEs) and/or cochlear microphonic (CM) and absent ABR. Given the diagnostic criteria, audiologists are often the professionals who perform these tests and subsequently identify ANSD for a patient. Appropriate evoked potential testing and accurate interpretation of the results are critical for identification of these patients and recommendation of appropriate intervention strategies and referrals.

Potential Sites of Lesion

The normal auditory system is a high-fidelity system designed to accurately convey multiple cues of a signal, including frequency, intensity, and timing information. Inner hair cells (IHCs) are the primary initial sensory transducers in this process, and finely timed neurotransmitter release stimulates action potentials in the auditory nerve (Palmer and Russell, 1986) and along the central auditory system, resulting in accurate perception of the stimulus. In ANSD, the possible sites of lesion include the IHCs (presynaptic), the auditory nerve dendrites and the auditory nerve axons (postsynaptic) (Berlin et al, 2005; Starr, Picton, Sininger, Hood, and Berlin, 1996; Starr, Sininger, and Pratt, 2000). Disruption of normal function in any of these structures may give rise to ANSD. Examples of presynaptic pathologies include missing IHCs (Amatuzzi et al, 2001) and dysfunction of synaptic proteins within the IHCs, such as otoferlin, which can interfere with neurotransmitter release (Rodríguez-Ballesteros et al, 2003, 2008; Varga et al, 2003). Postsynaptically, disease processes causing demyelination or axonal damage can interfere with conduction of action potentials and subsequently reduce the temporal synchrony, resulting in abnormal evoked potential responses (McDonald and Sears, 1970; Pareyson, Scaioli, Berta, and Sghirlanzoni, 1995). Temporal synchrony is particularly relevant in the perception of complex signals, such as speech and speech-in-noise, and the severity of temporal impairment has a direct relationship to deficits in speech perception performance (Rance, Cone-Wesson, Wunderlich, and Dowell, 2002; Rance, McKay, and Grayden, 2004; Zeng, Oba, Garde, Sininger, and Starr, 1999).

Candidacy for ANSD Testing

The ANSD evoked potential protocol should be implemented in all cases where there is no response to high-level (i.e., 80–90 dB nHL) alternating clicks or tone-burst ABR. Also, in infants or young children, ANSD may be suspected when there is a positive family history of ANSD or neonatal risk factors, such as anoxia, hyperbilirubinemia, premature birth, and exchange transfusion (Berlin et al, 1998, 2010; Miyamoto, Kirk, Renshaw, and Hussain, 1999; Rance et al, 1999; Shapiro, 2003; Starr et al, 1996, 2003; Starr, Sininger, and Pratt, 2000). It is particularly important to be aware of potential ANSD when there are concerns of hearing loss in a child who passed a newborn hearing screening (NHS) that used only OAE measures but not ABR. In older children or adults, it is possible to acquire late-onset ANSD in cases where there are sensorimotor neuropathies, such as Friedreich ataxia and Charcot-Marie-Tooth disease (Miyamoto et al, 1999; Starr et al, 1996, 2000, 2003). Speech perception in ANSD is often poorer than would be predicted by pure-tone thresholds, which can range from normal to profound (Berlin et al, 2010; Kraus et al, 2000; Kraus, Ozdamar, Stein, and Reed, 1984; Sheykholeslami, Kaga, and Kaga, 2001). Therefore, testing for ANSD should be completed in cases where there are concerns about speech perception regardless of audiometric threshold levels.

Improved auditory function over time in infants diagnosed with ANSD has been documented, particularly when there are risk factors such as low birth weight and hyperbilirubinemia (Attias and Raveh, 2007; Madden, Rutter, Hilbert, Greinwald, and Choo, 2002; Psarommatis et al, 2006). In these cases of "transient" ANSD, the appearance of ABR waveforms may be concurrent with improvements in audiometric thresholds. Observed changes in auditory function tend to emerge or be complete between 7 and 12 months of age; therefore, behavioral and objective testing for ANSD should be repeated until stability of auditory function is confirmed. Repeat ABR testing prior to cochlear implantation for children with ANSD is recommended.

Evoked Potentials for Diagnosis of ANSD

The minimum test battery for diagnosing ANSD includes OAEs and/or CM to test OHC function and ABR to test auditory nerve and brainstem function. Middle ear muscle reflexes (MEMRs) are another measure of neural synchrony and have diagnostic value as they are absent or elevated in ANSD; however, these should be confirmed by ABR (Berlin et al, 2005). Auditory steady-state responses (ASSRs) are not used in diagnosis of ANSD, as differences in stimulus and recording methods may result in present ASSRs while the ABR is absent. In addition, ASSR is not useful in predicting hearing thresholds in ANSD (Jafari, Malayeri, Ashayeri, and Farahani, 2009; Rance et al, 1998, 2005). The following sections specify the parameters and analyses of the diagnostic tests for ANSD. Prior to performing these tests, otoscopic examination and middle ear function must be confirmed, as would be routinely implemented in audiologic protocols.

Otoacoustic Emissions

OHC function can be measured using either transient evoked OAEs (TEOAEs) or distortion-product OAEs (DPOAEs). Exact parameters for stimulation level and criteria to determine normal OAE responses vary by clinic and type of equipment used. In general, to be considered present, the OAE response must be 4 to 6 dB above the noise floor, reproducible, and present across multiple frequencies/octave bands (Rance et al, 1999; Starr, Sininger, Nguyen, Michalewski, Oba, and Abdala, 2001).

OAEs are noninvasive and readily obtained from cooperative patients with normal middle ear function. They are therefore a useful clinical tool, although the presence of OAEs is not required to diagnose ANSD. OAEs are present in ~75% of patients with ANSD and are absent or questionable in the remaining patients (Berlin et al, 2010). In addition, OAEs can disappear over time independent of hearing aid use (Rodríguez-Ballesteros et al, 2003; Starr et al, 2000). A more stable measure of OHC function is the CM, and observation of the CM with absent ABR is the key diagnostic criterion for ANSD.

Cochlear Microphonic and Auditory Brainstem Response

Whereas OAEs measure the status of the cochlear amplifier arising from motile properties of the OHCs, the CM is electrical current generated by the OHCs as they depolarize and hyperpolarize in response to a stimulus. With single-polarity click stimuli, the propensity of the CM to follow a stimulus can lead to erroneous interpretation of the response. Specifically, the CM waveform may be mistaken for the ABR, and subsequently neural synchrony may be presumed when this is not the case. Berlin and colleagues (1998) established a protocol for differentiating the CM and ABR by comparing responses to positive and negative polarity clicks. Standard ABR stimulation rate, filter settings, and electrode montage should be used, as recommended earlier in this chapter. The following points are key considerations in the diagnostic protocol for ANSD.

Setup and Stimuli

Insert Earphones

Because the CM response follows the stimulus, it is important to differentiate between measurement of transducer stimulus artifact and the CM. When delivering the acoustic signal through tubal insert earphones, be sure to (1) separate transducer stimulus and the CM response over time, and (2) allow for recording of a trial to a single-polarity stimulus with the tube clamped (Rance et al, 1999; Starr et al, 2001).

When the tube is clamped, the acoustic signal is not reaching the ear at a level sufficient to elicit a response. If the response to a single-polarity stimulus disappears when the tube is pinched, then the response can be interpreted as physiologic. Conversely, if the response remains, it is most likely stimulus artifact.

High-Level Clicks of 80 to 90 dB HL

Levels of 80 to 90 dB HL are sufficient to observe the CM and determine dyssynchrony of the ABR. If the CM is observed at the onset of ABR threshold testing using a lower-intensity level (e.g., 50–60 dB), it would be advisable to fully characterize the CM at the recommended level.

Positive and Negative Polarity Clicks in Separate Trials

The CM waveform will show a reversal in polarity that follows the phase shift of the stimulus, whereas the ABR will not change in polarity. Summing the response waveforms for opposite polarity stimuli will cancel out the CM and reveal an absent ABR in ANSD. Alternating-polarity click stimuli will similarly cancel out the CM, and using such stimuli in isolation will miss an ANSD diagnosis. Conversely, software may allow recordings to alternating clicks, yet store positive and negative clicks in separate buffers for later analysis by single polarity.

Interpretation

Cochlear Microphonic

Factoring in the delay from insert earphones, latency of the initial CM peak occurs at ~0.4 msec and may persist for several milliseconds, as seen in **Fig. 16.6** (e.g., Berlin et al, 1998; Starr et al, 2001). The 180-degree phase shift in CM response follows the reversal in stimulus polarity for condensation and rarefaction clicks, which were measured in separate trials (waveforms are plotted on top of each other to illustrate the phase shift).

Auditory Brainstem Response

The ABR waveform is observable when the CM is canceled out either by mathematical summation of opposite polarity waveforms or by recording using alternating-polarity clicks (**Fig. 16.6** bottom two waveforms, respectively). In ANSD, the ABR waveform may be absent/flat or show poor morphology indicative of dyssynchrony at higher stimulation levels.

Analysis Note

Implementation of evoked potential ANSD testing has increased in recent years with awareness of the disorder. This diligence is to be celebrated and is of great benefit to patients with ANSD. We have noticed in our clinic, however, that referrals for ANSD have increased in cases where there is present CM but also present ABR, which is indicative of normal hearing (Starr et al, 2001). It is important to remember that the CM is present in normal hearing and mild hearing loss, and for an ANSD diagnosis, the ABR must be absent or abnormal.

Middle Ear Muscle Reflexes

MEMRs are absent (no response ≥110 dB HL) and/or elevated (>95 dB HL) in patients with ANSD (Berlin et al, 2005, 2010). Therefore, MEMRs can provide useful information that is readily obtained in the clinic. Caution must be exercised with infants, however, as high-frequency probe tones are used in this population, and the effects on MEMR thresholds are not established. When there is concern of hearing loss in a child with present OAEs, absent or elevated MEMRs warrant a follow-up diagnostic ABR evaluation with the ANSD protocol.

Magnetic Resonance Imaging in ANSD

The role of MRI in ANSD management has been under investigation. MRI is not required for the diagnosis of ANSD, and as mentioned, MRI studies are often normal in ANSD, particularly if the site of lesion is pre- or postsynaptic but below the resolution threshold of the MRI. The primary use of MRI in ANSD has been to determine whether there is auditory nerve deficiency, specifically, auditory nerve hypoplasia or aplasia. In a cohort of 51 children with ANSD, Buchman and colleagues (2006) found

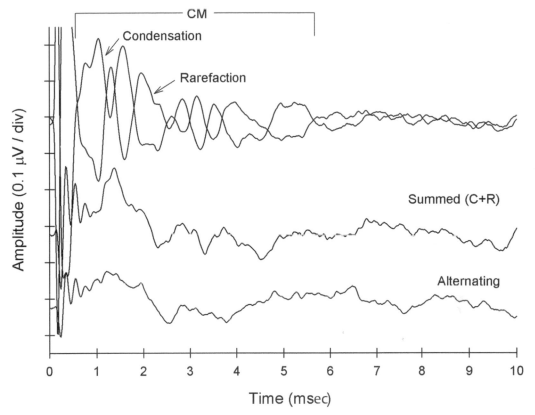

Fig. 16.6 ABR waveforms from a child with auditory neuropathy spectrum disorder (ANSD). The top two waveforms are responses to condensation (C) and rarefaction (R) click stimuli presented at 90 dB nHL, and the cochlear microphonic (CM) is apparent. The bottom two waveforms show the canceled CM resulting from summing of the waveforms or using alternating-polarity click stimuli.

that 4% presented with auditory nerve hypoplasia and 14% with auditory nerve aplasia by MRI. Patients with auditory nerve hypoplasia may benefit from amplification or cochlear implantation, although outcomes are variable (Buchman, Roush, Teagle, Brown, Zdanski, and Grose, 2006; Khan, Handzel, Burgess, Damian, Eddington, and Nadol, 2005). Auditory nerve aplasia contraindicates amplification and cochlear implantation. Recent evidence suggests, however, that the auditory nerve may innervate the cochlea via alternate anatomical pathways. This is referred to as apparent cochlear nerve aplasia, and in some cases responses

to auditory stimulation with a cochlear implant have been noted (Warren, Wiggins, Pitt, Harnsberger, and Shelton, 2010). Therefore, although MRI provides information regarding gross neural integrity in ANSD, it does not definitively characterize the potential for auditory responses with intervention. Audiologists should ensure that children are tested behaviorally and monitored closely for auditory responses. MRI results may be used when counseling families of children with auditory nerve deficiency to set realistic expectations and be fully informed of risks versus potential benefits of cochlear implantation.

Case Study 4: ANSD

B. is a 3-year-old boy diagnosed with a moderate hearing loss and ANSD, who is currently undergoing a second hearing aid trial. He has a significant birth history of twin-to-twin transfusion syndrome (surviving twin), was born at 29 weeks' gestation, and weighed 3 pounds, 2 ounces. He reportedly failed his NHS and received diagnostic ABR testing at 9 months of age after he could be safely sedated per clinical protocol. ABR testing revealed a present CM and absent ABR at 80 and 90 dB nHL bilaterally (right ear waveforms shown **Fig. 16.7**). TEOAEs were absent bilaterally. Behavioral thresholds obtained in the sound field at 10 months of age indicated a moderate to severe hearing loss, and ear-specific audiometric testing at 17 months revealed mild to moderate hearing loss (**Fig. 16.8**).

At 11 months, B. was fit bilaterally with Oticon Tego Pro (Oiticon Inc., Somerset, NJ) hearing aids using estimated real ear-to-coupler difference measures, and appropriate gain was suggested in the sound field. B. showed no indication of loudness intolerance. He was receiving 1 to 2 hours of aural habilitation services per week, and his therapist noted that since his hearing aid fitting, he had become "a very verbal child." At 16 months of age, he possessed the receptive-language skills typical of a 9-month-old and the expressive-language level of a 12-month-old. Therefore, he had made 3 months' progress in receptive language and 8 months' progress in expressive language over just a 4- to 5-month period. Despite these gains with amplification, B. was highly resistant to wearing the hearing aids and only wore them ~2 hours daily. During 8 months of hearing aid use, B. demonstrated responsiveness to sounds that were

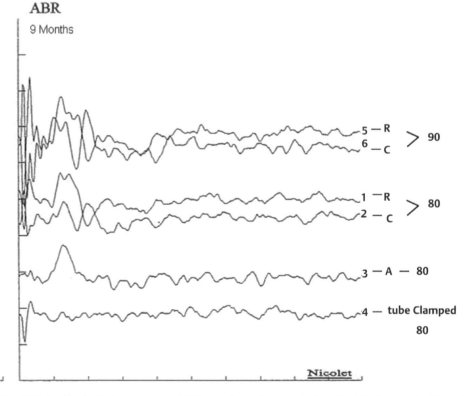

Fig. 16.7 Auditor brainstem response (ABR) waveforms for case study patient B. diagnosed with auditory neuropathy spectrum disorder (ANSD). Rarefaction (R), condensation (C), and alternating (A) click stimuli were presented at the levels indicated. Present cochlear microphonic (CM) and absent ABR are apparent. The tracing with the tube clamped is shown on the bottom.

Continued

similar with and without the hearing aids. Considering this and his increasing resistance to wearing hearing aids, a trial without amplification was subsequently undertaken. Initial observations without hearing aids indicated no regression or plateau in his auditory, speech, or language skills, and B. was reportedly more focused in therapy and cooperative at home.

B.'s progress without amplification and mild to moderate audiometric thresholds led to repeat ABR testing at 2 years of age to test whether the ANSD had resolved. The waveform again showed a present CM and absent ABR (right ear waveforms, **Fig. 16.9**), and the diagnosis of ANSD remained. B. continued receiving intensive therapy and close monitoring, and at 3 years of age speech and language delays began to emerge, as did difficulty perceiving and articulating high-frequency speech sounds and inattention. He was fit with hearing aids again and wears them consistently; his preschool teachers report significant improvements in his daily performance. We continue to monitor B.'s progress closely to determine whether evaluation for a cochlear implant should be recommended.

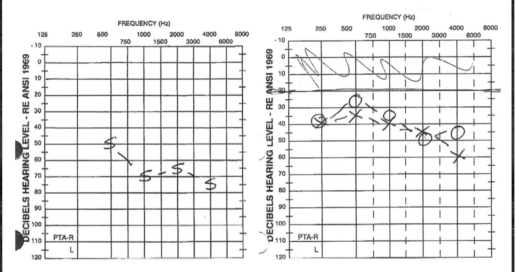

Fig. 16.8 Audiograms for patient B representing sound field results at 10 months of age (left) and ear-specific thresholds at 17 months of age (right)

Continued

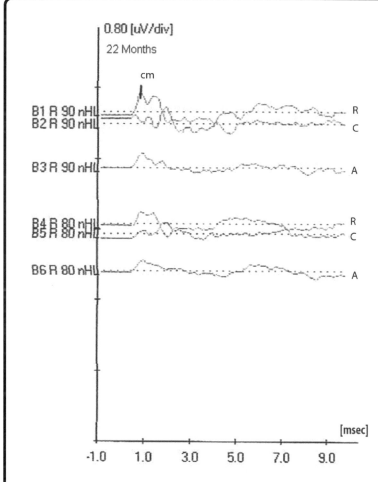

Fig. 16.9 Repeat auditory brainstem response (ABR) waveforms at 2 years of age. The present cochlear microphic and absent ABR persisted in this patient.

References

Amatuzzi, M. G., Northrop, C., Liberman, M. C., Thornton, A., Halpin, C., Herrmann, B., et al. (2001). Selective inner hair cell loss in premature infants and cochlea pathological patterns from neonatal intensive care unit autopsies. *Archives of Otolaryngology—Head and Neck Surgery*, *127*(6), 629–636. PubMed

American National Standards Institute (1969). American National Standard Specifications for Audiometers, ANSI S3.6-1969, New York, Acoustical Society of America.

Arriaga, M. A., Carrier, D., & Houston, G. D. (1995). False-positive magnetic resonance imaging of small internal auditory canal tumors: a clinical, radiologic, and pathologic correlation study. *Otolaryngology—Head and Neck Surgery*, *113*(1), 61–70. PubMed

Attias, J., & Raveh, E. (2007). Transient deafness in young candidates for cochlear implants. *Audiology and Neuro-Otology*, *12*(5), 325–333. PubMed

Bauch, C. D., & Olsen, W. O. (1990). Comparison of ABR amplitudes with TIPtrode and mastoid electrodes. *Ear and Hearing*, *11*(6), 463–467. PubMed

Bauch, C. D., Olsen, W. O., & Pool, A. F. (1996). ABR indices: Sensitivity, specificity, and tumor size. *American Journal of Audiology*, *5*, 97–104.

Berlin, C. I., Bordelon, J., St John, P., Wilensky, D., Hurley, A., Kluka, E., et al. (1998). Reversing click polarity may uncover auditory neuropathy in infants. *Ear and Hearing*, *19*(1), 37–47. PubMed

Berlin, C. I., Hood, L. J., Morlet, T., Wilensky, D., Li, L., Mattingly, K. R., et al. (2010). Multi-site diagnosis and management of 260 patients with auditory neuropathy/dys-synchrony (auditory neuropathy spectrum disorder). *International Journal of Audiology*, *49*(1), 30–43. PubMed

Berlin, C. I., Hood, L. J., Morlet, T., Wilensky, D., St. John, P., Montgomery, E., et al. (2005). Absent or elevated middle ear muscle reflexes in the presence of normal otoacoustic emissions: A universal finding in 136 cases of auditory neuropathy/dys-synchrony. *Journal of the American Academy of Audiology*, *16*(8), 546–553. PubMed

Brantberg, K. (1996). Easily applied ear canal electrodes improve the diagnostic potential of auditory brainstem response. *Scandinavian Audiology*, *25*(3), 147–152. PubMed

Buchman, C. A., Roush, P. A., Teagle, H. F., Brown, C. J., Zdanski, C. J., & Grose, J. H. (2006). Auditory neuropathy characteristics in children with cochlear nerve deficiency. *Ear and Hearing*, *27*(4), 399–408. PubMed

Bush, M. L., Jones, R. O., & Shinn, J. B. (2008). Auditory brainstem response threshold differences in patients with vestibular schwannoma: A new diagnostic index. *Ear, Nose, and Throat Journal*, *87*(8), 458–462. PubMed

Cashman, M. Z., Stanton, S. G., Sagle, C., & Barber, H. O. (1993). The effect of hearing loss on ABR interpretation: Use of a correction factor. *Scandinavian Audiology*, *22*(3), 153–158. PubMed

Cueva, R. A. (2004). Auditory brainstem response versus magnetic resonance imaging for the evaluation of asymmetric sensorineural hearing loss. *Laryngoscope*, *114*(10), 1686–1692. PubMed

Don, M., Elberling, C., & Maloff, E. (2009). Input and output compensation for the cochlear traveling wave delay in wide-band ABR recordings: Implications for small acoustic tumor detection. *Journal of the American Academy of Audiology*, *20*(2), 99–108. PubMed

Don, M., Kwong, B., Tanaka, C., Brackmann, D., & Nelson, R. (2005). The stacked ABR: A sensitive and specific screening tool for detecting small acoustic tumors. *Audiology & Neuro-Otology*, *10*(5), 274–290. PubMed

Don, M., Vermiglio, A. J., Ponton, C. W., Eggermont, J. J., & Masuda, A. (1996). Variable effects of click polarity on auditory brain-stem response latencies: Analyses of narrow-band ABRs suggest possible explanations. *Journal of the Acoustical Society of America*, *100*(1), 458–472. PubMed

Durrant, J. D., & Fowler, C. G. (1996). ABR protocols for dealing with asymmetric hearing loss. *American Journal of Audiology*, *5*(3), 5–6.

Elberling, C., & Don, M. (2008). Auditory brainstem responses to a chirp stimulus designed from derived band latencies in normal-hearing subjects. *Journal of the Acoustical Society of America*, *124*(5), 3022–3037. PubMed

Elberling, C., & Wahlgreen, O. (1985). Estimation of auditory brainstem response, ABR, by means of Bayesian inference. *Scandinavian Audiology*, *14*(2), 89–96. PubMed

Gorga, M. P., Kaminski, J. R., Beauchaine, K. L., Jesteadt, W., & Neely, S. T. (1989). Auditory brainstem responses from children three months to three years of age: normal patterns of response. *Journal of Speech and Hearing Research*, *32*(2), 281–288. PubMed

House, J. W., Bassim, M. K., & Schwartz, M. (2008). False-positive magnetic resonance imaging in the diagnosis of vestibular schwannoma. *Otology and Neurotology*, *29*(8), 1176–1178. PubMed

Jafari, Z., Malayeri, S., Ashayeri, H., & Farahani, M. A. (2009). Adults with auditory neuropathy: Comparison of auditory steady-state response and pure-tone audiometry. *Journal of the American Academy of Audiology*, *20*(10), 621–628. PubMed

Joseph, J. M., West, C. A., Thornton, A. R., & Herrmann, B. S. (1987, August). *Improved decision criteria for the evaluation of clinical ABRs*. Paper presented at the biennial meeting of the International Electric Response Study Group, Charlottesville, VA.

Khan, A. M., Handzel, O., Burgess, B. J., Damian, D., Eddington, D. K., & Nadol, J. B., Jr. (2005). Is word recognition correlated with the number of surviving spiral ganglion cells and electrode insertion depth in human subjects with cochlear implants? *Laryngoscope*, *115*(4), 672–677. PubMed

Kraus, N., Bradlow, A. R., Cheatham, M. A., Cunningham, J., King, C. D., Koch, D. B., et al. (2000). Consequences of neural asynchrony: A case of auditory neuropathy. *Journal of the Association for Research in Otolaryngology*, *1*(1), 33–45. PubMed

Kraus, N., Ozdamar, O., Stein, L., & Reed, N. (1984). Absent auditory brain stem response: Peripheral hearing loss or brain stem dysfunction? *Laryngoscope, 94*(3), 400–406. PubMed

Kurtz, I., & Steinman, A. (2005, February). *Kalman filtering in recording auditory evoked potentials.* Paper presented at the 28th midwinter meeting of the Association for Research in Otolaryngology.

Madden, C., Rutter, M., Hilbert, L., Greinwald, J. H., Jr., & Choo, D. I. (2002). Clinical and audiological features in auditory neuropathy. *Archives of Otolaryngology—Head and Neck Surgery, 128*(9), 1026–1030. PubMed

McDonald, W. I., & Sears, T. A. (1970). The effects of experimental demyelination on conduction in the central nervous system. *Brain, 93*(3), 583–598. PubMed

Miyamoto, R. T., Kirk, K. I., Renshaw, J., & Hussain, D. (1999). Cochlear implantation in auditory neuropathy. *Laryngoscope, 109*(2 Pt 1), 181–185. PubMed

Palmer, A. R., & Russell, I. J. (1986). Phase-locking in the cochlear nerve of the guinea-pig and its relation to the receptor potential of inner hair-cells. *Hearing Research, 24*(1), 1–15. PubMed

Pareyson, D., Scaioli, V., Berta, E., & Sghirlanzoni, A. (1995). Acoustic nerve in peripheral neuropathy: A BAEP study. *Electromyography and Clinical Neurophysiology, 35*(6), 359–364. PubMed

Psarommatis, I., Riga, M., Douros, K., Koltsidopoulos, P., Douniadakis, D., Kapetanakis, I., et al. (2006). Transient infantile auditory neuropathy and its clinical implications. *International Journal of Pediatric Otorhinolaryngology, 70*(9), 1629–1637. PubMed

Rance, G., Beer, D. E., Cone-Wesson, B., Shepherd, R. K., Dowell, R. C., King, A. M., et al. (1999). Clinical findings for a group of infants and young children with auditory neuropathy. *Ear and Hearing, 20*(3), 238–252. PubMed

Rance, G., Cone-Wesson, B., Wunderlich, J., & Dowell, R. (2002). Speech perception and cortical event related potentials in children with auditory neuropathy. *Ear and Hearing, 23*(3), 239–253. PubMed

Rance, G., Dowell, R. C., Rickards, F. W., Beer, D. E., & Clark, G. M. (1998). Steady-state evoked potential and behavioral hearing thresholds in a group of children with absent click-evoked auditory brain stem response. *Ear and Hearing, 19*(1), 48–61. PubMed

Rance, G., McKay, C., & Grayden, D. (2004). Perceptual characterization of children with auditory neuropathy. *Ear and Hearing, 25*(1), 34–46. PubMed

Rance, G., Roper, R., Symons, L., Moody, L. J., Poulis, C., Dourlay, M., et al. (2005). Hearing threshold estimation in infants using auditory steady-state responses. *Journal of the American Academy of Audiology, 16*(5), 291–300. PubMed

Rodríguez-Ballesteros, M., del Castillo, F. J., Martín, Y., Moreno-Pelayo, M. A., Morera, C., Prieto, F., et al. (2003). Auditory neuropathy in patients carrying mutations in the otoferlin gene (OTOF). *Human Mutation, 22*(6), 451–456. PubMed

Rodríguez-Ballesteros, M., Reynoso, R., Olarte, M., Villamar, M., Morera, C., Santarelli, R., et al. (2008). A multicenter study on the prevalence and spectrum of mutations in the otoferlin gene (*OTOF*) in subjects with nonsyndromic hearing impairment and auditory neuropathy. *Human Mutation, 29*(6), 823–831. PubMed

Selters, W. A., & Brackmann, D. E. (1977). Acoustic tumor detection with brain stem electric response audiometry. *Archives of Otolaryngology, 103*(4), 181–187. PubMed

Shapiro, S. M. (2003). Bilirubin toxicity in the developing nervous system. *Pediatric Neurology, 29*(5), 410–421. PubMed

Sheykholeslami, K., Kaga, K., & Kaga, M. (2001). An isolated and sporadic auditory neuropathy (auditory nerve disease): Report of five patients. *Journal of Laryngology and Otology, 115*(7), 530–534. PubMed

Sininger, Y. S. (1992). Establishing clinical norms for auditory brainstem response. *American Journal of Audiology, 1,* 16–18.

Starr, A., Michalewski, H. J., Zeng, F. G., Fujikawa-Brooks, S., Linthicum, F., Kim, C. S., et al. (2003). Pathology and physiology of auditory neuropathy with a novel mutation in the *MPZ* gene (Tyr145->Ser). *Brain, 126*(Pt 7), 1604–1619. PubMed

Starr, A., Picton, T. W., Sininger, Y., Hood, L. J., & Berlin, C. I. (1996). Auditory neuropathy. *Brain, 119*(Pt 3), 741–753. PubMed

Starr, A., Sininger, Y., Nguyen, T., Michalewski, H. J., Oba, S., & Abdala, C. (2001). Cochlear receptor (microphonic and summating potentials, otoacoustic emissions) and auditory pathway (auditory brain stem potentials) activity in auditory neuropathy. *Ear and Hearing, 22*(2), 91–99. PubMed

Starr, A., Sininger, Y. S., & Pratt, H. (2000). The varieties of auditory neuropathy. *Journal of Basic and Clinical Physiology and Pharmacology, 11*(3), 215–230. PubMed

Tanaka, H., Komatsuzaki, A. & Hentona, H. (1996). Usefulness of auditory brainstem responses at high stimulus rates in the diagnosis of acoustic neuroma. *Journal of Otorhinolaryngology and Related Specialties, 58*(4), 224–228.

Teagle, H. F., Roush, P. A., Woodard, J. S., Hatch, D. R., Zdanski, C. J., Buss, E., et al. (2010). Cochlear implantation in children with auditory neuropathy spectrum disorder. *Ear and Hearing, 31*(3), 325–335. PubMed

Varga, R., Kelley, P. M., Keats, B. J., Starr, A., Leal, S. M., Cohn, E., et al. (2003). Non-syndromic recessive auditory neuropathy is the result of mutations in the otoferlin (*OTOF*) gene. *Journal of Medical Genetics, 40*(1), 45–50. PubMed

Warren, F. M., III, Wiggins, R. H., III, Pitt, C., Harnsberger, H. R., & Shelton, C. (2010). Apparent cochlear nerve aplasia: To implant or not to implant? *Otology and Neurotology, 31*(7), 1088–1094. PubMed

Yagi, T., & Kaga, K. (1979). The effect of the click repetition rate on the latency of the auditory evoked brain stem response and its clinical use for a neurological diagnosis. *Archives of Oto-Rhino-Laryngology, 222*(2), 91–97. PubMed

Zeng, F. G., Oba, S., Garde, S., Sininger, Y., & Starr, A. (1999). Temporal and speech processing deficits in auditory neuropathy. *Neuroreport, 10*(16), 3429–3435. PubMed

Chapter 17

Evaluating Central Auditory Function and Brain-Related Injuries

Radhika Aravamudhan, Annette Hurley-Larmeu, and Tina M. Stoody

The assessment of central auditory function typically involves a test battery approach. However, each case is unique and requires the clinician to choose the most appropriate battery from the various behavioral tests available to increase sensitivity and efficiency of diagnosis. Clinicians must also decide whether they should include electrophysiologic testing in the test battery. The inclusion of electrophysiologic measures in the assessment of (central) auditory processing disorders (APDs) is a controversial topic. Electrophysiologic measures are recommended by the Working Group on Auditory Processing Disorders (American Speech-Language-Hearing Association, 2005) and the Task Force on the Diagnosis, Treatment, and Management of Children and Adults with Central Auditory Processing Disorder (American Academy of Audiology, 2010) when there is a suspected underlying neurologic disorder, to assess whether auditory neuropathy spectrum disorder (ANSD) is present, and/or in difficult-to-test children. Electrophysiologic tests in the APD evaluation may aid in the diagnosis or in the validation of behavioral test results (Bellis, 2003; Chermak and Musiek, 1997).

The addition of electrophysiologic tests to a behavioral test battery may provide useful information for possible gross site of dysfunction in the central auditory nervous system (CANS). Patients with CANS dysfunction may have other comorbidities, such as language, learning, or attention deficits, or they may have acquired a CANS dysfunction from an injury (e.g., head trauma). Electrophysiologic tests have been able to elucidate or provide objective evidence of CANS dysfunction in some patients (e.g., Cunningham, Nicol, Zecker, Bradlow, and Kraus, 2001; Fligor, Cox, and Nesathurai, 2002; Hall, Huangfu, Gennarelli, Dolinskas, Olson, and Berry, 1983). Despite the advantages of additional objective measures of central auditory function, it is still unclear which AEPs may be the most beneficial in APD evaluations. Hall (2007) reported that electrophysiologic measures were capable of identifying abnormalities in as few as 10% of children with APD using the auditory brainstem response (ABR) to as high as 40% using cortical event–related potentials (CERPs), such as the middle latency response (MLR) and the P300 response. There is also evidence in the literature that supports the use of middle and late AEPs to diagnose suspected APD in children diagnosed with learning disabilities (Purdy, Kelly, and Davies, 2002).

Support for the inclusion of electrophysiologic tests in the APD test battery is not held universally by researchers and clinicians in the field, particularly with pediatric populations (e.g., Jerger and Musiek, 2000; Katz et al, 2002). Katz and his colleagues (2002) argued that the extended test time and expense were not justified or warranted. The main reason for this is that some of the current tests lack specific norms and data to support their use in the diagnosis of APD. There is the further complication of maturational effects on the middle and late AEPs. Despite these drawbacks, we maintain that electrophysiologic tests can provide important objective evidence and a unique window to view the temporal firing of the CANS, and we recommend that they be considered for inclusion in APD assessment.

APD evaluations are commonly performed on pediatric populations, but many adult patients with closed head injuries resulting from motor vehicle accidents and veterans returning from U.S. military involvement are being referred to audiologists to be evaluated for both hearing loss and suspected auditory processing problems. Most patients suffering from head injury show signs of cognitive disturbances immediately following the injury, but our understanding of long-term effects of closed head injury on cognitive and auditory processing is not clear. Bergemalm and Lyxell (2005) investigated the possible signs of long-term cognitive and/or central auditory problems in people with closed head injury using a computer-based set of five cognitive tests and three central auditory tests. Even though many of the participants did not report any signs of cognitive or auditory impairment, 59% of them demonstrated cognitive shortcomings, and 58% demonstrated APD when tested using ABR, distorted speech audiometry (interrupted speech), and phase audiometry to test central auditory function.

Both behavioral and electrophysiologic test methods may be useful in helping to localize deficits or make assumptions about the affected underlying auditory mechanisms. The different levels of auditory processing can be classified as either encoding or decoding processes. According to Theunissen, Woolley, Hsu, and Fremouw (2004), encoding is the process by which a sound is transformed into neural activity. It can also be referred to as the process by which an acoustic signal is represented at the level of auditory neurons and the lower brainstem. Decoding is the process by which one makes sense of the neural representation of the signal. In other words, it is a process whereby patterns of neural activity take on perceptual meaning and therefore guide

behavioral responses to sounds. While evaluating the auditory–perceptual system, it is important to understand the process (encoding, decoding, or both) being tested and how a deficiency in each process may affect the test results. Most behavioral tests "stress" the auditory system by degrading the acoustic environment using various techniques, including the introduction of background or competing noise, use of filtering, and time compression. Behavioral tests may require multiple auditory processes, as well as other higher-order processes, such as attention, memory, and perception (Jirsa and Clontz, 1990). Therefore, behavioral tests may be confounded by learning, attention, fatigue, hearing sensitivity, cognition, developmental age, motivation, motor skills, language experience, and language impairments (Jerger and Musiek, 2000). Along with these factors, behavioral tests are generally unable to separate encoding and decoding processes. Hence, the results of behavioral test batteries most often reflect a breakdown in auditory processing but do not isolate whether or not the breakdown is specific to encoding or decoding processes (or both).

Electrophysiologic tests of the peripheral and central auditory pathways reflect neural functions and processes involved in the encoding of speech and nonspeech signals. One of the advantages of most electrophysiologic tests is that they do not require the patient to respond to a task. Rather, the patient is able to rest or sit quietly during testing. Most of these objective measures are not as influenced by nonauditory functions (cognition, language, motivation, etc.). Additionally, most electrophysiologic tests do not require attention. In some cases when attention is not required, patients may watch a movie (with controlled sound) or quietly read a book. The disadvantages of electrophysiologic testing is that it may be more time-consuming and some of the recordings may not yet be mature or may have large intrasubject variability. Many of these electrophysiologic tests lack published sensitivity and specificity measures in diagnosing APD both in adults and in children. This chapter gives an overview of some common electrophysiologic tests used in evaluating central auditory function, with examples of expected outcomes from each of these tests. For more information regarding recording and stimulus parameters for the AEPs discussed here, the reader is referred to Chapter 6 for ABR, Chapter 9 for MLR, and Chapter 10 for P300.

Controversial Point

The use of electrophysiologic tests for assessing APD has not been embraced because of the lack of normative data and because they have the potential to extend the test session unnecessarily. However, experience has shown that electrophysiologic tests can elucidate an otherwise borderline diagnosis and may detect subtle or medically critical neural abnormalities not picked up during behavioral testing.

◆ Auditory Brainstem Response

The ABR reflects the synchronous firing of neurons of the eighth cranial nerve (CN VIII) and lower brainstem structures (see Chapters 6 and 16). The aim of the ABR testing in the APD protocol is to evaluate the integrity of the auditory neurons (i.e., neurodiagnostic) rather than threshold estimation. This electrophysiologic recording provides information about the integrity of the lower central auditory pathways that are also involved in auditory processing and the requisite capabilities of the auditory system to encode information. Previous research investigations reporting ABR findings with APD have been conflicting. Early investigations have failed to pinpoint subject characteristics, for example, describing subjects "at risk" for APD or having "minimal brain dysfunction" (Sohmer and Student, 1978; Worthington, 1981; Worthington, Beauchaine, Peters, and Reiland, 1981); lack a description of the specific characteristics of the APD (Protti, 1983); or have not effectively described the criteria for wave latency abnormality of the ABR (Hall and Mueller, 1997). Although the ABR may be normal for most children with APD, it is a sensitive measure for neurologic disorders affecting the lower brainstem auditory pathway, including CN VIII. ABR waveforms are evaluated on the basis of several different diagnostic criteria, including absolute peak latencies, interpeak latencies, interaural latencies, and overall waveform morphology.

Peak amplitudes are not of great interest when evaluating ABR, although they may be smaller in patients with APD (Hurley, Hurley, and Homer, 2008; Mason and Mellor, 1984). It is also important to note that ABR amplitude is more variable than peak latency. However, clinicians should be aware that inherent noise conditions and other factors such as head size, the thickness of the skull, and electrode placement may affect the amplitude of the ABR.

Hall and Mueller (1997) reviewed ABR recordings for 102 pediatric patients with APD and found abnormal findings in ~10% of these individuals. They reported a greater percentage of abnormalities for the left auditory pathway than for the right auditory pathway. Despite these findings, the authors did not provide any explanation for the left versus right auditory pathway abnormality, and there was no information about the subjects' ages or their specific type of APD.

Response Analysis and Results

Early latency ABR responses merely reflect the auditory mechanism's ability to encode a transient signal (Brugge, 1975). Usually, ABR is within normal limits in individuals with APD. However the following are some differences that may be noted in the APD clinical population are:

- Poor repeatability of ABR waves
- Reduced amplitude for wave V
- Poorer morphology, depending on whether there is a significant neurologic cause
- Delayed wave V in masked conditions

The delay of wave V in masked conditions is thought to be a consequence of associated perceptual problems, related to backward masking (Kraus and Banai, 2007).

◆ BioMARK (Speech-Evoked Auditory Brainstem Response)

One of the newer, more promising electrophysiologic tests using speechlike stimuli was developed from the work of Kraus and colleagues (Kraus, McGee, Carrell, Zecker, Nicol, and Koch, 1996). Initially, this test was commercially introduced as BioMAP and later renamed BioMARK, both of which stand for Biological Marker of Audiology Processing. There has been increasing evidence that brainstem measures relating to encoding of speech information can provide further indications of auditory function as the brainstem neural response mimics the temporal characteristics of the speech signal presented. Much of the current literature refers to ABRs elicited by speech and other complex stimuli as cABR. Exciting new evidence suggests that cABR measurements can help differentiate auditory function in typically developing children from those with difficulty understanding speech in noise (Anderson, Skoe, Chandrasekaran, and Kraus, 2010; Chandrasekaran, Hornickel, Skoe, Nicol, and Kraus, 2009) and poor temporal processing skills (Johnson, Nicol, Zecker, and Kraus, 2007). At the present time, the BioMARK is no longer commercially available, but interested readers are referred to the Auditory Neuroscience Laboratory at Northwestern University for more information (Web Site: http://www.soc.northwestern.edu/brainvolts/).

Stimulus and Recording Parameters

The BioMARK test requires that the patient have a normal click-evoked ABR, showing normal synchronous firing of the auditory nerve. The patient preparation is the same as that for a single-channel neurodiagnostic ABR. Recommended electrode montage includes Cz to the right earlobe (or mastoid) with the forehead serving as the ground. A synthetic speech stimulus (/da/) is delivered to the right ear through ER-3A insert earphones. The left ear remains unoccluded. The patient is able to sleep or watch a video (with very low sound) and does not have to pay attention to the signal.

Response Analysis

The underlying assumption is that the response represents neural encoding of the temporal and spectral characteristics of the acoustic signal presented. Normative data have been established for the BioMARK, for the following age groups: patients aged from 3 to 4, 5 to 12, and 18 to 28 years. Although

the patient preparation and setup are very similar to neurodiagnostic ABR, the analysis of the BioMARK test is different. After averaging the waveforms, there are two peaks the clinician must mark (V and A), which reflect the response to the onset of the sound. Peak identification can be aided by comparison to the template waveform provided within the software. Once the clinician has picked and labeled the V and A waveform components, further analysis of the waveform is performed automatically by the AEP software by selecting the BioMARK analysis on the analysis menu. The analysis of the response includes comparing the temporal and spectral information represented at the level of the brainstem to the signal presented. The response is time locked to the signal, so the temporal envelope is matched for comparison of the response to the signal. The closer the match, the better the individual's auditory encoding capabilities.

Research Results

Several researchers have investigated the use of BioMARK on clinical populations. Cunningham and colleagues (2001) revealed that children with learning impairments show significantly different encoding of speech signal on BioMARK when compared with age-matched controls. Wible et al (2005) used speech auditory evoked potentials (AEPs) to investigate brainstem and cortical responses to the speech sound /da/ and /ga/ in 20 children. Results showed abnormal encoding of speech sounds in both brainstem and cortical processing measures in the language-impaired group. Kraus and Banai (2007) discussed the changes noted in cABR measures as a consequence of delayed perception of onset of speech sounds, examples of abnormal cortical representation of sound under temporal stress, and a reflection of difficulty in temporal resolution and temporal order judgment. Overall, if the signals are not represented correctly at the level of the brainstem, this can lead to further difficulty in speech perception abilities.

In summary, the BioMARK test is able to isolate temporal and spectral encoding problems in some children with APD or other language-based learning deficits. In turn, the BioMARK, along with other tests, can help in understanding the levels at which the problems exist and aid in recommending and/or implementing treatment options. An extensive tutorial by Skoe and Kraus (2010) can provide the reader with more information on the use of cABRs.

◆ Middle Latency Response

The middle latency response (MLR) was first reported by Geisler et al (1958) and occurs in the time following the ABR but before the late latency response (LLR), covering the range of 12 to 70 msec (Chapter 9). Each wave in the MLR is the result of the activation of multiple generator sites. The underlying auditory generators of the MLR include the thalamocortical pathway (Kileny, Paccioretti, and Wilson, 1987; Kraus, Ozdamar, Hier, and Stein, 1982; Ozdamar and Kraus, 1983), the planum temporale and superior temporal gyrus (Yvert, Crouzeix, Bertrand, Seither-Preisler, and Pantev, 2001; Yvert, Fischer, Bertrand, and Pernier, 2005), the reticular formation (Kraus, Kileny, and McGee, 1994), and the inferior colliculus (McGee, Kraus, Comperatore, and Nicol, 1991). Waves Na (15–20 msec) and Pa (25–35 msec) are most reliability recorded, whereas waves Nb (35–45 msec) and Pb (50–75 msec) are highly influenced by the reticular formation and certain stimulus and recording parameters.

The MLR recording can be a valuable tool in assessing the maturity of the central auditory pathway. Intersubject variability of the MLR is great in the pediatric population, so there are no normative latency and amplitude data available for very young children. It is important to note that the MLR does not reach adult maturity until around age 8 to 12 years. However, it is a significant finding if the MLR is absent (Chermak and Musiek, 1997).

Generally, waves Na and Pa are the only ones that are used diagnostically in APD assessments (Chermak and Musiek, 1997), providing amplitude and latency measures for interpretation. Amplitude may be a more sensitive measure than latency (Kileny, Paccioretti, and Wilson, 1987; Kraus et al, 1982; Scherg and Von Cramon, 1986).

For a neurodiagnostic MLR, it is important to record from electrode sites over both hemispheres. One would need at least two to four channels to perform MLR hemisphere–specific recordings. Hall (2007) recommends noninverting electrodes C3, C4, and Cz referenced to linked earlobes (or a noncephalic reference) with Fpz as ground. Another reference electrode option is the ipsilateral earlobe (e.g., Musiek, Charette, Kelly, Lee, and Musiek, 1999; Schochat, Musiek, Alonso, and Ogata, 2010). The choice of reference electrode montage appears to be a matter of personal preference.

Response Analysis and Results

MLR wave amplitude and morphology are more important clinically than latency. The amplitude of Pa is compared at different electrode sites (e.g. Cz, C3, and C4). Amplitude measures that are less than 50% compared with other electrode sites are diagnostically significant. If there is a lesion, the amplitude from the electrode closest to the lesion will be compromised. This reduced amplitude is referred to as an "electrode effect" (Musiek, Baran, and Pinheiro, 1994). This effect will be evident regardless of which ear is stimulated.

Other investigators have reported "ear effects," a reduction of the amplitude of the response when a specific ear is stimulated (Chermak and Musiek, 1997). An ear effect finding is not as diagnostically significant as an electrode effect (Kelly, Lee, Charette, and Musiek, 1996; Shehata-Dieler, Shimizu, Soliman, and Tusa, 1991) and may be minimized using linked earlobes. Although further research is needed, Schochat, Rabelo, and Loreti (2004) suggest that an ear effect is more likely to be found than an electrode effect in cases with APD.

MLR recordings have also been useful in documenting plasticity of the CANS or to assess the effectiveness of an auditory training program. Previous investigators have reported increased amplitude of the MLR after the patient has completed an intensive auditory training program (Morlet, Berlin, Norman, and Ray, 2003; Schochat, Musiek, Alonso, and Ogata, 2010). Although posttesting tends to show improvement in behavioral tests, the

MLR offers objective evidence of physiologic changes in the CANS.

◆ P300

P300 is a cortical and cognitive response that is a manifestation of strategies used by the auditory system in selective attention (Chapter 10). Even though the generator sites for P300 are not exclusive to the auditory cortex (e.g., there are contributions from the frontal cortex, centroparietal cortex, and hippocampus), most of the changes detected in P300 have been very useful in identifying APD.

Response Analysis and Results

The recording equipment will include separate averaged waveforms for both the frequent and infrequent stimuli. The P300 is present only within the infrequent average, whereas the P1, N1, P2, and N2 are seen in both frequent and infrequent averaged responses. If the patient is unable to attend to, or to detect the difference between the standard (frequent) and oddball (infrequent) stimuli used in the oddball paradigm, the P300 is significantly reduced in amplitude and significantly prolonged in latency.

Jirsa and Clontz (1990) compared P300 responses of children with APD and normal age-matched controls. The children with APD had significantly reduced amplitudes and prolonged latencies. Similar changes in P300 (i.e., longer latency and smaller amplitude) have been observed in children with dyslexia when compared with age-matched controls. (Jirsa, 1992; Mazzotta and Gallai, 1992). In addition to latency and amplitude changes, the overall morphology of the wave was also significantly different between the two groups. This study illustrates the diagnostic value of P300. Jirsa (1992) investigated whether the P300 could be used to reflect behavioral changes resulting from therapeutic intervention in a group of children with APD. A significant decrease in P300 latency and a significant increase in P300 amplitude were noted following a structured treatment program.

> **Special Consideration**
>
> Even though current electrophysiologic measures are not able to replace the behavioral test battery for APDs, current research suggests that they can provide useful information about the neurophysiology and integrity of the auditory system.

◆ Case Studies

The remainder of this chapter briefly summarizes some case studies of patients who help demonstrate the use of AEPs in APD evaluations and treatment. The following AEPs are included: ABR, BioMARK, MLR, and P300. **Table 17.1** summarizes the case history, behavioral test results, and AEP test results for all of the cases presented.

ABR Case Studies

In most children with APD, the ABR will be unremarkable; however, this test takes just a few minutes and provides valuable information about the integrity of the CANS. Many of the children with APD have predisposing risk factors that can affect the latency of the ABR, such as a protracted history of otitis media and hyperbilirubinemia. **Figure 17.1** provides some examples of ABR waveforms recorded in children referred for APD testing. In panel A there is a typical ABR recording from an 11-year-old boy. Although his electrophysiologic testing was within normal limits, he was diagnosed with APD, specifically an integration deficit, after results from a behavioral test battery included a left ear deficit on dichotic digits (double pairs) testing, as well as reduced performance on pitch pattern testing in the left ear. This individual receives academic resource services through the school. In panel B, the ABR waveforms from a 7-year-old boy with a history of protracted middle ear infections with four sets of pressure equalization tubes and infantile jaundice are displayed. Numerous atypical results within the comprehensive APD behavioral test battery were found (**Table 17.1**) that led to a diagnosis of

Table 17.1   Summary of Behavioral and Electrophysiologic Test Results for Case Studies

Case History and Diagnosis	Auditory Figure Ground	Filtered Speech	Time-Compressed Speech	Dichotic Digits Double Pair	Pitch Pattern Test	Phonemic Synthesis Test	Masking Level Difference	AEP Test and Results
11-year-old boy APD (integration deficit) Dyslexia	WNL	WNL	WNL	* Left ear deficit	* left ear for verbal response	DNT	WNL	ABR (WNL)
7-year-old boy APD (decoding deficit) PE tubes	*	*	*	* Bilateral deficit	WNL	*	*	ABR (delayed latencies) BioMARK (abnormal)
7-year-old girl Negative for APD Spinal bifida, hydrocephalus	WNL	WNL	WNL	WNL	WNL	DNT	DNT	ABR (delayed wave V for the left ear)
9-year-old girl APD (decoding deficit) Expressive/receptive language disorder	*	*	*	* Bilateral deficit	WNL	*	WNL	BioMARK (asymmetric response)
14-year-old boy ANSD	*	*	*	WNL	DNT	DNT	WNL	MLR (WNL) P300 (WNL)
10-year-old boy History of seizures APD (decoding deficit)	*	*	*	* Right ear deficit	*	*	DNT	MLR (electrode effect: reduced amplitude on right side) P300 (WNL)
Young adult girl Negative for APD	WNL	WNL	WNL	WNL	WNL	WNL	WNL	P300
9-year-old boy Initial diagnosis of APD	*	*	*	WNL	WNL	*	WNL	P300 (low-amplitude response)
9-year-old boy After computer-based auditory training therapy	WNL	V/NL	*	WNL	WNL	WNL	WNL	P300 (higher response amplitude)

Abbreviations: ABR, auditory brainstem response; AEP, auditory evoked potential; ANSD, auditory neuropathy spectrum disorder ; APD, auditory processing disorder; DNT, did not test; MLR, middle latency response; PE, pressure equalization; WNL, within normal limits.

*Atypical performance.

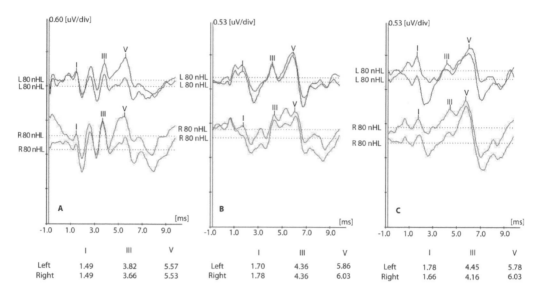

	I	III	V
Left	1.49	3.82	5.57
Right	1.49	3.66	5.53

	I	III	V
Left	1.70	4.36	5.86
Right	1.78	4.36	6.03

	I	III	V
Left	1.78	4.45	5.78
Right	1.66	4.16	6.03

Fig. 17.1 Auditory brainstem response (ABR) case examples. These waveforms were collected to supplement behavioral test data during auditory processing disorder (APD) evaluations for (**A**) an 11-year-old with integration deficits, (**B**) a 7-year-old with a history of otitis media, and decoding deficits, and (**C**) a 7-year-old with a history of hydrocephalus and a mild receptive language disorder.

decoding characteristics of APD. In addition to the behavioral test findings, his ABR latencies were slightly delayed. In panel C, waveforms were recorded from a 7-year-old girl referred for APD assessment. The case history also included spinal bifida and a history of hydrocephalus with shunt placement. A slightly delayed wave V is noted for the left ear. Behavioral test findings were not consistent with an APD diagnosis, although she was diagnosed with a mild receptive language disorder. She receives academic support services both privately and through the school system.

BioMARK Case Studies

A BioMARK (displayed as BioMAP in this case) calculated waveform and algorithm printout is displayed in **Fig. 17.2**. This recording is from a 7-year-old boy who had a normal ABR, but the BioMARK results were abnormal. The Bio-MARK findings were consistent with behavioral test results that were atypical in several instances, resulting in a diagnosis of decoding characteristics of APD (**Table 17.1**). This child is receiving speech-language therapy services and is also participating in an afterschool auditory training program.

Although the recommended clinical protocol is to record the BioMARK from the right ear only, we routinely record the BioMARK from both ears to examine interaural differences. Interestingly, we have found asymmetric recordings in some individuals. Displayed in **Fig. 17.3** are the symmetrical click-evoked right and left ABRs and BioMARK waveforms. The BioMARK algorithm was normal for the right ear (algorithm =1) and abnormal for the left ear (algorithm =10). This asymmetry is very interesting and unusual. This objectively reflects differences in the monaural pathway's ability to encode speech. This 9-year-old girl had a severe expressive and receptive language disorder. She was also diagnosed with decoding characteristics of APD, based on the behavioral test battery (**Table 17.1**). She is receiving speech-language therapy and resource services at school.

MLR Case Studies

Recording the MLR in young children can be a challenge because of developmental changes. A normal MLR is shown in **Fig. 17.4**; the amplitude of Na-Pa is compared across electrode sites and found to be very similar. This MLR was recorded

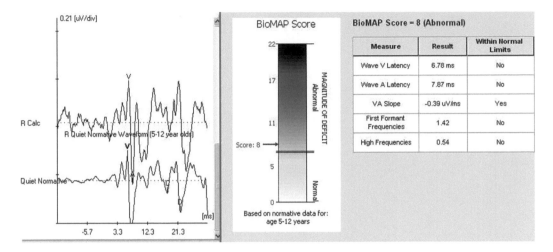

Fig. 17.2 BioMARK (shown here as BioMAP) analysis example. A calculated BioMARK waveform is shown on the left side of the figure, and the corresponding BioMARK score and test analysis summary table algorithm are shown on the right.

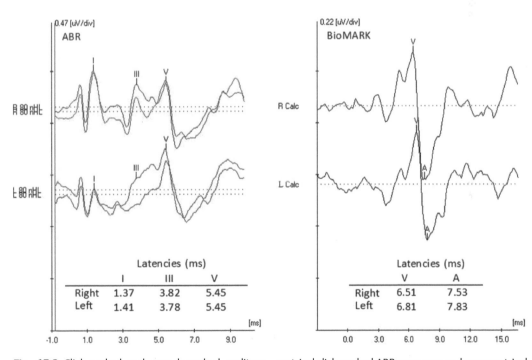

Fig. 17.3 Click-evoked and speech-evoked auditory brainstem response (ABR). This patient exhibited symmetrical click-evoked ABR responses and asymmetrical responses to speech stimuli.

from a 14-year-old boy patient with ANSD. Individuals with ANSD typically present with absent or grossly abnormal ABR results; however, middle and late auditory evoked responses can remain unaffected, as is seen here with a clear electrode effect.

An abnormal MLR is displayed in **Fig. 17.5.** Shown are summed MLR responses from two

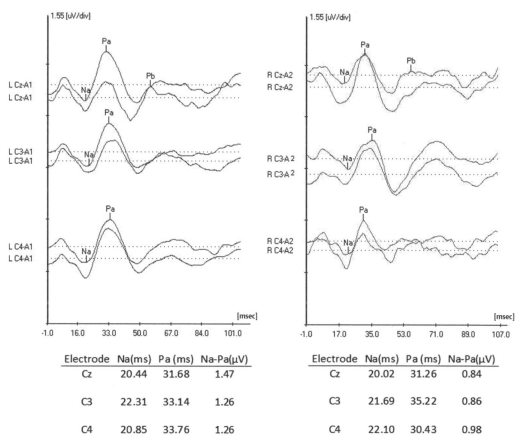

Electrode	Na(ms)	Pa (ms)	Na-Pa(µV)
Cz	20.44	31.68	1.47
C3	22.31	33.14	1.26
C4	20.85	33.76	1.26

Electrode	Na(ms)	Pa (ms)	Na-Pa(µV)
Cz	20.02	31.26	0.84
C3	21.69	35.22	0.86
C4	22.10	30.43	0.98

Fig. 17.4 A middle latency response (MLR) recording representing typical or "normal" latency and amplitude values.

individual sweeps for each electrode site with right and left stimulation. This recording is from a 10-year-old boy with a history of seizures over the right temporal lobe. The amplitude of the MLR from C4 is less than 50% in comparison to the other electrodes, which is consistent with pathology over the right hemisphere. Interestingly, the ABR and P300 recordings were normal. Based on behavioral and electrophysiologic results, this child was diagnosed with decoding characteristics of APD (**Table 17.1**) and is receiving private speech language therapy and reading tutoring, as well as resource services through the school.

P300 Case Examples

When using P300 in the clinic, it is important to remember that the P300 response is highly variable across individuals. Previous reports have found significant group differences for many disordered populations, but for individuals this evoked potential should not be used as the only diagnostic tool. However, if incorporated into an appropriate test battery, the P300 recording can add support to behavioral APD test results. The presence of the P300 response is not necessarily an indicator of absence of pathology. Rather, groups with pathologic conditions typically have delayed latencies and/or reduced amplitudes compared with groups of "normal" individuals. A normal P300 recording is depicted on the left-hand side of **Fig. 17.6.** This recording was obtained from the same patient with ANSD discussed in the preceding section. Latencies and amplitudes were similar for the right and left ears. The top traces are the responses to the standard (frequent) stimuli,

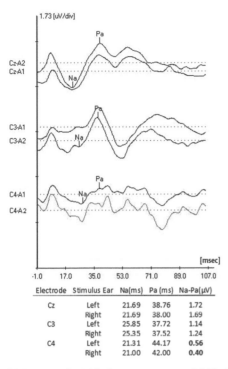

Electrode	Stimulus Ear	Na(ms)	Pa (ms)	Na-Pa(µV)
Cz	Left	21.69	38.76	1.72
	Right	21.69	38.00	1.69
C3	Left	25.85	37.72	1.14
	Right	25.35	37.52	1.24
C4	Left	21.31	44.17	0.56
	Right	21.00	42.00	0.40

Fig. 17.5 Atypical middle latency response (MLR). An electrode effect is shown here with significantly reduced amplitudes recorded over the right hemisphere (C4) compared to left hemisphere (C3).

and the bottom traces are the responses to the oddballs (infrequent stimuli).

Just as the presence of a P300 response is not always an indicator of absence of pathology, an absent P300 is not always indicative of auditory dysfunction. On the right-hand side of **Fig. 17.6,** no P300 was recorded with left ear stimulation. This individual does not have any academic difficulties or auditory processing concerns and is excelling academically in a graduate degree program. This case demonstrates that a diagnosis of APD cannot be based on an absent P300. However, electrophysiologic recordings may be used to support or validate behavioral test results.

In addition to being used as diagnostic indicators of pathology, electrophysiologic measures can serve as a means to measure progress within a treatment program. Pre- and post-treatment P300 recordings are shown from a 9-year-old boy who completed a computer-mediated auditory training program are shown in **Fig. 17.7.** Improvements were also seen on behavioral tests of APD. This improvement reflects the plasticity of the CANS.

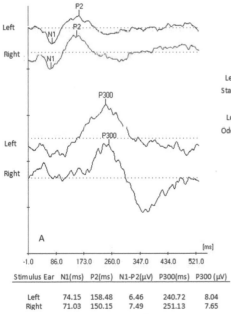

Stimulus Ear	N1(ms)	P2(ms)	N1-P2(µV)	P300(ms)	P300 (µV)
Left	74.15	158.48	6.46	240.72	8.04
Right	71.03	150.15	7.49	251.13	7.65

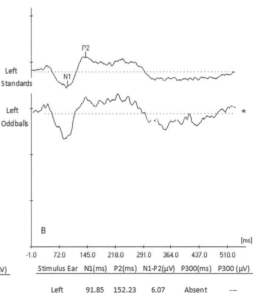

Stimulus Ear	N1(ms)	P2(ms)	N1-P2(µV)	P300(ms)	P300 (µV)
Left	91.85	152.23	6.07	Absent	---

Fig. 17.6 P300 case examples. **(A)** The left top traces are for standard stimuli, and the bottom traces are for oddball stimuli. Robust P300 responses were recorded for target stimuli in both ears. **(B)** The recording from the left ear only shows that the averaged waveforms for both standards and oddballs are devoid of the P300 response. However, this absence was not an indication of auditory processing disorders in this case (see text).

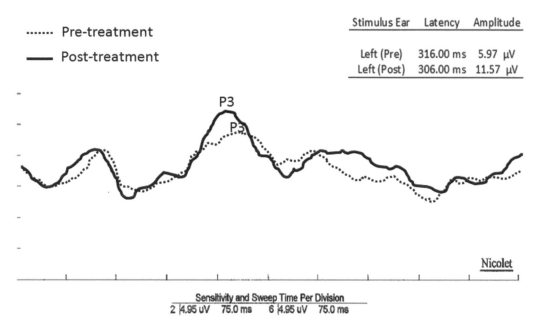

Stimulus Ear	Latency	Amplitude
Left (Pre)	316.00 ms	5.97 µV
Left (Post)	306.00 ms	11.57 µV

Sensitivity and Sweep Time Per Division
2 |4.95 uV 75.0 ms 6 |4.95 uV 75.0 ms

Fig. 17.7 Improvement in the P300 response. Auditory evoked potentials indicate a treatment effect for a computer-based auditory training program with increased P300 amplitude after treatment.

◆ Summary

This chapter presented evidence to support the use of AEP testing to supplement typical behavioral test batteries used in diagnosis of auditory processing disorders. While findings may be of limited value when used in isolation, the data obtained from AEP recordings when used in addition to behavioral measures, will serve to strengthen/support behavioral findings. AEPs may also be used as a tool to evaluate physiologic changes after treatment/remediation therapies.

References

American Academy of Audiology. (2010). *American Academy of Audiology clinical practice guidelines: Diagnosis, treatment and management of children and adults with central auditory processing disorder.* Available from http://www.audiology.org/resources/documentlibrary/

American Speech-Language-Hearing Association. (2005). (Central) auditory processing disorders. Available from http://www.asha.org/policy/

Anderson, S., Skoe, E., Chandrasekaran, B., & Kraus, N. (2010). Neural timing is linked to speech perception in noise. *Journal of Neuroscience, 30*(14), 4922–4926. PubMed

Bellis, T. (2003). *Assessment and management of central auditory processing disorders in the educational setting: From science to practice* (2nd ed.). San Diego: Singular Publishing Group.

Bergemalm, P. O., & Lyxell, B. (2005). Appearances are deceptive? Long-term cognitive and central auditory sequelae from closed head injury. *International Journal of Audiology, 44*(1), 39–49. PubMed

Brugge, J. (1975). Progress in neuroanatomy and neurophysiology of auditory cortex. In E. Eagles (Ed.), *The nervous system: Human communication and its disorder* (Vol. 3, pp. 97–111). New York: Raven Press.

Chandrasekaran, B., Hornickel, J., Skoe, E., Nicol, T. G., & Kraus, N. (2009). Context-dependent encoding in the human auditory brainstem relates to hearing speech in noise: Implications for developmental dyslexia. *Neuron, 64*(3), 311–319. PubMed

Chermak, G. D., & Musiek, F. E.(1997). *Central auditory processing disorders: New perspectives.* San Diego: Singular Publishing Group.

Cunningham, J., Nicol, T., Zecker, S. G., Bradlow, A., & Kraus, N. (2001). Neurobiologic responses to speech in noise in children with learning problems: Deficits and strategies for improvement. *Clinical Neurophysiology, 112,* 758–767.

Fligor, B. J., Cox, L. C., & Nesathurai, S. (2002). Subjective hearing loss and history of traumatic brain injury exhibits abnormal brainstem auditory evoked response: A case report. *Archives of Physical Medicine and Rehabilitation, 83*(1), 141–143. PubMed

Geisler, C. D., Frishkopf, L. S., & Rosenblith, W. A. (1958). Extracranial responses to acoustic clicks in man. *Science, 128*(3333), 1210–1211. PubMed

Hall, J. W., III, Huangfu, M., Gennarelli, T. A., Dolinskas, C. A., Olson, K., & Berry, G. A. (1983). Auditory evoked responses, impedance measures, and diagnostic speech audiometry in severe head injury. *Otolaryngology—Head and Neck Surgery, 91*(1), 50–60. PubMed

Hall, J. W., III, & Mueller, H. G., III. (1997). *Audiologist's desk reference* (Vol. 1). San Diego: Plural Publishing.

Hall, J. W., III. (2007). *New handbook of auditory evoked responses.* Boston: Allyn & Bacon.

Hurley, A., Hurley, R. M., & Homer, E. (2008, November). *Behavioral and electrophysiological evidence of CANS plasticity after auditory training.* Platform presentation at the ASHA convention, Chicago.

Jerger, J., & Musiek, F. (2000). Report of the Consensus Conference on the diagnosis of auditory processing disorders in school-aged children. *Journal of the American Academy of Audiology, 11*(9), 467–474. PubMed

Jirsa, R. E., & Clontz, K. B. (1990, Jun). Long latency auditory event-related potentials from children with auditory processing disorders. *Ear and Hearing, 11*(3), 222–232. PubMed

Jirsa, R. E. (1992). The clinical utility of the P3 AERP in children with auditory processing disorders. *Journal of Speech and Hearing Research, 35*(4), 903–912. PubMed

Johnson, K. L., Nicol, T. G., Zecker, S. G., & Kraus, N. (2007). Auditory brainstem correlates of perceptual timing deficits. *Journal of Cognitive Neuroscience, 19*(3), 376–385. PubMed

Katz, J., DeConde-Johnson, C., Brander, S., Delagrange, T., Ferre, J., King, J., et al.. (2002). Clinical and research concerns regarding the 2000 auditory processing disorders consensus report and recommendations. *Audiology Today, 14*(2), 14–17.

Kelly, T., Lee, W., Charette, L., & Musiek, F. (1996, March). Middle latency evoked response sensitivity and specificity. Paper presented at the annual meeting of the American Auditory Society, Salt Lake City, UT.

Kileny, P. R., Paccioretti, D., & Wilson, A. F. (1987). Effects of cortical lesions on middle-latency auditory evoked responses (MLR). *Electroencephalography and Clinical Neurophysiology, 66*(2), 108–120. PubMed

Kraus, N., & Banai, K (2007). Auditory processing malleability: Focus on language and music. *Current Directions in Psychological Science, 16*(2), 105–109.

Kraus, N., Kileny, P., & McGee, T.(1994). Middle latency auditory evoked potentials. In J. Katz (Ed.), *Handbook of clinical audiology* (4th ed., pp. 387–405). Baltimore: Lippincott Williams & Wilkins.

Kraus, N., McGee, T. J., Carrell, T. D., Zecker, S. G., Nicol, T. G., & Koch, D. B. (1996). Auditory neurophysiologic responses and discrimination deficits in children with learning problems. *Science, 273*(5277), 971–973. PubMed

Kraus, N., Ozdamar, O., Hier, D., & Stein, L. (1982). Auditory middle latency responses (MLRs) in patients with cortical lesions. *Electroencephalography and Clinical Neurophysiology, 54*(3), 275–287. PubMed

Mason, S. M., & Mellor, D. H. (1984). Brain-stem, middle latency and late cortical evoked potentials in children with speech and language disorders. *Electroencephalography and Clinical Neurophysiology, 59*(4), 297–309. PubMed

Mazzotta, G., & Gallai, V. (1992). Study of the P300 event-related potential through brain mapping in phonological dyslexics. *Acta Neurologica, 14*(3), 173–186. PubMed

McGee, T., Kraus, N., Comperatore, C., & Nicol, T. (1991). Subcortical and cortical components of the MLR generating system. *Brain Research, 544*(2), 211–220. PubMed

Morlet, T., Berlin, C. I., Norman, M., & Ray, M. (2003). Fast ForWord™: Its scientific basis and treatment effects on the human efferent auditory system. In C. I. Berlin & T. G. Weyand (Eds.), *The brain and sensory plasticity: Language acquisition and hearing* (pp. 129–148). New York: Delmar Learning.

Musiek, F. E., Baran, J. A., & Pinheiro, M. L. (1994). *Neuroaudiology case studies.* San Diego: Singular Publishing Group.

Musiek, F., Charette, L., Kelly, T., Lee, W., & Musiek, E. (1999). Hit and false-positive rates for the middle latency response in patients with central nervous system involvement. *Journal of the American Academy of Audiology, 10*(3), 124–132.

Ozdamar, O., & Kraus, N. (1983). Auditory middle-latency responses in humans. *Audiology, 22*(1), 34–49. PubMed

Protti, E. (1983). Brainstem auditory pathways and auditory processing disorders. In E. Lasky & J. Katz (Eds.), *Central auditory processing disorders* (pp. 117–139). Baltimore, MD: University Park Press.

Purdy, S. C., Kelly, A. S., & Davies, M. G. (2002). Auditory brainstem response, middle latency response, and late cortical evoked potentials in children with learning disabilities. *Journal of the American Academy of Audiology, 13*(7), 367–382. PubMed

Scherg, M., & Von Cramon, D. (1986). Evoked dipole source potentials of the human auditory cortex. *Electroencephalography and Clinical Neurophysiology, 65*(5), 344–360. PubMed

Schochat, E., Musiek, F. E., Alonso, R., & Ogata, J. (2010). Effect of auditory training on the middle latency response in children with (central) auditory processing disorder. *Brazilian Journal of Medical and Biological Research, 43*(8), 777–785. PubMed

Schochat, E., Rabelo, C. M., & Loreti, R. C. D. A. (2004). Sensitivity and specificity of middle latency potential. *Revista Brasileira de Otorrinolaringologia (English Ed.), 70*(3), 353–358.

Shehata-Dieler, W., Shimizu, H., Soliman, S. M., & Tusa, R. J. (1991). Middle latency auditory evoked potentials in temporal lobe disorders. *Ear and Hearing, 12*(6), 377–388. PubMed

Skoe, E., & Kraus, N. (2010). Auditory brain stem response to complex sounds: A tutorial. *Ear and Hearing, 31*(3), 302–324. PubMed

Sohmer, H., & Student, M. (1978). Auditory nerve and brain-stem evoked responses in normal, autistic, minimal brain dysfunction and psychomotor retarded children. *Electroencephalography and Clinical Neurophysiology, 44*(3), 380–388. PubMed

Theunissen, F. E., Woolley, S. M., Hsu, A., & Fremouw, T. (2004, June). Methods for the analysis of auditory pro-

cessing in the brain. *Annals of the New York Academy of Sciences, 1016,* 187–207. PubMed

Wible, B., Nicol, T., & Kraus, N. (2005, February). Correlation between brainstem and cortical auditory processes in normal and language-impaired children. *Brain, 128*(Pt 2), 417–423. PubMed

Worthington, D. (1981). *ABR in special populations.* Paper presented at the ABR Workshop, Cleveland, Ohio.

Worthington, D., Beauchaine, K., Peters, J., & Reiland, J. (1981, November). *Abnormal ABRs in children with severe speech/language delays.* Paper presented at the American Speech Language and Hearing Association Convention, Los Angeles, CA.

Yvert, B., Crouzeix, A., Bertrand, O., Seither-Preisler, A., & Pantev, C. (2001). Multiple supratemporal sources of magnetic and electric auditory evoked middle latency components in humans. *Cerebral Cortex, 11*(5), 411–423. PubMed

Yvert, B., Fischer, C., Bertrand, O., & Pernier, J. (2005). Localization of human supratemporal auditory areas from intracerebral auditory evoked potentials using distributed source models. *NeuroImage, 28*(1), 140–153. PubMed

Chapter 18

Surgical Applications of Auditory Evoked Potentials

Gayle E. Hicks

The acquisition of auditory evoked potentials (AEPs) during surgery is one of the most challenging intraoperative monitoring (IOM) procedures. Compared with other electrophysiologic modalities, AEPs are more affected by physiologic and environmental artifacts because of their size, frequency content, and, in the case of middle latency and cortical responses, sensitivity to anesthesia. Much of the contaminating noise in the operating room (OR) is high frequency in nature, such as electrocautery devices, the minute voltage given off by metal instruments, and patient electromyographic (muscle) artifact. Although most patients are deeply anesthetized, those surgeries where assessment of the auditory system is indicated typically involve monitoring of motor cranial nerves in the same anatomical vicinity as the auditory nerve. Minute muscle tension can occur even with a deeply anesthetized patient. Without the use of muscle-relaxing agents, these small potentials can contaminate an auditory brainstem response (ABR) acquired from needle electrodes placed on the head.

The crossover to acquiring AEPs from the clinic to the OR is a wide gap. In the clinic, the audiologist has control of the environment, electrode configuration, and placement of the transducers and usually has enough time to make any necessary adjustments to optimize the recording. Because of the equipment and personnel required to provide surgical services, the addition of the evoked potential equipment and a technologist or clinician can be problematic. In optimum situations, the OR has enough space for equipment and the personnel who operate them. However, that is not often the case (**Fig. 18.1**).

In the clinic, the AEP system usually has a permanent location, and the patient is situated to accommodate the testing environment. In the OR, the AEP equipment and clinician must adapt to the environment. The initial arrangement of the recording equipment is crucial. If the equipment is set up in an area that is inconvenient to other aspects of the patient's care, it might be necessary to move it during the surgery. The circulating nurse is responsible for the OR suite and is a good individual to ask where to locate the evoked potential equipment. Optimally, the equipment and operator are arranged within clear view of the anesthesiologist and his or her monitoring systems. The patient's temperature, blood pressure, and in some cases anesthetic levels, are usually displayed on a monitor at standing eye level on or above the anesthesia cart. Tracking changes in these values is important to distinguish iatrogenic (i.e. physician induced) from anesthetic changes.

During the surgery, electrophysiologic monitoring equipment needs to be a safe distance from the patient, operating surgeon, and sterile field. Most IOM systems are supplied with

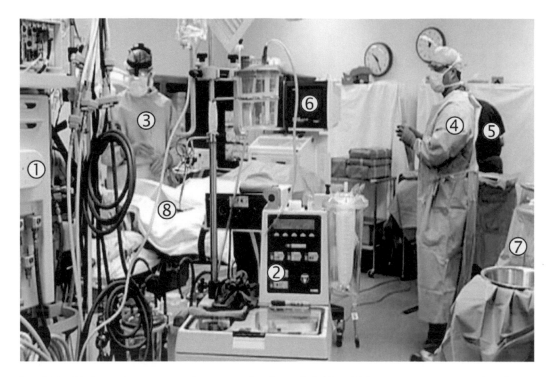

Fig. 18.1 This figure demonstrates the personnel and equipment necessary for surgery: (1) anesthesia cart, (2) cell saver, (3) surgeon, (4) scrub technologist, (5) circulating nurse, (6) fluoroscopic radiograph screen, (7) sterile field, and (8) patient. Not seen: anesthesiologist, perfusionist, assisting surgeon, fluoroscopic radiograph machine, electrocautery systems, evoked potential equipment, and operator.

cables that can be strung a safe distance from the sterile field. If monitoring is performed using a machine not specifically designed for the OR, cable extensions may be needed. In cases where AEPs are requested for diagnostic purposes to be performed prior or subsequent to a minor surgical procedure (e.g., placement of pressure equalization [PE] tubes), this is not as important an issue.

Once the IOM equipment has been set up, the cables to the preamplifier and stimulus delivery devices (i.e., insert earphones) should be arranged to avoid any traffic areas. This is mostly a safety issue for the surgeons, nurses, and surgical technologists that need clear access to the patient and sterile field. Additionally, heavy equipment such as radiograph machines and microscopes are moved toward and away from the patient, depending on the stage of surgery. If stimulating and preamplifier cables are in the path of one of these machines, they could impede their movement and/or become damaged themselves.

The preamplifier (recording electrode input) should be placed near the patient's head but arranged to allow access during the surgical procedure. Again, the circulating nurse or surgical technologist is the best source for deciding where to place the preamplifier. Usually the side opposite the sterile instrument field (a table where sterile surgical instruments are organized) is the optimum location. If the preamplifier is placed too close to the patient, it may be in the surgeon's way, and access to it may be difficult in the event of a technical issue. If it is placed too far from the patient, the electrodes on the patient could be stretched or dislodged, and the additional distance may result in greater interference from electromagnetic fields (EMFs), which are airborne signals emitted from other equipment in the OR. Another consideration is protecting the preamplifier and stimulating devices from fluids such as prepping washes, irrigation, and blood. For additional protection, these devices can be wrapped with small clear plastic drapes available in the OR.

Arrangement of the AEP equipment depends greatly on the desired information. The most widely used applications of AEPs in the OR fall into three main categories: diagnostic, hearing preservation, and brainstem assessment. Other AEPs have been studied as methods for evaluating the depth of anesthesia.

◆ AEPs in Anesthetized Patients

The appropriate use of AEPs in anesthetized patients is determined by the information desired, the type of surgical procedure, and the anesthetic requirements. As with most sensory evoked potentials, the more proximal the response generators are to the central nervous system (CNS), the greater the anesthetic effects. The N1 peak of the auditory cortical response exhibits a gradual decrease in amplitude during sleep (Campbell and Colrain, 2002) and is abolished during general anesthesia (Horn, Pilge, Kochs, Stockmanns, Hock, and Schneider, 2009; Plourde and Picton, 1991). The middle latency response (MLR) and its derivative, the 40-Hz auditory steady-state response (ASSR), show significant changes in normal-hearing anesthetized patients that include latency onset, phase, and amplitude at suprathreshold levels. (Davies, Mantzaridis, Kenny, and Fisher, 1996; Dutton, Smith, Rampil, Chortkoff, and Eger, 1999; Horn et al, 2009; Schraag, Flaschar, Schleyer, Georgieff, and Kenny, 2006; Tooley, Greenslade, and Prys-Roberts, 1996; Tooley, Stapleton, Greenslade, and Prys-Roberts, 2004). The focus of these studies is to ascertain the viability of the MLR and ASSR as methods for determining depth of anesthesia. Little information is available on the effects of anesthesia on threshold assessment of the MLR and ASSR.

Although some anesthesia-related changes have been reported in the averaged auditory brainstem response (ABR), the effects are negligible for suprathreshold responses (Doufas, Wadhwa, Shah, Lin, Haugh, and Sessler, 2004; Purdie and Cullen, 1993; Scheller, Daunderer, and Pipa, 2009; Smith and Mills, 1989). Other authors indicate that combining agents (e.g., nitrous oxide and halogenated agents) affects both the latency and the amplitude of the ABR, which might be an issue when performing threshold assessment under general anesthesia (Sloan, Sloan, and Rogers, 2010). In anesthetized gerbils, a threshold increase was reported as high as 8 dB compared with unanesthetized animals (van Looij, Liem, van der Burg, van der Wees, De Zeeuw, and van Zanten, 2004). Regardless, the ABR, as well as otoacoustic emissions (OAEs) (Guven et al, 2006), in anesthetized patients are excellent tools to assess the sensitivity of the peripheral auditory mechanisms, function of the eighth cranial nerve (CN VIII) during surgeries of the cerebellopontine angle (CPA), and, to a limited extent, brainstem function.

Of much greater concern when acquiring ABRs in anesthetized patients is the effect of temperature. As temperature is decreased, there is prolongation of latencies and interpeak intervals and a decrease in the amplitude of all waves to temperatures lower than 34°C (93.2°F) (Markand, Warren, Mallik, and Williams, 1990). At core temperatures lower than 30°C (86°F), the ABR may become unreliable or absent (Rodriguez, Edmonds, Auden, and Austin, 1999).

◆ Hearing Assessment by AEPs in the Operating Room

Some difficult-to-test patients cannot be safely sedated in the clinic for purposes of acquiring AEPs. These include toddlers and the developmentally delayed. Young children who exhibit behavior suggesting hearing impairment may not respond adequately to safely prescribed sedation, such as chloral hydrate, for testing purposes. Many of these children have chronic otitis media and often require tympanostomy (placement of PE tubes in the eardrum) under a general anesthetic. The older developmentally delayed child, teen, or adult often receives dental care under general anesthesia. These are opportunities to perform an AEP test safely and quickly.

When scheduling an AEP test during a minor surgical or dental procedure, the surgical center or OR must be notified to allow for the additional room and anesthesia time to perform the test. Surgery schedules are extremely tight because of the cost of the OR suite, anesthesia, and personnel time, and the need to provide efficient and timely service to all scheduled patients. The request for the additional time required to perform the AEP must come from the patient's physician and be coordinated with the surgeon or dentist, the surgery center or OR, and the anesthesiologist. Requesting much more than 15 minutes of OR time may be met with some resistance, so be prepared to defend the need for more. However, with good planning and proper supplies, 15 minutes should be adequate to obtain the necessary information from an anesthetized patient.

Certain surgery centers and many ORs located in hospitals have requirements for non-employee personnel to access patient care areas. These requirements may include a copy of your professional license, allied health certification in basic life support (American Heart Association BLS Healthcare Provider Card), copy of your current vaccination records, and verification of a tuberculosis (TB) test within the last year. Prior to arriving at the surgery center or OR, contact the Nursing Supervisor about these issues.

Pearl

Clinicians should allow plenty of time prior to the patient's scheduled procedure to change into scrubs, clean and set up the equipment, and prepare supplies. OR schedules are dynamic and can change quickly. Without advanced preparation to account for the unpredictable nature of the OR schedule, the opportunity to evaluate the patient may pass.

A diagnostic AEP performed in an OR must be done as quickly as possible. The testing will usually occur subsequent to the planned surgical or dental procedure. With otologic surgeries, ask the surgeon if any solutions, antibiotics or topical analgesics will be placed in the ear following the procedure. Accurate AEP testing requires a dry ear canal, and insertion of medications may produce a false-positive finding. Use subdermal needle electrodes, as they can be applied quickly and provide matched impedances immediately. Reusable subdermal electrodes

must be packaged, sterilized, and ready for use. Disposable subdermal electrodes are available but slightly increase the cost of the test. Clean the forehead, mastoids, and vertex with an alcohol wipe, and insert the electrodes parallel to and just under the skin, making sure the entire area of the needle is beneath the skin's surface. Exposure of the needle can produce unwanted artifacts. Never insert a subdermal needle electrode perpendicular to the surface of the skin. It is not necessary, but you may want to tape the hub and wire of the electrode to the skin as a precautionary measure.

Four needle electrodes are recommended: one for each mastoid (inverting electrode for each test ear), the vertex (noninverting electrode), and the forehead as the ground or common. Braid or tie several knots in the four electrode lead wires to prevent tangling and improve the process of common mode rejection. Insert receivers are preferred because once placed they need no further adjustment. Have a plan of approach based on previous attempts at evaluating the patient in the clinic. If the patient's previous test attempts suggest at least a moderate-to-severe hearing loss, start testing at more intense levels (e.g., 80 dB nHL [normal hearing level]) with a fast rate that is not a harmonic of 60 Hz cycle (odd-ending numbers, e.g., 33, 37, or 43/s); otherwise, choose a stimulus level suspected to be suprathreshold. Quickly determine the presence of a response based on a 2:1 signal-to-noise ratio (SNR). If the response (i.e., wave V of the ABR) appears to be twice that of the surrounding, nonreplicating noise, quickly move onto the next intensity level. In the case of an ABR, a wave V response to a click that exceeds 0.2 µV should require only 500 to 1000 sweeps in an anesthetized patient to meet 2:1 SNR criteria. Obtaining responses near or at threshold requires more averages to meet the signal-to-noise criteria taking up most of the allotted test time. If other types of AEPs (e.g., tone burst ABRs) are planned, prioritize the frequencies by their importance and follow a planned protocol.

Figure 18.2 is an example of a click ABR intensity study acquired from an anesthetized child. The traces comprising the 60-dB nHL (normal hearing level) response were averaged with 500 and 600 sweeps. The 40-dB nHL response traces were with 900 and 1000 sweeps. The three traces at 35-dB nHL were averaged

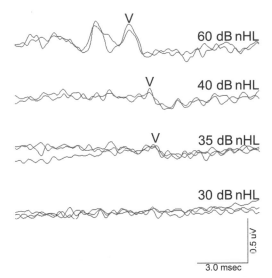

V   60 dB nHL

V   40 dB nHL

V   35 dB nHL

30 dB nHL

0.5 uV

3.0 msec

Fig. 18.2 Shown are four replicated auditory brainstem response (ABR) studies collected in an operating room following a surgical procedure unrelated to the auditory system. Each study is labeled by the click intensity delivered through insert earphones at a rate of 37.3/s. The acquisition montage was Cz (vertex) to the ipsilateral mastoid. Total number of combined averages for the two to three traces per response is 1100, 1900, 4950, 6000 for intensities 60-, 40-, 35-, and 30-dB nHL (normal hearing level) studies, respectively.

with 1600 to 1700 sweeps. At 30-dB nHL, however, there was no reliable response averaged with 2000 sweeps. The total test time was slightly longer than 6 minutes. Had the test protocol been set to include 2000 sweeps for each intensity level, the test would have taken nearly 10 minutes. Although 4 additional minutes does not sound like much time, it increases the cost of the test significantly when you include the OR time.

◆ Hearing Preservation by AEPs during Surgery

Several surgical procedures can place hearing at risk. The most common surgical procedures where hearing preservation is a priority are infratentorium exposure for removing a tumor in the internal auditory canal and/or CPA, microvascular decompression of CN V and VII for relief of trigeminal neuralgia (tic de la rue syndrome),

and hemifacial spasm (HFS) (Fritz, Schäfer, and Klein, 1988; Ma, Li, Cao, and Chen, 2010; Huang, Chang, and Hsu, 2009; Park, Hong, Hong, Cho, Chung, and Ryu, 2009). Damage to CN VIII can occur during these and related types of surgeries (Fröhling, Schlote, and Wolburg-Buchholz, 1998; Hatayama, Sekiya, Suzuki, and Iwabuchi, 1999; McLaughlin, Jannetta, Clyde, Subach, Comey, and Resnick, 1999; Mom, Telischi, Martin, Stagner, and Lonsbury-Martin, 2000). During these procedures, it is difficult to predict when tearing (avulsion) or cutting has occurred because once a change in the AEP is detected, permanent damage may have already taken place. However, compression and/or stretching from retraction can be detected quickly enough to alert the surgeon and make any appropriate maneuvers to prevent permanent damage to the nerve. Ischemic damage can also occur with compression or traction on the acoustic artery. In some situations, the differentiation between a stretch on the CN VIII or acoustic artery is not evident, but both conditions may be reversed with early detection of AEP changes. **Figure 18.3** is an example of the changes that can occur with retraction on the cerebellum to visualize the brainstem and CN VII during a microvascular decompression of CN VII for treatment of HFS.

In preparation for recording AEPs during a craniotomy, good protocol is to have the surgeon define the incision and surgical field. With a middle or posterior fossa approach, the mastoid on the side of surgery may not be accessible for electrode placement. Alternate montages include the earlobe or anterior to the tragus at the juncture of the lobule and the upper jaw. Either will give excellent recordings, but the latter may be more secure and less likely to become dislodged. Insert receivers are required for delivery of the stimuli. Foam tips are not the best method of coupling the receiver tube to the ear canal. These tips can work their way out of the canal over time and affect the stability of the response. Custom-fit earmolds are best, but universal earmolds that come in a variety of sizes work equally well (e.g., Doc's Promolds, International Aquatic Trades, Inc., Santa Cruz, CA). A custom earmold or universal earmold secures itself by locking in place under the helix, tragus, and antitragus and will accommodate the standard receiver tube that comes with most insert earphones. With the

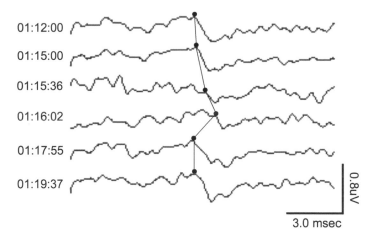

01:12:00

01:15:00

01:15:36

01:16:02

01:17:55

01:19:37

0.8 μV

3.0 msec

Fig. 18.3 The traces shown were acquired during a microvascular decompression of the eighth nerve (CN VIII) for treatment of hemifacial spasm. Each trace is labeled by the time acquired subsequent to the surgical incision, and the wave V peak is shown by the trend plot. Between traces 01:15:00 and 01:15:36, retraction was placed on the cerebellum to expose CN VIII at the brainstem. Between traces 01:16:02 and 01:17:55, the retractor was removed.

recording electrode, earmold, and tubing in place, the outer ear should be prepped with an adhesive liquid, such as tincture of benzoin, and then covered with a small plastic adhesive drape (e.g., Tegaderm). Not only will this help to secure the earpiece, inverting (reference) needle electrode, and, in some cases, electrocochleography (ECochG) electrode, it will also keep moisture from entering the ear canal during prepping.

differences in morphology of individual peaks, with some latency differences, particularly for wave I. These differences may be critical in a diagnostic situation, but for the purposes of monitoring the integrity of the hearing mechanism during craniotomies, these differences are incidental.

Standard electrode placement at vertex (i.e., Cz) and the contralateral mastoid is usually allowed. It is strongly advised to record from the ear contralateral to the surgery. In the event a

> **Pitfall**
>
> Standard insert earphone foam tips are vulnerable to slippage and moisture during surgery. Thus, it is recommended that custom or universal earmolds with sound delivery be used. These special earmolds can lock themselves into the concha area and form a protective barrier. A small amount of adhesive liquid can help.

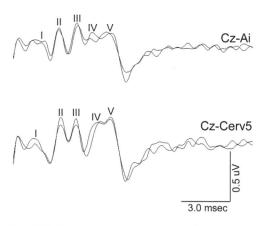

Cz-Ai

Cz-Cerv5

0.5 uV

3.0 msec

If the AEP system allows multiple channels of acquisition, place an electrode at the back of the neck as an additional reference or inverting channel. A vertex-to-posterior neck montage yields ABRs that are as reliable as those from the mastoid. **Figure 18.4** reflects a two-channel ABR using reference electrodes placed at the lobule-jaw junction and at the back of the neck approximately at the fifth cervical vertebra. Evident in the responses are subtle

Fig. 18.4 The two displayed auditory brainstem responses were recorded simultaneously using two channels of acquisition from an anesthetized patient. The responses are labeled by the acquisition montage: vertex to the lobule–jaw junction ipsilateral to the stimulated ear (Cz-Ai) and vertex to the back of the neck approximately at the fifth cervical vertebrae (Cz-Cerv5). Click intensity was 80 dB nHL, and the click rate was 17.7/s.

significant change occurs in the response from the surgical ear, an unaltered response from the nonsurgical ear confirms the absence of most technical issues (particularly if both include the Cz-Cerv5 channel) and the changes are related most likely to a CN VIII compromise and not brainstem conduction. Special care needs to be taken with securing the vertex electrode. Once the patient is draped, access to the patient's head will be impossible. A skin staple is an effective means of securing electrodes on the scalp where there is hair.

Unlike diagnostic AEPs, where the critical information is in the smallest response observed at or near physiologic threshold, surgical AEPs focus on a robust response to a preset intense stimulus. To observe small changes in the AEPs, alerting the potential for damage to the auditory nerve, acquisition of well-defined peaks with excellent SNR (>2:1) is imperative. In a patient with normal hearing, a 70- to 80-dB nHL stimulus intensity is typical. In patients with sensorineural hearing loss, more intense stimuli may be required. To detect changes quickly in an AEP, the required number of averages needs to be as little as necessary to record a reliable response (~500 sweeps). At a rate of ~17/s, 2000 sweeps will take about 2 minutes. That is a long time to wait if a retractor has compromised the nerve or its vascular supply (**Fig. 18.3**). One strategy for early detection of evoked potential changes during surgical manipulation of related structures is to determine the number of sweeps required to meet the 2:1 SNR. If a much greater number of sweeps is suddenly required, and the recording conditions are unchanged, this may be an early sign that the peaks are shifting, resulting in averaging the same peak (usually wave V) with progressively increasing phase shifts. In that situation, it is best to start a new average to confirm a shift of the peaks rather than continue with averaging an already poor response.

During critical stages of a surgery (opening the dura, placing retractors, moving vessels, and tumor dissection), an expedient turnover rate of the ABR is vital to preventing permanent hearing damage. Most surgeries of this nature are done with a microscope that often has output to a slave video monitor. Make sure a clear view of the monitor is available for observing the surgical intervention.

The primary peaks of interest when recording the ABR for hearing preservation are waves I, III, and V. Many patients receiving surgical treatment of a CPA tumor do not exhibit all of these peaks. To ensure accurate recording during surgery, a preoperative ABR should be performed. Although the ABR may appear slightly different in the anesthetized patient, a baseline ABR performed in the clinic will alert the surgical neurophysiologist (or audiologist) to any possible technical or pathophysiologic issues. If the initial ABR is of poor quality, monitoring may be of little value to the surgeon and the decisions he or she may be required to make during the surgical procedure.

Any technical issues related to placement of recording and stimulating devices must be resolved prior to application of the surgical prep. The first recordings should be acquired prior to this so that technical problems can be resolved without contaminating the surgical field. Recording of any electrophysiologic data during exposure is difficult because of interference from electrocautery devices, drilling, and other surgical instrument–related artifacts. Subsequent to the incision, the stability of the ABR must be established prior to opening the dura and exposing the offending mass or vessel (Gouveris and Mann, 2009). Opening the dura and exposing CN VIII to air and irrigation can produce delays in the ABR peaks that may not be predicted by the patient's core temperature. Therefore, collecting responses during and after exposure of intradural structures is imperative prior to any retraction or manipulation of these structures.

Many authors report on the sensitivity and importance of specific ABR peaks in the preservation of hearing during CPA surgeries

(Colletti, Fiorino, Mocella, and Policante, 1998; Matthies and Samii, 1997; Møller, 1995). However, the focus of the intraoperative changes in the ABR is determined by the patient's individual data and the reliability of the individual ABR peaks. Baseline data that demonstrate reliable waves I, III, and V can help discern the status of the peripheral or most distal ABR components (wave I or N1) and those reflecting more proximal activity (waves III and V). Any sudden changes in the ABR peaks that cannot be accounted for by temperature, blood pressure, or extra axial influences (e.g., drilling on the skull) should be reported to the surgeon. Additionally, iatrogenic changes of the operative side should not be reflected in the contralateral ear ABR.

The ABR exhibits high sensitivity, but in some cases where the baseline response is poorly defined, there can be poor specificity (high false-positive rate) for predicting a postoperative hearing deficit (Colletti et al, 1998). In addition to scalp-recorded AEPs, recording from an electrode placed at or near the brainstem or CN VIII may provide greater specificity for estimating hearing preservation during CPA craniotomies (Cueva and Hicks, 2003). To record these potentials, a specially designed electrode is placed by the surgeon at or near the CN VIII root entry zone to the brainstem. Using the previously placed vertex electrode as the active amplifier input (+) and the direct cranial nerve/brainstem electrode as the reference amplifier input (–), a large AEP may be observed within 10 to 20 sweeps of a click stimulus. If this type of recording is planned, include an electrode extension in the montage arrangement and position it to easily connect with the direct recording electrode. The problems associated with this type of recording include inadvertent movement of the electrode with surgical manipulation, lack of clear access to the CN VIII root entry zone, and interference of the electrode with the surgeon's intervention. However, this type of recording provides exceptional information, particularly where the scalp ABR is abnormal and poorly defined.

The cochlear microphonic (CM) and summating potential (SP) are generated in response to cochlear activation by an acoustic stimulus. They are not typically monitored during surgery, although the presence of an SP is consistent with the presence of cochlear perfusion.

The vascular supply to the cochlea is the internal auditory (labyrinthine) artery, which may arise directly from the basilar artery or as a branch of the anteroinferior cerebellar artery (AICA) (Blumenfeld, 2002). Surgeries requiring access to the CPA place both of these arteries at risk secondary to cerebellar retraction or compression of the vessels. Significant obstruction of the blood supply to the cochlea results in sudden and irreversible deafness signaled by loss of the ABR and ECochG, whereas changes in the ABR only would suggest CN VIII damage (Attias, Nageris, Ralph, Vajda, and Rappaport, 2008; Noguchi, Komatsuzaki, and Nishida, 1999; Schlake et al, 2001).

◆ Brainstem Assessment by AEPs during Surgery

The ABR can provide a wealth of information related to the conduction of activity via its associated brainstem pathways. Often surgeries that place the brainstem structures at risk involve compromise to their blood supply. The arterial supply to the brainstem is complex and includes input from the posterior cerebral artery (PCA), basilar artery, vertebral arteries, cerebellar arteries (superior, anteroinferior, and posteroinferior), and labyrinthine artery. The internal auditory (labyrinthine) artery supplies the cochlea and labyrinth. This small artery usually arises as a branch of the AICA or may branch directly from the basilar artery (Blumenfeld, 2002). Both of these arteries branch from the inferior region of the basilar artery, which courses along the inferior to superior borders of the anterior surface of the pons. Additionally, the AICA and, to some extent, the posteroinferior cerebellar artery (PICA) are the primary arterial supply to the nuclei critical to auditory and vestibular function. These nuclei are arranged in the dorsal-lateral pons anterior to the fourth ventricle. Any surgery involving the area around the pontine medullary junction or CPA has the potential for compromising the flow of oxygenated blood critical to auditory and vestibular function. By extrapolation, other brainstem structures may also suffer compromise and include the facial nerve (CN VII), spinal trigeminal nucleus and tract (CN V), cerebellar peduncles, and spinothalamic tract. However, any brainstem structures caudal to the root entry zone of CN VIII have alternate arterial inputs, and their function would not be adequately reflected by any changes in an AEP.

Surgeries involving the areas surrounding or near the brainstem may not always be adequately monitored via AEPs. These might include masses of the fourth ventricle, basilar tip aneurysms, and arteriovenous malformations (AVMs) of the brainstem. The vestibular nuclei are located along the dorsal surface of the brainstem near the floor of the fourth ventricle. However, the auditory nuclei and pathways course more laterally. Thus, using the ABR to predict compromise to the brainstem structures during a surgery involving entry to the fourth ventricle may result in false-negative findings.

Somatosensory evoked potentials (SSEPs) reflect the conduction of proprioceptive sensory fibers (Ia) that enter the spinal cord via the dorsal columns and ascend to the cuneatus and gracile nuclei (upper and lower extremity, respectfully) within the medulla, where these pathways cross and project to the contralateral thalamus via the medial lemniscus. From the thalamus, these crossed pathways send sensory information to the primary sensory cortex located in the lateral (upper extremity) and medial (lower extremity) areas of the postcentral gyrus. The N13 response is a far-field brainstem potential reflecting activity from the medulla whose primary arterial supply is the vertebral and anterior spinal arteries. The next scalp-recorded potentials are a series of cortical responses (e.g., N20). Any iatrogenic event affecting the conduction of electrophysiologic activity of the medial lemniscal system and/or its subsequent thalamocortical projections will result in the loss of the cortical response. The structures involved in this system receive oxygenated blood from various sources. In particular, the medial lemniscal pathways (projection from the medullary nuclei to the thalamus)

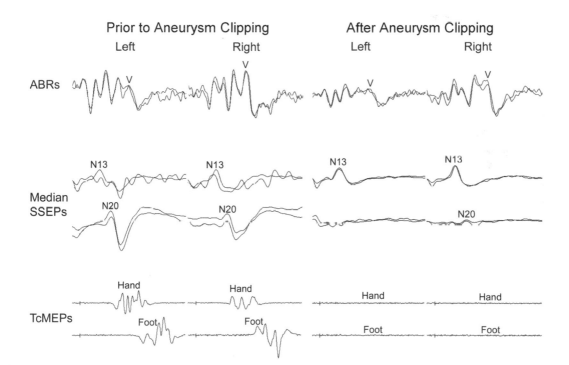

Fig. 18.5 Exhibited are multimodality recordings obtained from a patient undergoing clipping of a basilar artery aneurysm. Traces for three modalities (auditory brainstem responses [ABRs], somatosensory evoked potential [SSEP], and transcranial motor evoked potential [TcMEP]) are shown. Those responses recorded before clipping the aneurysm are shown on the left and after clipping the aneurysm on the right. Following clipping of the aneurysm, the ABRs exhibit few changes, but there are noted changes in the cortical SSEPs (N20) and TcMEPs.

that ascend via the medial brainstem near the pontine-medullary junction are perfused by the vertebral and basilar arteries.

Transcranial motor evoked potentials (TcMEPs) are evoked by passing a voltage across the head, activating axonal conduction that descends directly to the designated lower motor neurons in the spinal cord. These axons pass through several structures whose arterial supply varies depending on the level within the central nervous system. At the brainstem, these axons pass through the anterior pons and make up the pyramids. Like the brainstem pathways of the SSEPs, the pyramidal tracts are perfused by the vertebral and basilar arteries.

Aneurysms or AVMs of the basilar artery may or may not involve direct blood supply to the peripheral and brainstem pathways of the auditory system. The basilar artery via the paramedian branches supplies oxygenated blood to the medial and anterior brainstem structures. Most critically, the basilar artery is the primary arterial supply to the anterior pons through which the corticospinal and cortical bulbar tracts (pyramidal tract) pass. Selective compromise to the basilar artery and/or its paramedian branches may show no significant change in an AEP but result in severe postoperative consequences for the patient.

Figure 18.5 shows the electrophysiologic data from a patient with a large basilar tip aneurysm. The baseline IOM data shown on the left exhibit well-defined ABRs, upper extremity SSEPs, and TcMEPs from the upper and lower extremities. The same data series collected subsequent to clipping the aneurysm are shown on the right. Although the ABRs are slightly reduced in amplitude compared with the baseline data, all the components are well defined and easily identified, indicating good function for those pathways responsible for that particular evoked potential. However, notice the significant change in the upper extremity SSEPs. Both extremities exhibit the cervicomedullary response (N13) that is generated within the most caudal region of the brainstem. However, no cortical response (N20) is observed to left-side stimulation, and the response to right-side stimulation is significantly reduced. In addition, the TcMEPs are absent from all extremities.

◆ Multimodality Neurophysiologic Intraoperative Monitoring

Although AEPs can be of significant utility as a method of monitoring hearing function and areas of the brainstem during surgeries of the ear and craniotomies of the infratentorial compartment, rarely are they recorded in isolation (particularly in the latter situation). Any surgery with the possible risk of compromising CN VIII or its ascending brainstem pathways will most likely require monitoring of nearby CN and brainstem structures. In addition to the auditory system, CN monitoring during infratentorial surgeries involves the efferent system. Most of the cranial nerves (with the exception of CN I, II, and VIII) are responsible for motor function; therefore, electromyography (EMG) is used to monitor their function. Unlike sensory evoked responses (e.g., ABR and SSEP), EMG is monitored in real time much like electronystagmography (ENG). Electrodes (usually subdermal) are placed over muscles of the face, head, and/or neck (and sometimes shoulder for CN XI). These electrodes provide a continuous survey of the state of the associated nerves. Depolarization of axons within a motor nerve occurs secondary to mechanical, thermal, or electrical influences. These axons conduct to their associated muscles activating muscle fibers at the neuromuscular junction. The compound muscle action potential (CMAP) generated is large in comparison to the averaged AEP (20–100 μV as compared with 0.5–1.0 μV).

Recording EMG may be as a continuous "free-run" manner and/or may be captured to a triggering event. Triggering events include increase in the voltage of the normally silent EMG and direct stimulation of the associated CN by the surgeon via a handheld probe. The EMG events are appraised by the experienced clinician according to their amplitude, morphology, and duration.

The CMAP may also be recorded to activation of the CNS. Unlike activation of axons in a peripheral nerve, evoking EMG centrally requires the activation of the lower motor neurons in the brainstem or spinal cord. Instigating an action potential at the lower motor neuron requires specific input from the upper motor neurons. A standard electrophysiologic method for centrally evoked EMG is the TcMEP described earlier in this chapter. Only IOM equipment with U.S. Food and Drug Administration (FDA) approval should be used in acquiring TcMEPs. Additionally, advanced knowledge by the operating clinician is critical to the proper and safe implementation of this procedure.

◆ Documentation and Medical Legal Issues

Documentation of electrophysiologic data and corresponding anesthetic, surgical, and technical events is vital to proper patient care and has medical-legal bearing on the monitoring clinicians' participation in that care. Any information collected from a patient (as out-patient or in-patient) becomes a part of the medical record and is potentially available for review by a patient's advocate. The documentation of information collected in the acquisition of electrophysiological data during surgery includes data reliability and a written record of events that coincide with the data. Determining data reliability by individual observers is dependent on their subjective assessment of visually inspected waveforms. This method can exhibit profound interobserver disagreement (Elberling and Don, 1984). Mathematical methods for determining waveform reliability as a measure of the SNR have been investigated, but the application of these processes has limited clinical value (Don, Elberling, and Waring, 1984; Silva, 2009). Experienced clinicians will typically look for a signal (or replicated waveform) with amplitudes that are approximately twice that of the surrounding background noise (2:1 SNR), whereas inexperienced clinicians will disregard SNR and typically identify any repeatable peaks occurring within a predictable latency range as responses (Hicks, 2008). The latter method of peak identification leads to erroneous results, with the potential for serious consequences to the patient. Prior to entering the operating room as a provider of electrophysiologic monitoring, the clinician needs to devise a method of determining, reporting, and scientifically defending reliability measures for the collected data. Indices for reporting response reliability may include SNR, morphology, and stability (or instability).

> **Pitfall**
>
> Inexperienced clinicians have a tendency to rely only on the repeatability of peaks within a predictable latency range. Instead, clinicians should focus more on a response that is at least twice the size of the surrounding background noise.

The written log should include statements on reliability and the presence of abnormality of the collected data. Additionally, the log needs to include critical surgical events, such as incision, drilling, irrigation, and retraction. These comments should coincide with other patient data, such as temperature, anesthetic levels, and blood pressure. Any changes in the data reported to the surgeon need to be included in the log, as well as the surgeon's acknowledgment. Most manufacturers of IOM equipment allow typed input of these data that can be referenced during and after the surgical procedure. If not, prepare your own IOM log, such as those shown in **Fig. 18.6**.

System:		Patient:		
Location:		DOB:		Age:
Date of Service		MR#:		Sex:

Neurophysiological Intraoperative Monitoring Report

TIME	Arrival:		Start:		Stop:		Total Hours: 0:00
NIOM Clinician:						NIOM System:	
Anesthesiologist:			Agents:				
Surgeon(s):							
Reason for Surgery:							
Surgical Procedure:							

CPT/Data	Montage/Recording Site	Stimulation	Baseline Results/Comments

BASELINE DATA	Temp:	BP(MBP):	%Agent(s):
Evoked Potential			
Scale			
Peak(s)			
Value			

Pertinent History and Report of Results   Height: Weight:

Continued

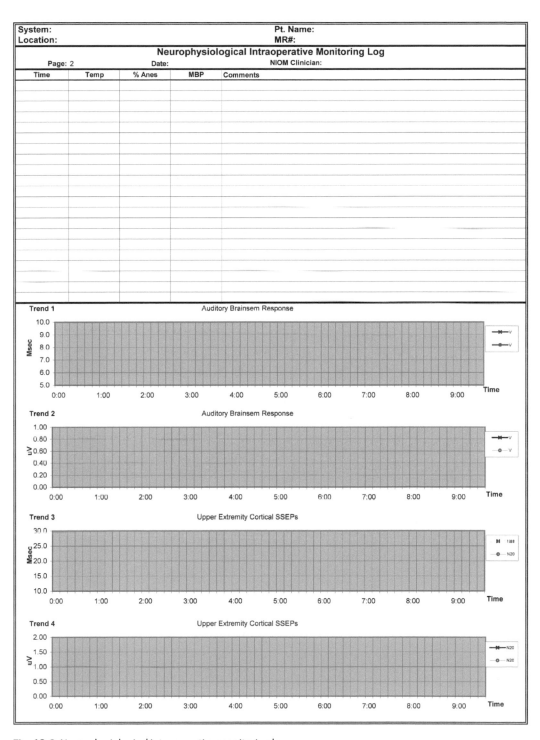

Fig. 18.6 Neurophysiological intraoperative monitoring log.

◆ Summary

The acquisition of AEPs during surgery is considered one of the more challenging IOM procedures. Audiologists should be prepared for the transition of AEP testing from the clinic to OR, which will require specialized training, orientation, and a high level of technical and professional skill. In the OR, there are numerous personnel, patient, and surgical access considerations. Communication will be critical prior to, during, and following all surgeries. In addition to IOM of auditory structures during surgery, audiologists may also find that their specialized training leads them to the assessment of other structures including muscles and cranial nerves.

References

Attias, J., Nageris, B., Ralph, J., Vajda, J., & Rappaport, Z. H. (2008). Hearing preservation using combined monitoring of extra-tympanic electrocochleography and auditory brainstem responses during acoustic neuroma surgery. *International Journal of Audiology, 47*(4), 178–184. PubMed

Blumenfeld, H. (2002). *Neuroanatomy through clinical cases.* Sunderland, MA: Sinauer Associates.

Campbell, K. B., & Colrain, I. M. (2002). Event-related potential measures of the inhibition of information processing: II. The sleep onset period. *International Journal of Psychophysiology, 46*(3), 197–214. PubMed

Colletti, V., Fiorino, F. G., Mocella, S., & Policante, Z. (1998). ECochG, CNAP and ABR monitoring during vestibular schwannoma surgery. *Audiology, 37*(1), 27–37. PubMed

Cueva, R. A., & Hicks, G. E. (2003). Neurophysiologic monitoring in otologic/neurotologic surgery. In M. E. Glasscock & A. G. Gulya (Eds.), *Glasscock-Shambaugh surgery of the ear* (pp. 315–324). Hamilton, Ontario: BC Decker.

Davies, F. W., Mantzaridis, H., Kenny, G. N. C., & Fisher, A. C. (1996). Middle latency auditory evoked potentials during repeated transitions from consciousness to unconsciousness. *Anaesthesia, 51*(2), 107–113. PubMed

Don, M., Elberling, C., & Waring, M. (1984). Objective detection of averaged auditory brainstem responses. *Scandinavian Audiology, 13*(4), 219–228. PubMed

Doufas, A. G., Wadhwa, A., Shah, Y. M., Lin, C. M., Haugh, G. S., & Sessler, D. I. (2004). Block-dependent sedation during epidural anaesthesia is associated with delayed brainstem conduction. *British Journal of Anaesthesia, 93*(2), 228–234. PubMed

Dutton, R. C., Smith, W. D., Rampil, I. J., Chortkoff, B. S., & Eger, E. I., II. (1999). Forty-hertz midlatency auditory evoked potential activity predicts wakeful response during desflurane and propofol anesthesia in volunteers. *Anesthesiology, 91*(5), 1209–1220. PubMed

Elberling, C., & Don, M. (1984). Quality estimation of averaged auditory brainstem responses. *Scandinavian Audiology, 13*(3), 187–197. PubMed

Fritz, W., Schäfer, J., & Klein, H. J. (1988). Hearing loss after microvascular decompression for trigeminal neuralgia. *Journal of Neurosurgery, 69*(3), 367–370. PubMed

Fröhling, M. A., Schlote, W., & Wolburg-Buchholz, K. (1998). Nonselective nerve fibre damage in peripheral nerves after experimental thermocoagulation. *Acta Neurochirurgica, 140*(12), 1297–1302. PubMed

Gouveris, H., & Mann, W. (2009). Association between surgical steps and intraoperative auditory brainstem response and electrocochleography waveforms during hearing preservation vestibular schwannoma surgery. *European Archives of Oto-Rhino-Laryngology, 266*(2), 225–229. PubMed

Guven, S., Tas, A., Adali, M. K., Yagiz, R., Alagol, A., Uzun, C., et al. (2006). Influence of anaesthetic agents on transient evoked otoacoustic emissions and stapedius reflex thresholds. *Journal of Laryngology and Otology, 120*(1), 10–15. PubMed

Hatayama, T., Sekiya, T., Suzuki, S., & Iwabuchi, T. (1999). Effect of compression on the cochlear nerve: A short- and long-term electrophysiological and histological study. *Neurological Research, 21*(6), 599–610. PubMed

Hicks, G. E. (2008, May). *Response identification strategies of experienced readers from the somatosensory evoked potential (SSEP).* Paper presented at the 19th annual meeting of the American Society for Neurophysiologic Monitoring, Chicago.

Horn, B., Pilge, S., Kochs, E. F., Stockmanns, G., Hock, A., & Schneider, G. (2009). A combination of electroencephalogram and auditory evoked potentials separates different levels of anesthesia in volunteers. *Anesthesia and Analgesia. 108*(5), 1512–1521. PubMed

Huang, B. R., Chang, C. N., & Hsu, J. C. (2009). Intraoperative electrophysiological monitoring in microvascular decompression for hemifacial spasm. *Journal of Clinical Neuroscience, 16*(2), 209–213. PubMed

Ma, Z., Li, M., Cao, Y., & Chen, X. (2010). Keyhole microsurgery for trigeminal neuralgia, hemifacial spasm and glossopharyngeal neuralgia. *European Archives of Oto-Rhino-Laryngology, 267*(3), 449–454. PubMed

Markand, O. N., Warren, C., Mallik, G. S., & Williams, C. J. (1990). Temperature-dependent hysteresis in somatosensory and auditory evoked potentials. *Electroencephalography and Clinical Neurophysiology, 77*(6), 425–435. PubMed

Matthies, C., & Samii, M. (1997). Management of vestibular schwannomas (acoustic neuromas): The value of neurophysiology for intraoperative monitoring of auditory function in 200 cases. *Neurosurgery, 40*(3), 459–466, discussion 466–468. PubMed

McLaughlin, M. R., Jannetta, P. J., Clyde, B. L., Subach, B. R., Comey, C. H., & Resnick, D. K. (1999). Microvascular decompression of cranial nerves: lessons learned after 4400 operations. *Journal of Neurosurgery, 90*(1), 1–8. PubMed

Møller, A. R. (1995). *Intraoperative neurophysiologic monitoring.* Luxembourg: Harwood Academic Publishers, pp. 45–126.

Mom, T., Telischi, F. F., Martin, G. K., Stagner, B. B., & Lonsbury-Martin, B. L. (2000). Vasospasm of the internal auditory artery: Significance in cerebellopontine angle surgery. *American Journal of Otology, 21*(5), 735–742. PubMed

Noguchi, Y., Komatsuzaki, A., & Nishida, H. (1999). Cochlear microphonics for hearing preservation in vestibular schwannoma surgery. *Laryngoscope, 109*(12), 1982–1987. PubMed

Park, K., Hong, S. H., Hong, S. D., Cho, Y. S., Chung, W. H., & Ryu, N. G. (2009). Patterns of hearing loss after microvascular decompression for hemifacial spasm. *Journal of Neurology, Neurosurgery, and Psychiatry, 80*(10), 1165–1167. PubMed

Plourde, G., & Picton, T. W. (1991). Long-latency auditory evoked potentials during general anesthesia: N1 and P3 components. *Anesthesia and Analgesia, 72*(3), 342–350. PubMed

Purdie, J. A., & Cullen, P. M. (1993). Brainstem auditory evoked response during propofol anaesthesia in children. *Anaesthesia, 48*(3), 192–195. PubMed

Rodriguez, R. A., Edmonds, H. L., Jr., Auden, S. M., & Austin, E. H., III. (1999). Auditory brainstem evoked responses and temperature monitoring during pediatric cardiopulmonary bypass. *Canadian Journal of Anaesthesia, 46*(9), 832–839. PubMed

Scheller, B. C., Daunderer, M., & Pipa, G. (2009). General anesthesia increases temporal precision and decreases power of the brainstem auditory-evoked response-related segments of the electroencephalogram. *Anesthesiology, 111*(2), 340–355. PubMed

Schlake, H. P., Milewski, C., Goldbrunner, R. H., Kindgen, A., Riemann, R., Helms, J., et al. (2001). Combined intraoperative monitoring of hearing by means of auditory brainstem responses (ABR) and transtympanic electrocochleography (ECochG) during surgery of intra- and extrameatal acoustic neurinomas. *Acta Neurochirurgica, 143*(10), 985–995, discussion 995–996. PubMed

Schraag, S., Flaschar, J., Schleyer, M., Georgieff, M., & Kenny, G. (2006). The contribution of remifentanil to middle latency auditory evoked potentials during induction of propofol anesthesia. *Anesthesia and Analgesia, 103*(4), 902–907. PubMed

Silva, I. (2009). Estimation of postaverage SNR from evoked responses under nonstationary noise. *IEEE Transactions on Bio-Medical Engineering, 56*(8), 2123–2130. PubMed

Sloan, T., Sloan, H., & Rogers, J. (2010). Nitrous oxide and isoflurane are synergistic with respect to amplitude and latency effects on sensory evoked potentials. *Journal of Clinical Monitoring and Computing, 24*(2), 113–123. PubMed

Smith, D. I., & Mills, J. H. (1989). Anesthesia effects: auditory brain-stem response. *Electroencephalography and Clinical Neurophysiology, 72*(5), 422–428. PubMed

Tooley, M. A., Greenslade, G. L., & Prys-Roberts, C. (1996). Concentration-related effects of propofol on the auditory evoked response. *British Journal of Anaesthesia, 77*(6), 720–726. PubMed

Tooley, M. A., Stapleton, C. L., Greenslade, G. L., & Prys-Roberts, C. (2004). Mid-latency auditory evoked response during propofol and alfentanil anaesthesia. *British Journal of Anaesthesia, 92*(1), 25–32. PubMed

van Looij, M. A., Liem, S. S., van der Burg, H., van der Wees, J., De Zeeuw, C. I., & van Zanten, B. G. (2004). Impact of conventional anesthesia on auditory brainstem responses in mice. *Hearing Research, 193*(1–2), 75–82. PubMed

Chapter 19

Vestibular Evoked Myogenic Potentials

Matthew Wester

One man's artifact is another's dependent measure.

—Goff, Allison, and Vaughn (1978)

The vestibular evoked myogenic potential (VEMP) is a sound-evoked muscle response associated with the vestibulocollic reflex (VCR). The function of the VCR is to keep the head stable while the body is moving. The commonly accepted anatomical pathway of the VEMP response is the saccule, the inferior vestibular division of the eighth cranial nerve (CN VIII), the vestibular nuclei of the brainstem, the ipsilateral descending vestibulospinal tracts to CN XI, and the sternocleidomastoid (SCM) muscle (Colebatch and Halmagyi, 1992; Colebatch, Halmagyi, and Skuse, 1994; Halmagyi and Colebatch, 1995; Itoh et al, 2001; Murofushi, Halmagyi, Yavor, and Colebatch, 1996; Murofushi, Shimizu, Takegoshi, and Cheng, 2001; Robertson and Ireland, 1995).

A VEMP is a signal-averaged recording of the inhibition in electromyographic (EMG) activity of a contracted SCM in response to an acoustic stimulus in the ipsilateral ear, resulting in a waveform with a positive peak (P1) at ~13 msec and a negative peak (N1) at ~23 msec in normal subjects. In contrast and complement to tests of the vestibulo-ocular reflex (VOR), such as caloric testing and rotary chair, the VEMP measures the VCR and the integrity of its unique peripheral and central vestibular system anatomy **(Table 19.1)** and thus can contribute to a more complete evaluation of a patient's vestibular system. It has been found to be clinically useful in contributing diagnostic information for various otologic disorders, such as superior canal dehiscence (SCD), Meniere disease, vestibular schwannoma/acoustic neuroma, and vestibular neuritis.

The main strength of the VEMP test is that it measures the function of a unique portion of vestibular anatomy as compared with other vestibular tests. The VEMP can be present regardless of the degree of sensorineural hearing loss, as it does not depend on cochlear function and has been shown to be present in individuals with profound sensorineural hearing loss (Ackley and Tamaki, 2003). Therefore, it can be helpful in assessing at least a portion of CN VIII function in cases in which there is excessive sensorineural hearing loss that prevents obtaining an auditory brainstem response (ABR). There are a few limitations inherent in VEMP testing. First, conductive hearing loss also confounds interpretation of results. Because the VEMP response is based on a high level of sound pressure reaching the saccule, a normally functioning outer and middle ear system is required to allow a sufficiently high level to reach the saccule when the stimulus is transmitted through the external auditory canal. A conductive hearing loss or middle ear dysfunction will typically result in an absent or reduced (lower amplitude and/or higher threshold) response. Another potential challenge with VEMP testing is inconsistent or insufficient SCM contraction in some patients, which can be a confounding variable when

Table 19.1 Anatomical Pathways of VOR and VEMP Tests

VOR Tests: Caloric, Rotary Chair	VEMP
VOR	VCR
Horizontal semicircular canal	Saccule
Superior vestibular nerve	Inferior vestibular nerve
Ascending neural path to eye muscles	Descending neural path to SCM muscle

Abbreviations: SCM, sternocleidomastoid; VCR, vestibulocollic reflex; VEMP, vestibular evoked myogenic potential; VOR, vestibulo-ocular reflex.

comparing and interpreting VEMP amplitude from side to side in a single patient as well as from patient to patient. Currently, there is a lack of standardized testing procedures and corresponding normative values, as different clinics and research sites have developed their own testing parameters and methods.

More recent areas of research are focusing on VEMP elicited by bone conduction (BC-VEMP), as well as VEMP measured at the eye muscle (ocular VEMP, or oVEMP) by both air- and bone-conducted stimuli, although these tests are not yet commonly used clinically. With the advent of oVEMP, traditional VEMP has been relabeled as cervical VEMP, or cVEMP (Rosengren, Welgampola, and Colebatch, 2010). In this chapter, which focuses on clinical use of VEMP, the term *VEMP* indicates an air-conducted cVEMP.

◆ Testing Methodology

Patient Position

Because the VEMP response represents an inhibition of EMG activity, elicitation of the response requires continuous contraction of the SCM muscle during measurement. This can be accomplished in several ways: The patient can lie supine with head unturned and lift the head for simultaneous activation of both SCM muscles on each side of the neck; the patient can lie in a 30-degree supine position with the head turned fully away from the ear being stimulated and then lift the head, activating the SCM muscle ipsilateral to the upward-facing ear; or the patient can sit upright and turn the head to one side to activate the SCM muscle ipsilateral to the forward-facing ear.

Because the VEMP response has been shown to be largely ipsilateral (Colebatch et al, 1994; Murofushi et al, 1996; Wilson et al, 1995), some practitioners have proposed a bilateral SCM contraction method in which VEMP is measured on both sides simultaneously with a two-channel evoked potential recording system and bilateral acoustic stimulation. The benefit of the bilateral contraction method is a reduction in test time; in the unilateral SCM contraction method, a separate measurement for each side is required.

Pitfall

SCM contraction is usually maximized when the patient lifts the head only 1 or 2 inches off the headrest. Lifting the head too high can reduce SCM contraction strength. Care must be taken to ensure the patient is lifting the head using the neck muscles only and not lifting the torso or shoulders.

Electrode Preparation and Montage

Because the VEMP response is a myogenic potential of a large amplitude, obtaining very low electrode impedance is not as crucial as it is in ABR and other neurogenic potential testing. Thus, it is not necessary to scrub the skin at the electrode placement sites. Cleaning the skin with an alcohol wipe so that it is free of any oil or makeup is sufficient preparation for electrode placement. VEMP is recorded with the active electrode on the middle or upper third of the SCM; the reference electrode is in an electrically indifferent location, such as the forehead (Fpz), chin, or dorsum of the hand; and a ground electrode typically on the forehead. When the reference electrode is placed on the SCM and the active electrode on an electrically indifferent location, the result is a reversed-polarity waveform, with P1 being downward and N1 being upward. Whether P1 is recorded as upward or downward does not affect the validity or accuracy of the test results. Buckingham et al (2008) found that different reference electrode locations produced different amplitudes, with the sternum producing the largest (amplitude) responses, the dorsum of the hand producing the smallest, and the forehead (Fpz) producing amplitudes in between. Reference effects, however, were eclipsed by large variability across sessions. Rosengren et al (2010) recommend placing the reference electrode at the sternum.

Table 19.2 Recording and Stimulus Parameters

Amplifier gain	5000x
Filter	10–1500 Hz
Recording window	50–100 msec
Number of sweeps	60–200
Artifact rejection	Off
Type	500 Hz tone burst
Level	95 dB nHL (125 dB SPL)
Rate	5 per second
Rise/fall	2 cycles
Plateau	0 cycles
Gating	Blackman

Abbreviations: nHL, normal hearing level; SPL, sound pressure level.

Pearl

If a VEMP response is abnormally low, try adjusting the placement of the electrode on the SCM, making sure it is placed on the most prominent part of the belly of the muscle, then re-recording a VEMP response. This may entail moving the electrode either laterally so that it sets directly on the "ridge" of the muscle or slightly higher or lower vertically on the belly of the muscle. Proper electrode placement is important to record an accurate VEMP response.

Recording and Stimulus Parameters

The VEMP response is typically recorded using a 10-Hz high-pass and 1000- to 2000-Hz low-pass filter, amplified 5000 times, over a 50- to 100-msec window and averaged from 60 to 200 sweeps. The stimulus to evoke the VEMP response is typically a low-frequency (500 Hz) tone burst or click. Several studies (Janky and Shepard, 2009; Rosengren, Govender, and Colebatch, 2009; Todd, Cody, and Banks, 2000) have demonstrated that a 500-Hz tone burst is a more effective stimulus than a click for evoking a VEMP response. It is delivered at a high level (95 dB nHL [normal hearing level], or 125 dB SPL [sound pressure level]) through air-conduction earphones, typically insert earphones. It is important that insert earphones are properly and fully inserted in the external ear canal to ensure that proper sound pressure level (SPL) reaches the saccule through the outer and middle ear. SPL will decrease in a larger space, as occurs when insert earphones are not placed deeply in the external ear canal. The 500-Hz tone burst is usually presented at a repetition rate of 5/s. It typically has a rise and fall of 1 or 2 cycles, with 0 or 1 cycle of plateau and a Blackman gating envelope. **Table 19.2** gives an overview of a typical VEMP recording and stimulus protocol.

Pitfall

For patients with Tulio phenomenon, the high-level stimulus may cause vertigo. Be alert to this possibility to minimize patient discomfort.

Procedure

After preparing the skin at the electrode placement sites, placing the electrodes, and inserting the earphone in the test ear, the high-level stimulus and recording are turned on, and the patient contracts the ipsilateral SCM muscle. Stimulus, contraction, and recording are continued until at least 60 sweeps are averaged, and a waveform judged to be a valid response is recorded. A valid waveform should have P1 ~12 to 16 msec and N1 ~23 to 27 msec. Amplitudes typically range from 60 to 500 μV. The stimulus and recording are turned off, the patient relaxes the SCM muscle and rests briefly, and the process is repeated as needed to collect at least two waveforms that are roughly matched in latency and amplitude at the initial high level of stimulus. The stimulus is decreased by 5 dB nHL, and the process is repeated. As the stimulus level is decreased, amplitude should also decrease. Latency should remain relatively stable. The stimulus is repeatedly decreased in 5 dB nHL steps until a waveform with stable latency can no longer be recorded. The lowest stimulus level at which a response is judged to be present is considered the VEMP threshold. The entire process is then repeated, with the stimulus and electrodes placed on the other side.

◆ Test Interpretation

Measurement Parameters

The three parameters of a VEMP recording that may be diagnostically useful are threshold, amplitude, and latency. VEMP threshold is defined as the lowest stimulus level at which a VEMP response can be identified (distinct P1 and N1 peaks without shifts in latency as compared with the high-stimulus level VEMP). Threshold has been seen to increase with age (Ochi and Ohashi, 2003; Welgampola and Colebatch, 2001). VEMP amplitude is a P1-N1 peak-to-peak amplitude measure. Amplitude decreases with decreases in stimulus intensity, as well as with decreases in the strength of muscle contraction. Amplitude has also been seen to decrease with age (Basta et al, 2005, 2007). Latency is the most stable parameter of the three, as it is not affected by muscle tension or stimulus intensity, and it may not be affected by age, although that has not been consistently demonstrated in the literature (Basta et al, 2005; Lee, Cha, Jung, Park, and Yeo, 2008; Su, Huang, Young, and Cheng, 2004; Welgampola and Colebatch, 2001; Zapala and Brey, 2004).

Normative Values

Normative values for VEMP parameters have been published (Basta et al, 2005; Zapala and Brey, 2004). However, variations in procedures and stimulus and recording parameters from site to site may affect normative values; therefore, it is recommended that each clinic obtain its own norms for its own test procedures and parameters. Age-related norms for VEMP amplitude and threshold are needed, as VEMP responses have been shown to become reduced (decreased amplitude and increased threshold) or absent with age in normal subjects (Basta et al 2005, 2007; Janky and Shepard, 2009; Lee et al, 2008; Ochi and Ohashi, 2003; Su et al, 2004; Welgampola and Colebatch, 2001; Zapala and Brey, 2004).

Latency

Absolute normative latency values typically range from 12 to 16 msec for P1 and 23 to 27 msec for N1. Latencies greater than 20 and 30 msec for P1 and N1, respectively, are typically considered abnormally prolonged. Interaural latency differences greater than 3.5 msec for each of the VEMP components are considered abnormal (Zapala and Brey, 2004).

Amplitude

The range of normal values for amplitude is large, typically from 60 to 500 μV (or sometimes larger), depending on the strength of muscle contraction and the age of the patient (with larger amplitudes commonly seen in younger patients). Amplitude also varies with intensity of stimulus, strength of muscle contraction, amount of cutaneous tissue over the SCM, age of the patient, and electrode placement (Ochi, Ohashi, and Nishino, 2001; Sheykholeslami, Murofushi, and Kaga, 2001). Amplitude asymmetry is calculated as (right amplitude − left amplitude)/(right amplitude + left amplitude) × 100. Because of the wide range of normal amplitudes, only large asymmetries from ear to ear are considered significant. Zapala and Brey's (2004) normative data, collected without SCM muscle contraction monitoring, suggest an amplitude asymmetry from ear to ear must be greater than 47% to be considered abnormally asymmetric.

Amplitude asymmetry values less than ~40% are generally considered normal. Because of the high variability of absolute amplitude values from patient to patient, absolute amplitude norms may be less useful.

Monitoring SCM muscle contraction may improve VEMP amplitudes by maximizing muscle contraction and validate ear-to-ear VEMP amplitude symmetry comparisons by ensuring symmetric muscle contraction (Stoody, Guy, Bright, and Erdbruegger, n.d.; Vanspauwen, Wuyts, and Van de Heyning, 2006). Vanspauwen and colleagues (2006) suggested using a blood pressure cuff to help patients maintain optimal SCM contraction and equalize contraction from side to side, thus improving overall VEMP reliability and reducing ear-to-ear amplitude variability. In this method, a blood pressure cuff is inflated to a base pressure of 20 mm Hg. The patient holds the cuff against the upward-facing cheek and lifts the head, achieving and trying to maintain a pressure of ~40 mm Hg while the VEMP is being recorded. One potential problem with this method is that some patients elevate the pressure in the cuff by pushing it or squeezing it with their hands instead of pushing against it with their heads. Measuring the baseline tonic EMG level of the contracted SCM prior to stimulation and having the patient maintain a baseline level of ~30 to 50 µV throughout the recording is another method of monitoring SCM contraction (Akin, Murnane, Panus, Caruthers, Wilkinson, and Proffitt, 2004). Some evoked potential recording systems are capable of this and also include a device that alerts the patient and tester (through lights) that a sufficient level of contraction has been achieved, although as of this writing, these devices are not available in the United States because of issues with U.S. Food and Drug Administration (FDA) approval. Rectified or normalized amplitude measures take into account average EMG activity throughout the recording, mathematically eliminating it, thus leaving just the amount of inhibition. As long as a minimum muscle contraction of ~40 µV is achieved, rectified/normalized amplitude responses should be comparable from ear to ear (Welgampola and Colebatch, 2005). Rectified/normalized amplitude measures require equipment set up to record ongoing EMG activity and the VEMP response. Some evoked potential systems are capable of this, but again they currently are not available in the United States.

Threshold

Because VEMP thresholds increase with age (Janky and Shepard, 2009), age-related norms are needed. In normal populations younger than 60 years, an average threshold is typically ~80 dB nHL. Because of the variability of VEMP threshold owing to factors such as patient age and strength of muscle contraction, it is problematic to determine an absolute threshold value that qualifies as significantly elevated. However, many clinics use lower than 70 dB nHL as a cutoff value for a significantly reduced VEMP threshold. When a VEMP response is present at stimulus levels of 65 dB nHL or greater, an abnormally low VEMP threshold may be considered. Threshold asymmetry between the ears is perhaps a stronger method to interpret threshold results with asymmetries of 15 dB or greater considered clinically significant. As with amplitude asymmetry, monitoring of SCM contraction to ensure equal contraction from side to side strengthens the interpretability of threshold asymmetry.

♦ Disorders and Corresponding Common VEMP Results

Peripheral Otologic Disorders

Endolymphatic Hydrops/Early Meniere Disease

In early stage Meniere disease, enhanced amplitude in the affected ear can be seen and is thought to be due to saccular distention (Young, Wu, and Wu, 2002). VEMP threshold can also be abnormally low in early stage Meniere disease (Rauch, Zhou, Kujawa, Guinan, and Herrmann, 2004). Current research indicates that in some cases, Meniere disease can affect the optimal frequency of the VEMP response in the affected ear (Janky and Shepard, 2009; Lin et al, 2006; Rauch et al, 2004). Janky and Shepard (2009) found in some Meniere ears that, VEMP responses were greatest with 1000-Hz tone bursts instead of with 500-Hz tone bursts, as is seen in normal ears. Meniere patients who also experience crisis of Tumarkin (drop attacks) were more likely to exhibit the upward shift in optimal frequency of VEMP stimulation. As Meniere disease progresses (advanced Meniere disease), VEMP responses are more likely either to be absent or to have reduced amplitude and/or increased threshold in the affected ear. This is thought to be due to increased damage to the saccule as the disease progresses.

Superior Canal Dehiscence Syndrome

Abnormally low VEMP threshold (<70 dB nHL) and enhanced VEMP amplitude on the affected side, sometimes accompanied by a low-frequency air–bone gap with normal tympanograms and acoustic reflexes, are the common findings in SCD. There is no upper limit of normal for amplitude, so enhanced amplitude is typically determined by a comparison with the other ear. SCD can be bilateral, but it is often worse in one ear, so ear-to-ear symmetry comparisons for threshold and amplitude can be useful. If a patient has active, symptomatic bilateral SCD, one would expect low thresholds and large amplitudes in both ears, but this finding may also be seen in young patients without vestibulopathy. Clinical correlation by computed tomography (CT) scan is required to confirm the diagnosis of SCD.

Enlarged Vestibular Aqueduct

This disorder has been seen to result in significantly lower VEMP thresholds and enhanced VEMP amplitudes compared with the nonaffected ear, along with congenital sensorineural hearing loss, which helps to distinguish it from SCD (Sheykholeslami, Schmerber, Habiby Kermany, and Kaga, 2004).

Retrocochlear Disorders of the Eighth Cranial Nerve

Vestibular Neuritis

In some cases of vestibular neuritis, delayed latencies, reduced amplitudes, or absent responses can be seen in the affected ear if the inferior portion of CN VIII is affected. Halmagyi

et al (2002) and Iwasaki et al (2005) proposed the existence of inferior vestibular neuritis. (See the case studies section in this chapter for an example.) However, in many cases, vestibular neuritis spares the inferior vestibular nerve and affects only the superior vestibular nerve (Ochi and Ohashi, 2003). This is thought to be due to the longer, narrower bony canal that the superior vestibular nerve passes through as compared with the shorter, wider bony canal the inferior vestibular nerve passes through (Goebel, O'Mara, and Gianoli, 2001), so VEMPs are often normal in the ear with vestibular neuritis (Manzari, Tedesco, Burgess, and Curthoys, 2010).

Vestibular Schwannoma

If the inferior portion of the vestibular nerve is affected by a vestibular schwannoma, the VEMP response may be delayed in latency, reduced in amplitude, or absent on the affected side. VEMP response can be normal if the inferior portion of the vestibular nerve is not affected by the lesion. VEMP, in conjunction with caloric and pure tone, acoustic reflex threshold, and ABR testing, can be helpful in determining which portions of CN VIII are affected by the lesion, as each of the three portions of CN VIII are assessed separately (Takeichi, Sakamoto, Fukuda, and Inuyama, 2001).

Bell Palsy/Ramsay Hunt Syndrome

Much like vestibular neuritis, Bell palsy/Ramsay Hunt syndrome, a typically unilateral cranial nerve disorder that involves CN VIII, among others, may result in delayed latencies, reduced amplitudes, or absent responses in the affected ear (Lu and Young, 2003).

Central Nervous System Disorders

Central nervous system (CNS) disorders related to demyelinization or ischemia of the brainstem, such as multiple sclerosis, spinocerebellar degeneration, and brainstem stroke, may also affect VEMP responses, as the VEMP response pathway includes the caudal portion (medulla) of the brainstem. By contrast, ABR and caloric pathways are through the rostral part of the brainstem, the pons and midbrain. Therefore, the combined use of VEMP, calorics, and ABR testing improves differential diagnosis of the location of brainstem lesions (Chen and Young, 2003). When VEMP responses are affected by a CNS disorder, results are typically delayed latencies or absent responses (Rosengren, Nogajski, Cremer, and Colebatch, 2007).

Basilar artery migraine has been shown to affect VEMP responses with delayed latencies or absent responses (Liao and Young, 2004). Reduced amplitudes have also been reported in patients with migraine (Allena, Magis, De Pasqua, Schoenen, and Bisdorff, 2007).

◆ Case Studies

Case 1: Bell Palsy

A 77-year-old woman had a sudden onset of right-sided facial droop, inability to close her right eye or raise her right forehead, and right hearing loss with vertigo and imbalance. Her test results included a recent-onset sensorineural hearing loss in the right ear, a 4, 5, 6 surface-dependent pattern on computerized dynamic posturography (CDP) testing, a left-beating head-shake nystagmus, a left-beating static positional nystagmus, and a complete absence of response to caloric testing in the right ear. VEMP results indicated right ear latencies that were prolonged and asymmetric compared with left ear latencies, which were within normal limits (**Fig. 19.1**). The amplitudes between the right and left ears were symmetric. The patient was diagnosed with right-sided Bell palsy, a disorder related to herpes simplex virus and/or varicella zoster virus affecting the facial and/or auditory cranial nerves, typically unilaterally (Murakami, Mizobuchi, Nakashiro, Doi, Hato, and Yanagihara, 1996). Based on these test results, both the superior and inferior vestibular portions, as well as the auditory portion of CN VIII, were affected by the lesion.

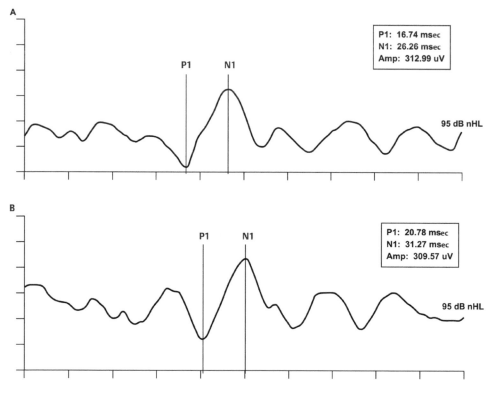

Fig. 19.1 Bell palsy. (**A**) Normal latencies in the left ear. (**B**) Prolonged latencies in the right ear.

Case 2: Superior Canal Dehiscence

A 30-year-old woman had a 2-year history of Tulio phenomenon in the left ear; that is, she became dizzy when exposed to loud sounds, particularly a baby crying to her left. An otolaryngologic physical examination was negative for any abnormalities. Her audiogram indicated a low frequency "relative" air–bone gap in the left ear: normal air conduction and extremely low masked bone-conduction thresholds (thought to be due to the "third window" effect) (**Fig. 19.2**). Tympanograms were normal, and acoustic reflexes were present in both ears. VEMP results were normal in the right ear, whereas the left VEMP threshold was low (65 dB nHL) and asymmetric (15 dB nHL difference) compared with the right ear. Additionally, VEMP amplitude asymmetry ratio was 34%, with the left response larger than the right, although still within normal limits for symmetry (**Fig. 19.3**). High-resolution CT scan indicated bilateral thinning of the bone over both superior semicircular canals, with the left dehiscence worse than the right.

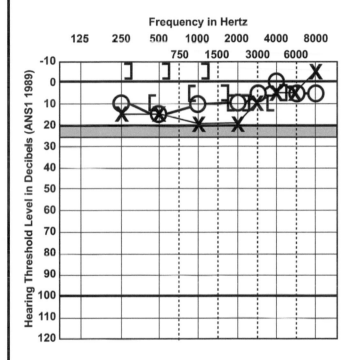

Fig. 19.2 Audiogram of superior canal dehiscence (SCD). Low frequency "relative" air–bone gap in the left ear is seen.

Continued

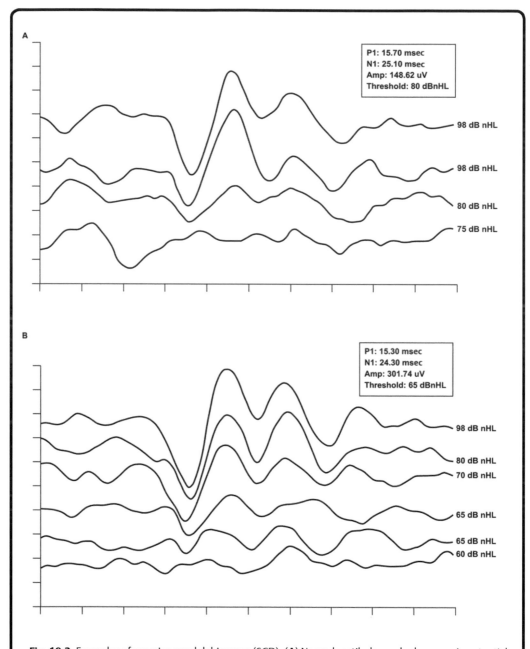

A

P1: 15.70 msec
N1: 25.10 msec
Amp: 148.62 uV
Threshold: 80 dBnHL

98 dB nHL

98 dB nHL

80 dB nHL

75 dB nHL

B

P1: 15.30 msec
N1: 24.30 msec
Amp: 301.74 uV
Threshold: 65 dBnHL

98 dB nHL

80 dB nHL

70 dB nHL

65 dB nHL

65 dB nHL

60 dB nHL

Fig. 19.3 Examples of superior canal dehiscence (SCD). (**A**) Normal vestibular evoked myogenic potential (VEMP) threshold (80 dB nHL [normal hearing level]) in the right ear. (**B**) Abnormally low (65 dB nHL) and asymmetric (15 dB difference between ears) vestibular evoked myogenic potential (VEMP) threshold in the left ear.

Case 3: Vestibular Schwannoma

A 53-year-old man presented had a recent decrease in hearing in the left ear and increase in tinnitus without vertigo or dizziness (**Fig. 19.4**). Caloric testing revealed a complete absence of response from the left ear and a normal response from the right ear, consistent with a lesion affecting the superior division of the left vestibular nerve. VEMP testing indicated normal and symmetric latencies, symmetric amplitudes, and symmetric thresholds in both ears, indicating the inferior division of the left vestibular nerve was not affected (**Fig. 19.5**). High-resolution T2-weighted magnetic resonance imaging (MRI) scan with fast spin echo revealed a 6 mm left vestibular schwannoma. ABR was not completed. Combining the audiogram, caloric, and VEMP test results indicated that the site of lesion was the superior division of the vestibular portion and the auditory portion of CN VIII; the function of the inferior division of the vestibular portion of CN VIII was intact.

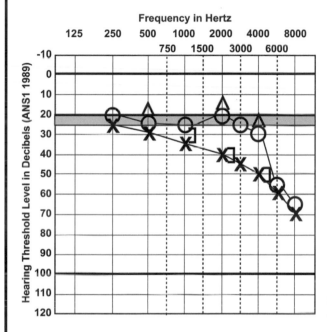

Fig. 19.4 Audiogram of a patient with a left side vestibular schwannoma.

Continued

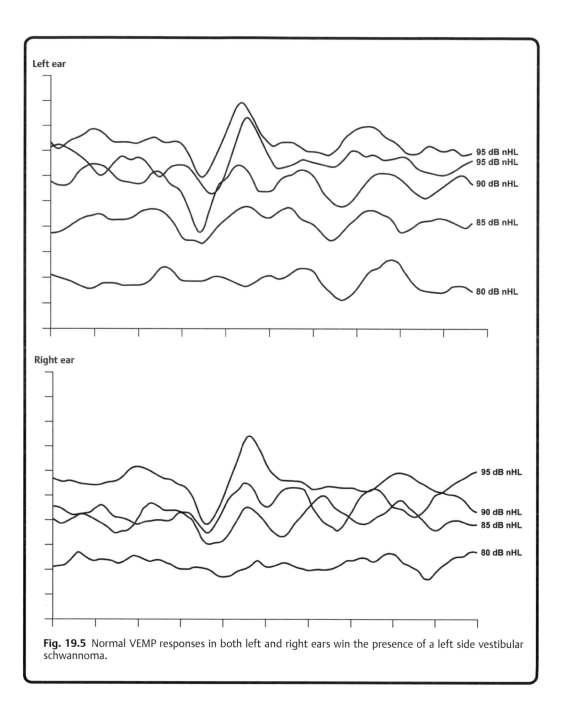

Left ear

95 dB nHL
95 dB nHL

90 dB nHL

85 dB nHL

80 dB nHL

Right ear

95 dB nHL

90 dB nHL
85 dB nHL

80 dB nHL

Fig. 19.5 Normal VEMP responses in both left and right ears win the presence of a left side vestibular schwannoma.

Case 4: Vestibular Schwannoma #2

A 57-year-old woman had a known right vestibular schwannoma diagnosed 8 years earlier. A recent hearing test indicated a symmetric mild to moderate sensorineural hearing loss in both ears. Previous vestibular test results were unknown. An MRI showed a 2-mm schwannoma in the right ear. Recently, the patient reported right otalgia and episodes of dizziness and imbalance without true vertigo. She denied changes in hearing. Caloric testing was within normal limits of symmetry at 19% weakness in the right ear. VEMP results were in agreement on MRI with reduced amplitude and increased threshold in the right ear and a normal response in the left ear (**Fig. 19.6**). ABR testing was not completed.

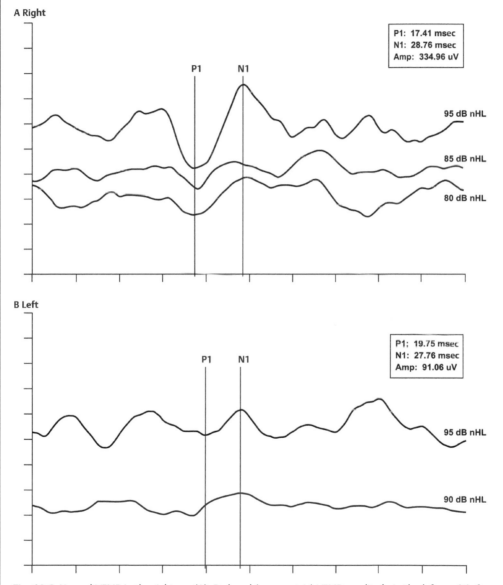

Fig. 19.6 Normal VEMP in the right ear (A). Reduced (asymmetric) VEMP amplitude in the left ear (B), for a patient with a lesion on the left CN VII.

Case 5: Inferior Vestibular Neuritis

A 49-year-old woman reported episodic positional vertigo, with episodes months apart. Test results included normal caloric testing, normal posturography, normal ABR, and symmetric hearing thresholds within normal limits. On MRI, a 3-mm lesion on the left CN VII, initially thought to be a vestibular schwannoma, was detected. The left ear VEMP response was delayed in latency and reduced in amplitude relative to the right ear (**Fig. 19.7**). The patient was seen 7 months later. She had not had any recurrence of vertigo, and her balance had improved by her own report. VEMP latencies on the left had returned to normal, and latencies and amplitudes were no longer asymmetric (**Fig. 19.8**). Caloric testing was still normal. The lesion was no longer seen on MRI. As the lesion disappeared, the diagnosis changed from vestibular schwannoma to suspected vestibular neuritis that resolved. As caloric and audiometric testing were both normal, and the VEMP was abnormal, only the inferior division of the vestibular portion of CN VIII was affected by the lesion. This case, along with others in the literature, supports the existence of vestibular neuritis that affects only the inferior vestibular portion and spares the auditory and superior vestibular portions of CN VIII, as well as the theory that VEMP response can recover in cases of inferior vestibular neuritis.

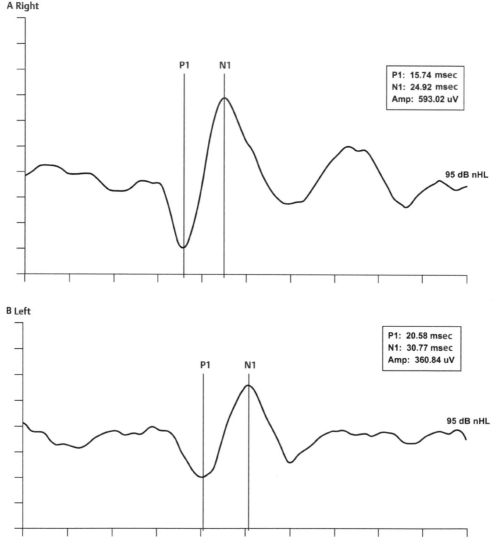

A Right

P1   N1

P1: 15.74 msec
N1: 24.92 msec
Amp: 593.02 uV

95 dB nHL

B Left

P1: 20.58 msec
N1: 30.77 msec
Amp: 360.84 uV

P1   N1

95 dB nHL

Fig. 19.7 VEMP testing for a patient with left side inferior vestibular neuritis. Normal VEMP in the right ear (A). VEMP with delayed latencies and reduced amplitudes in the left ear (B).

Continued

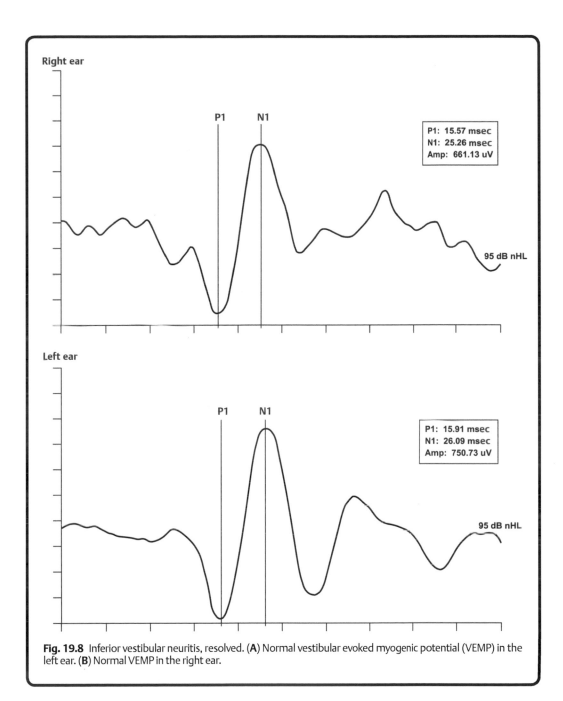

Right ear

P1   N1

P1: 15.57 msec
N1: 25.26 msec
Amp: 661.13 uV

95 dB nHL

Left ear

P1   N1

P1: 15.91 msec
N1: 26.09 msec
Amp: 750.73 uV

95 dB nHL

Fig. 19.8 Inferior vestibular neuritis, resolved. (**A**) Normal vestibular evoked myogenic potential (VEMP) in the left ear. (**B**) Normal VEMP in the right ear.

References

Ackley, R., & Tamaki, C. (2003). *Application of VEMP to deaf and HoH patients: A clinical study.* Paper presented at the national convention of the American Speech-Language and Hearing Association Chicago.

Akin, F. W., Murnane, O. D., Panus, P. C., Caruthers, S. K., Wilkinson, A. E., & Proffitt, T. M. (2004). The influence of voluntary tonic EMG level on the vestibular-evoked myogenic potential. *Journal of Rehabilitation Research and Development, 41*(3B), 473–480. PubMed

Allena, M., Magis, D., De Pasqua, V., Schoenen, J., & Bisdorff, A. R. (2007). The vestibulo-collic reflex is abnormal in migraine. *Cephalalgia, 27*(12), 1424. PubMed

American National Standard Institute. (1989). *American National Standard Specification for audiometers* (ANSI S3.6-1989). New York: Author.

Basta, D., Todt, I., & Ernst, A. (2005). Normative data for P1/N1-latencies of vestibular evoked myogenic potentials induced by air- or bone-conducted tone bursts. *Clinical Neurophysiology, 116*(9), 2216–2219. PubMed

Basta, D., Todt, I., & Ernst, A. (2007). Characterization of age-related changes in vestibular evoked myogenic potentials. *Journal of Vestibular Research, 17*(2–3), 93–98. PubMed

Buckingham, J. M., Zapala, D. A., Hibbitts, K. G., Hawkins, D. B., Pratt, T. L., Seymour, M. K., et al. (2008). *VEMP amplitude and latency variability by montage over time.* Paper presented at the meeting of the American Auditory Society, Scottsdale, AZ.

Chen, C. H., & Young, Y. H. (2003). Vestibular evoked myogenic potentials in brainstem stroke. *Laryngoscope, 113*(6), 990–993. PubMed

Colebatch, J. G., & Halmagyi, G. M. (1992). Vestibular evoked potentials in human neck muscles before and after unilateral vestibular deafferentation. *Neurology, 42*(8), 1635–1636. PubMed

Colebatch, J. G., Halmagyi, G. M., & Skuse, N. F. (1994). Myogenic potentials generated by a click-evoked vestibulo-collic reflex. *Journal of Neurology, Neurosurgery, and Psychiatry, 57*(2), 190–197. PubMed

Goebel, J. A., O'Mara, W., & Gianoli, G. (2001). Anatomic considerations in vestibular neuritis. *Otology & Neurotology, 22*(4), 512–518. PubMed

Goff, W. R., Allison, T., & Vaughn, H. G. (1978). The functional neuroanatomy of event related potentials. In E. Callaway, P. Tueting, & S. H. Koslow (Eds.), *Event related potentials in man* (pp. 1–79). New York: Academic Press.

Halmagyi, G. M., Aw, S. T., Karlberg, M., Curthoys, I. S., & Todd, M. J. (2002). Inferior vestibular neuritis. *Annals of the New York Academy of Sciences, 956*, 306–313. PubMed

Halmagyi, G. M., & Colebatch, J. G. (1995). Vestibular evoked myogenic potentials in the sternocleidomastoid muscle are not of lateral canal origin. *Acta Oto-Laryngologica Supplement, 520*(1), 1–3.

Itoh, A., Kim, Y. S., Yoshioka, K., Kanaya, M., Enomoto, H., Hiraiwa, F., et al. (2001). Clinical study of vestibular-evoked myogenic potentials and auditory brainstem responses in patients with brainstem lesions. *Acta Oto-Laryngologica. Supplementum, 545,* 116–119. PubMed

Iwasaki, S., Takai, Y., Ito, K., & Murofushi, T. (2005). Abnormal vestibular evoked myogenic potentials in the presence of normal caloric responses. *Otology and Neurotology, 26*(6), 1196–1199. PubMed

Janky, K. L., & Shepard, N. (2009). Vestibular evoked myogenic potential (VEMP) testing: normative threshold response curves and effects of age. *Journal of the American Academy of Audiology, 20*(8), 514–522. PubMed

Lee, S. K., Cha, C. I., Jung, T. S., Park, D. C., & Yeo, S. G. (2008). Age-related differences in parameters of vestibular evoked myogenic potentials. *Acta Oto-Laryngologica, 128*(1), 66–72. PubMed

Liao, L. J., & Young, Y. H. (2004). Vestibular evoked myogenic potentials in basilar artery migraine. *Laryngoscope, 114*(7), 1305–1309. PubMed

Lin, M. Y., Timmer, F. C., Oriel, B. S., Zhou, G., Guinan, J. J., Kujawa, S. G., et al. (2006, Jun). Vestibular evoked myogenic potentials (VEMP) can detect asymptomatic saccular hydrops. *Laryngoscope, 116*(6), 987–992. PubMed

Lu, Y. C., & Young, Y. H. (2003). Vertigo from herpes zoster oticus: Superior or inferior vestibular nerve origin? *Laryngoscope, 113*(2), 307–311. PubMed

Manzari, L., Tedesco, A. R., Burgess, A. M., & Curthoys, I. S. (2010). Ocular vestibular-evoked myogenic potentials to bone-conducted vibration in superior vestibular neuritis show utricular function. *Otolaryngology—Head and Neck Surgery, 143*(2), 274–280. PubMed

Murakami, S., Mizobuchi, M., Nakashiro, Y., Doi, T., Hato, N., & Yanagihara, N. (1996). Bell palsy and herpes simplex virus: Identification of viral DNA in endoneural fluid and muscle. *Annals of Internal Medicine, 124*(1, Pt 1), 27–30. PubMed

Murofushi, T., Halmagyi, G. M., Yavor, R. A., & Colebatch, J. G. (1996). Absent vestibular evoked myogenic potentials in vestibular neurolabyrinthitis: An indicator of inferior vestibular nerve involvement? *Archives of Otolaryngology—Head and Neck Surgery, 122*(8), 845–848. PubMed

Murofushi, T., Shimizu, K., Takegoshi, H., & Cheng, P. W. (2001). Diagnostic value of prolonged latencies in the vestibular evoked myogenic potential. *Archives of Otolaryngology—Head and Neck Surgery, 127*(9), 1069–1072. PubMed

Ochi, K., & Ohashi, T. (2003). Age-related changes in the vestibular-evoked myogenic potentials. *Otolaryngology—Head and Neck Surgery, 129*(6), 655–659. PubMed

Ochi, K., Ohashi, T., & Nishino, H. (2001). Variance of vestibular-evoked myogenic potentials. *Laryngoscope, 111*(3), 522–527. PubMed

Rauch, S. D., Zhou, G., Kujawa, S. G., Guinan, J. J., & Herrmann, B. S. (2004). Vestibular evoked myogenic potentials show altered tuning in patients with Ménière's disease. *Otology and Neurotology, 25*(3), 333–338. PubMed

Robertson, D. D., & Ireland, D. J. (1995). Vestibular evoked myogenic potentials. *Journal of Otolaryngology, 24*(1), 3–8. PubMed

Rosengren, S. M., Govender, S., & Colebatch, J. G. (2009). The relative effectiveness of different stimulus waveforms in evoking VEMPs: Significance of stimulus energy and frequency. *Journal of Vestibular Research, 19*(1–2), 33–40. PubMed

Rosengren, S. M., Nogajski, J. H., Cremer, P. D., & Colebatch, J. G. (2007). Delayed vestibular evoked responses to the eyes and neck in a patient with an isolated brainstem lesion. *Clinical Neurophysiology, 118*(9), 2112–2116. PubMed

Rosengren, S. M., Welgampola, M. S., & Colebatch, J. G. (2010). Vestibular evoked myogenic potentials: Past, present and future. *Clinical Neurophysiology, 121*(5), 636–651. PubMed

Sheykholeslami, K., Murofushi, T., & Kaga, K. (2001). The effect of sternocleidomastoid electrode location on vestibular evoked myogenic potential. *Auris, Nasus, Larynx, 28*(1), 41–43. PubMed

Sheykholeslami, K., Schmerber, S., Habiby Kermany, M., & Kaga, K. (2004). Vestibular-evoked myogenic potentials in three patients with large vestibular aqueduct. *Hearing Research, 190*(1–2), 161–168. PubMed

Stoody, T.M., Guy, H., Bright, K.E., & Erdbruegger, D. (n.d.). *Effects of blood pressure cuff levels on VEMP responses.* Manuscript in preparation.

Su, H. C., Huang, T. W., Young, Y. H., & Cheng, P. W. (2004). Aging effect on vestibular evoked myogenic potential. *Otology & Neurotology, 25*(6), 977–980. PubMed

Takeichi, N., Sakamoto, T., Fukuda, S., & Inuyama, Y. (2001). Vestibular evoked myogenic potential (VEMP) in patients with acoustic neuromas. *Auris Nasus Larynx, 28,* S39–41.

Todd, N. P., Cody, F. W. J., & Banks, J. R. (2000). A saccular origin of frequency tuning in myogenic vestibular evoked potentials? Implications for human responses to loud sounds. *Hearing Research, 141*(1–2), 180–188. PubMed

Vanspauwen, R., Wuyts, F. L., & Van de Heyning, P. H. (2006). Improving vestibular evoked myogenic potential reliability by using a blood pressure manometer. *Laryngoscope, 116*(1), 131–135. PubMed

Welgampola, M. S., & Colebatch, J. G. (2001). Vestibulocollic reflexes: Normal values and the effect of age. *Clinical Neurophysiology, 112*(11), 1971–1979. PubMed

Welgampola, M. S., & Colebatch, J. G. (2005). Characteristics and clinical applications of vestibular-evoked myogenic potentials. *Neurology, 64*(10), 1682–1688. PubMed

Wilson, V. J., Boyle, R., Fukushima, K., Rose, P. K., Shinoda, Y., Sugiuchi, Y., et al. (1995). The vestibulocollic reflex. *Journal of Vestibular Research, 5*(3), 147–170. PubMed

Young, Y. H., Wu, C. C., & Wu, C. H. (2002). Augmentation of vestibular evoked myogenic potentials: an indication for distended saccular hydrops. *Laryngoscope, 112*(3), 509–512. PubMed

Zapala, D. A., & Brey, R. H. (2004). Clinical experience with the vestibular evoked myogenic potential. *Journal of the American Academy of Audiology, 15*(3), 198–215. PubMed

Chapter 20

Patient Preparation, Orientation, and Data Collection

Tina M. Stoody

Competence in collection of auditory evoked potentials (AEPs) begins with proper preparation and an ability to adapt quickly to unforeseen situations during data collection. Before testing, it is important to prepare both the patient and yourself for the session. Knowledge of procedures related to patient preparation is a skill set specified within the guidelines for competencies in AEP measurement (American Speech-Language-Hearing Association, 2003). Items related to patient preparation that will be discussed in this chapter include sedation and anesthesia considerations, instruction and explanation of test procedures, and skin preparation for electrode application. Once the patient is properly prepared, efficient and appropriate data collection is essential for a successful test session. The ability to troubleshoot quickly and adapt to problems that may arise is a skill that is acquired with experience. This chapter provides an overview of what to do before, during, and after an electrophysiologic test session focusing on patient preparation and data collection.

◆ Clinician Preparation

Case History Review

Preparation for an electrophysiologic test session begins with a thorough case history review. A seasoned clinician will enter into a test session well equipped with key details about the patient coming in for testing, such as age, the referral source, reason for the referral, and other pertinent health-related information. Normative data are dependent on the patient's age, so knowing the age is important for appropriate interpretation of test results. The referral source is needed so that clinical reports are sent promptly to the proper individual/location. If the reason for the evaluation is a follow-up for a newborn hearing screening referral, there is likely paperwork that will need to be filed with the appropriate agency. For example, in the state of Colorado, the clinician is required to submit results to the Colorado Hearing Program in the state health department. More information on documentation for newborn hearing referrals can be found in Chapter 13. Other pertinent health-related information is medications or conditions that might affect testing. If the patient is generally not alert or is taking medication that affects the central nervous system in any way, these could affect test results or possibly be contraindications to testing. If the clinician is employed at a facility where sedated testing is performed, then chart review to determine the need for sedation is important so that the appropriate medical personnel are present to administer the sedative and monitor the patient.

Patient Instructions before Testing

Occasionally, electrophysiologic testing takes place without prior scheduling. In such cases, there is no opportunity to instruct patients ahead of time about the testing. However, it is more typical that an electrophysiologic testing session is scheduled ahead of time, as the patient is often referred from an outside agency, which provides the clinician an opportunity to prepare the patient for the upcoming session. The testing facility may have a prepared sheet, which can be given to the patient by either the audiologist or the office staff, that explains the test being scheduled and provides key instructional information. These instructions will depend on the specific test being ordered and the age of the client. For example, the instructions for an adult will be much different from those given to a parent of a newborn. Instructions for a pediatric test with sedation will be different from those for a test without sedation. Refer to **Figs. 20.1** and **20.2** for examples of patient instructions.

Supplies and Equipment

Electrophysiologic testing can be somewhat daunting for patients, even with instructional sheets or brochures given ahead of time. It is helpful to have all necessary supplies out and ready, as well as equipment up and running, before testing is scheduled to being. This includes having patient information entered into the computer and having the appropriate testing protocol parameters programmed and selected. It can sometimes be challenging to obtain all the desired information during a test session, especially with a pediatric patient, who may become too fussy for testing. Audiologists need to be efficient with their time, and fumbling with computer applications to input patient data and alter test protocols can take away from valuable test time. In addition, it helps to have supplies neatly arranged and ready for use. The clinician should ensure that an adequate amount of supplies is available, including transducers, electrodes, alcohol wipes, cotton-tipped applicators, gauze pads, conductive paste/gel, tape, and abrasive skin preparation liquid, before the patient arrives. More details regarding use of these supplies are found later in this chapter. Having everything ready ahead of time not only will make the patient feel more at ease but will also help the test session to run in a more timely fashion.

XYZ AUDIOLOGY CLINIC

ABR TEST INSTUCTIONS

You have been scheduled for an auditory brainstem response (ABR) test. This test will evaluate the function of the pathway from the ear to the brainstem by measuring brain waves produced when the ear hears sounds. The ABR is a painle ss procedure and does not require the use of any needles.

In order to achieve the bes test results please follow these simple instructions: t

- Dress comfortably.
- Do not apply makeup, lotions, or creams to your face on the day of the test.
- Do not wear any earrings.
- Try to avoid caffeine, nicotine, or other stimulants on the day of the test.
- Continue to take your medications as prescribed.

If you have any questions regarding the test procedure or these instructions please contact our office at XXX-XXXX.

Fig. 20.1 Sample adult patient instruction sheet.

XYZ AUDIOLOGY CLINIC

Instructions For Parents Preparing for an ABR

Your baby has been scheduled for a specialized hearing test. The test is called an auditory brainstem response test (ABR). It is a safe and painless test for your baby. In order to collect the information we need, your baby will need to sleep during the test. We will need your cooperation to help make the test session a success. To prepare for the test it will help if you do the following:

WHEN SCHEDULING THE TEST:

Note when your baby normally naps during the day and try to schedule the test for that time.

AT HOME THE DAY OF THE APPOINTMENT

- Please wake your baby earlier than normal and don't let him/her go back to sleep.
- Feed your baby a light meal. **Please do NOT feed your child until right before the appointment time**. A full stomach will help your child sleep during the test.

BRING THE FOLLOWING TO THE APPOINTMENT

- Enough formula or milk to feed your baby a larger meal.
- Extra formula milk, or juice just in case more is needed.
- Extra diapers, pacifier, and comfortable blanket
- If your baby likes to sleep in a carrier, car seat, or stroller, bring it along.

AT THE CLINIC

- Please arrive for the appointment at least 15 minutes early to allow time to settle in and get your baby comfortable.
- When settled into the test room, you will be asked to feed the baby and let him/her fall asleep.
- Testing will begin when the baby is quiet and sleeping.

We realize that it is difficult to deprive your child of sleep and food; however, this will lead to a successful procedure and allows the audiologist to obtain the most reliable results. If you have any questions regarding the test or these instructions please call the clinic at XXX-XXXX.

Fig. 20.2 Sample pediatric patient instruction sheet, without sedation.

◆ Patient Preparation

Patient Orientation

You will want to orient the patient (i.e., explain the upcoming test procedure), or the parents if you are testing an infant, once you have brought the patient to the testing area. The best data are typically taken from a calm patient, so spending some time explaining what to expect and will usually make your patient less anxious and provide you a better opportunity to collect clean waveforms. Children will often follow their parents' lead. If the parents are calm, the child is likely to be calm as well. If the parents are nervous, the child will pick up on these cues. Keep in mind that, although you may perform this testing on a fairly regular basis, the testing may seem very technical and foreign to your patient. The thought of having electrodes attached can be scary to some patients. It is for this reason that I often refer to the electrodes as "sensors" or "wires" during instructions to avoid the fear of electric shock associated with the term *electrodes*. Depending on the reason for the testing, some patients may be very worried about the test results, including the possibility of a diagnosis of hearing loss in an infant or a possible tumor in an adult. By discussing the procedure with the patient thoroughly in layperson's terms and answering questions up front, you can put many concerns about the testing to rest. Common concerns are fear of electric shock and concern that the test will be uncomfortably loud and painful. Therefore, it is especially important to make it clear to the patient that the testing you will be performing is routine for all ages (infants to adults), that there is no risk or threat from the electrodes or acoustic stimulus, and that for nonsedated testing there are no side effects (except for some minor skin irritation from electrode application materials or tape). Although certain aspects of instructions will vary slightly for different procedures, the core instructions are relatively similar for all electrophysiologic tests (**Fig. 20.3**).

For the population of patients who are unable to maintain a quiet, relaxed state, successful test sessions may be accomplished with sedation to calm the patient and optimize data acquisition. Medication of patients for electrophysiologic test procedures requires collaboration between the audiologist and other medical professionals. Clinicians who perform testing on sedated/anesthetized patients will need to work with physicians in the development of protocols to ensure patient comfort and safety (see Chapter 14). There are complex factors that can expose patients to risk or harm with respect to sedation or topical anesthesia. These factors need to be appreciated by the clinician. Keep in mind that administering any medications to achieve a desired patient state (i.e., calming/quieting a patient for auditory brainstem response [ABR] recording) is a medical procedure that is not in the scope of practice for audiologists. Therefore, these testing situations will require a physician prescription, as well as physician administration, monitoring, and availability in case of emergency situations that may arise (American Speech-Language-Hearing Association, 1992). In the case of a sedated test, medical personnel performing and monitoring the anesthesia can provide additional information to patients about the possible risks associated with sedation.

Electrode Application

Proper electrode application takes a bit of practice, but once the skill is mastered, it will save time and keep patient anxiety to a minimum. The experienced clinician should be able to secure electrodes with minimal discomfort

---

Audiologist: "To prepare you for the testing first I am going to clean three areas of skin with alcohol, one spot on your forehead and your earlobes (or mastoids). Next I will be using a liquid to clean off any remaining oils or skin cells. The liquid is gritty so it may scratch a little or feel like sandpaper when I use it, but it won't be painful. Any excess liquid will be wiped off with a guaze pad. Once the skin has been cleaned I will be placing sensors on each of these areas. The sensors will have some cream (or gel) in them to help with the connection to your skin. A piece of paper tape will be used to keep the sensors in place. Once the sensors are in place, small foam plug earphones will be placed in your ears. You will hear clicking sounds that sound similar to a jackhammer. The sounds are supposed to be loud but many people actually fall asleep during testing. You don't need to respond to the sounds at all, your job is simply to close your eyes and relax. When the testing is completed I will remove the sensors and help you clean any remaining cream/gel. Do you have any questions?"

Fig. 20.3 Sample script of verbal instructions for evoked potentials testing.

to the patient. In addition, he or she should be able to obtain low electrode impedances (<5000 Ω [ohms] for individual electrodes and <2000 Ω difference between electrodes) upon initial application. Accurate placement of electrodes is also important such that the clinician is consistent with electrode placement from one patient to the next (e.g., in accordance with the 10–20 system). Keep in mind that there are many different "techniques" that clinicians develop as this skill is mastered. I present some tips and personal preferences in this chapter that have been helpful, but they are not the only way to place electrodes.

Different types of electrodes are available that can be broadly categorized as disposable or reusable. Disposable electrodes have the added benefit of being pretreated with electrode gel and adhesive, but this benefit comes at a financial expense. In the past, many clinics I worked in overwhelmingly chose to use reusable electrodes because of the added cost of disposables with the exception of certain procedures, such as the vestibular evoked myogenic potential (VEMP). However, several clinics have switched to disposable electrodes, incurring an added expense as a trade-off for the ease of use as well as reduced potential for hygeine problems. Disposable electrodes either come connected with a cable or have a snap connection to a separate cable. Reusable electrodes most often used during evoked

response measurement include disk electrodes, cup electrodes, ear clip electrodes, and TIPtrodes, which require a special connector to insert transducers. These different electrode types are depicted in (**Fig. 20.4**).

The supplies required for electrode application and their individual purposes are listed in **Table 20.1.** There are six basic steps involved in electrode application: (1) clean the skin, (2) abrade the skin, (3) apply conductive gel or paste to the electrode (except in the case of disposable electrodes already pretreated with gel), (4) apply the electrode to the appropriate site, (5) secure the electrode (typically involves taping the electrode), and (6) collect and secure all electrode leads and plug them into the head box. Of course, the sites where the electrodes are applied and the specific electrodes that are used will vary slightly from one test procedure to the next. **Figure 20.5** provides a visual of the electrode application for a single-channel ABR test.

Some clinicians prefer to go through each of the steps for one electrode site before moving on to the next, whereas others complete each step for all electrode sites before moving to the next step. Each method is perfectly acceptable; I prefer to go through each step across all electrode sites (i.e., clean all sites and then apply electrodes at each site, rather than apply the first electrode, then prepare the site for the second). One instance when it may be helpful to prepare one site at a time is when electrode

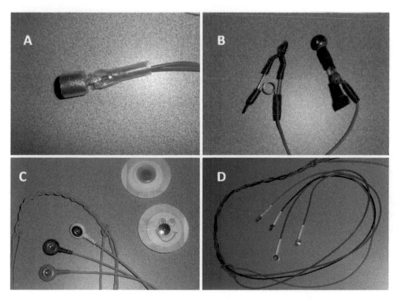

Fig. 20.4 Sample of different electrode types for electrophysiologic testing, including (**A**) TIPtrode with insert earphone connector, (**B**) earlobe electrodes, (**C**) disposable "snap connector" electrodes, and (**D**) reusable disk electrodes.

Table 20.1 Electrode Application Supplies

Supplies	Purpose
Alcohol and/or alcohol pads	Remove dirt, oil, makeup, and other cosmetic substances from the skin
Abrasive liquid (e.g., NuPrep)	Abrade skin to remove oils and dead skin cells
Conductive paste or gel	Improve connection between skin and electrode
Square gauze pads	Application of abrasive liquid and wiping excess liquid from patient Application of alcohol if alcohol pads are not used
Cotton-tipped applicators	Application of abrasive liquid
Tape (surgical or medical grade)	Secure electrodes to skin
Cotton balls	Help secure electrodes to "hairy" electrode sites, such as Cz Can be used to apply alcohol instead of gauze

sites are covered with hair. Keeping a finger in place where the scalp has been abraded can help ensure that electrodes are placed properly (as it may be difficult to visually locate the area that was scrubbed). In this instance, a cotton ball rather than tape can help keep an electrode in place. Once the electrode has been placed on the scalp, a cotton ball can be pressed firmly on top for a solid connection.

Another question often asked is, which material is best for increased conductivity: gel or paste? Disposable electrodes are typically pretreated with gel. It has been my experience that gel works well with certain types of electrodes, such as tympanic membrane electrodes, ball electrodes, and TIPtrodes.

Special Consideration

A simple search on the Internet reveals that some brands of gel are specially formulated for sensitive skin, so you may want to experiment with different types of electrode gel if skin sensitivity is a concern. Conductive paste may cause more of a skin reaction than expected. One commonly used brand of conductive paste cautions users regarding patients with a history of skin allergy or sensitivity to cosmetics and lotions.

Conductive paste works well with disk electrodes attached to scalp locations for testing, as it adheres to the skin well and forms a nice seal. It has also been my experience that it is particularly helpful to use enough paste so that it keeps the electrode in place throughout the recording session (**Fig. 20.5**). There have been instances where too little paste was used, and the result was an electrode that slipped quite a bit, even when tape was applied. This can be very frustrating, particularly when reapplication of electrodes agitates an otherwise calm pediatric patient.

Pearl

If initial impedance values for reusable electrodes are too high, first try firmly pressing on the electrode for a few seconds. This will strengthen the seal between the electrode and the skin via the conductive paste and is usually enough to lower impedances into the acceptable range. However, if you are using disposable electrodes that are already pre-gelled, do not press down on the middle of the electrode, as that can cause the gel to be pressed out, ruining the adhesive. High impedances will result if a tight seal is not maintained.

One of the most common errors that inexperienced clinicians will encounter during electrode application is poor electrode impedances. The first thing the clinician can try to lower impedance values is to apply some pressure to electrode sites. If this method is unsuccessful, the clinician did not properly prepare the skin,

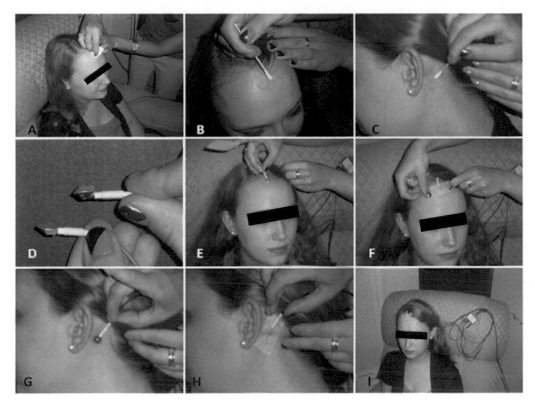

Fig. 20.5 Six-step process in electrode application for a single-channel auditory brainstem response (ABR) test. (**A**) Wipe areas with alcohol pad. (**B,C**) Abrade these areas. (**D**) Apply conductive gel or paste to electrodes (the top electrode has an adequate amount of paste; the bottom electrode may not have enough for an optimal connection). (**E,G**) Apply the electrode to the appropriate site. (**F,H**) Secure the electrode with tape. (**I**) Collect and secure all electrode leads behind the ear and plug them into the head box.

resulting in the need to repeat the entire electrode application procedure. You can save test time and patient frustration by abrading the skin properly the first time; it is okay to scrub the skin enough to make it red. The flushed skin will also aid in electrode placement; if you cannot see where you have scrubbed when placing the electrode, chances are you may not have scrubbed hard enough. The goal is to thoroughly cleanse the skin, so vigorous scrubbing is required, so long as the patient does not bleed. Most adults will tolerate this as long as details regarding the procedure have been provided ahead of time. Unfortunately, many infants will fuss regardless of how gentle the clinician is. Therefore, it is much easier for everyone involved to avoid being "too gentle" when applying electrodes so that the procedure does not have to be repeated. In my experience, repetitive electrode application procedures can cause

more discomfort, especially in areas where skin tends to be a bit thinner or more sensitive, such as the mastoid region.

> ### Pearl
>
> The skin on the head of an individual who is bald is often a bit thicker than average and requires the clinician to be a little more vigorous when preparing placement of scalp electrodes.

Although there are no side effects to evoked potential testing itself, dermatologic reactions can occur in response to electrode application materials, particularly electrode paste/gel and tape. I have had some patients report mild itching, stinging, or burning in response to electrode application. It is important to be aware of the ingredients of substances that will be coming into contact with your patients. Of particular concern are electrode-conducting substances that include calcium as an ingredient. There is a condition called calcinosis cutis (calcification of the skin) that can occur when the skin is exposed to substances containing calcium. There are several documented cases of calcinosis cutis occurring after electroencephalographic testing, including ABR (Guillod, Hauser, Ruffieux, Masouyé, and Harms, 2002; Mancuso, Tosti, Fanti, Berdondini, Mongiorgi, and Morandi, 1990; Puig, Rocamora, Romaní, Saavedra, and Alomar, 1998; Schoenfeld, Grekin, and Mehregan, 1965; Wiley and Eaglstein, 1979; Zurbuchen, LeCoultre, Calza, and Halpérin, 1996). To minimize the risk for the rare occurrence of calcinosis cutis, it is important to thoroughly clean the skin following testing, avoid skin abrasions during electrode application preparation, try to minimize test time, and use calcium-free electrode preparation materials (Puig et al, 1998).

◆ Data Collection

Initial training on electrophysiologic data collection often occurs with students testing one another. It cannot be emphasized enough that collecting data on young adult patients with normal hearing in a laboratory or classroom setting is far different from and much less challenging than performing these tests in the clinic on patient populations with much more varied responses. Therefore, it is helpful for novice clinicians to develop a test strategy for data collection. This strategy will depend on the reason for testing. For example, is the patient being referred for a neurodiagnostic evaluation or for threshold estimation? **Table 20.2** provides a general summary of reasons for referral and the AEP tests appropriate for each. See Chapters 12 to 19.

In an optimal test environment, the clinician will have the ability to collect all the data he or she wants. However, conditions are rarely optimal; sometimes there are problems related to the equipment, environment, or patient state that prevent complete data collection. Knowing the reason for referral can help the clinician decide what the most important information to obtain will be. For example, in the case of an infant hearing evaluation, an optimal evaluation would be a full ABR wave V threshold search for clicks and low- and high-frequency tone bursts in both ears. When the testing does not proceed as planned, it is time for some clinical decision making. The audiologist needs to prioritize and decide what information should be collected and what may be sacrificed. To make this determination, the following questions need to be answered: Is there more than one test required for this session? In which order or sequence will testing be performed? Which ear is going to be tested first? Should I complete all testing for one ear first

Table 20.2 Auditory Evoked Potential Test Selection Based on Common Referrals

Reason for Referral	Auditory Evoked Potential Test
Threshold estimation after inability to obtain behavioral threshold information	ABR, ASSR
Follow-up from newborn hearing screening	ABR, ASSR
Rule out retrocochlear pathology	ABR
Meniere disease workup	ECochG
Differential diagnosis of ANSD	ABR and ECochG
APD evaluation	MLR, ALR, P300
Vestibular assessment for cochlear implant candidacy or suspected balance disorder	VEMP

Abbreviations: ABR, auditory brainstem response; ALR, auditory late response; ANSD, auditory neuropathy spectrum disorder; APD, auditory processing disorder; ASSR, auditory steady-state response; ECochG, electrocochleography; MLR, middle latency response; VEMP, vestibular evoked myogenic potential.

or alternate between ears? What step size for intensity should be used during threshold search? Having a plan before the test session will increase testing speed, which is critical for successful test sessions in most instances, as well as reduce potential frustration.

With a proper plan in place, there are a few other items the beginning clinician should consider for a successful test session. Noise is usually the biggest challenge to overcome. Low electrode impedances will reduce biological noise, but there are other sources of electrical noise that should be minimized throughout the test session. The clinician should ensure that the only pieces of equipment turned on within the test room are those necessary for testing. If there are other pieces of equipment, such as computers or fans, turn them off. Often lights can interfere with recording and are best left off, if possible. (This will also aid in relaxing the patient for evoked potentials that are not affected by sleep.) Muscle activity can also be an issue for longer evoked potentials (e.g., postauricular muscle artifact obscuring the middle latency response), so it is important to be sure the patient is not tensing any muscles and is in a position that fosters relaxation. Do not forget that eyeblinks can be mistaken for or obscure waveform components of cortical event–related potentials (refer to Chapter 10 for more information on eyeblink artifact). Electrode wires can be braided to help reduce electrical noise. Braiding the wires is thought to reduce the magnetic flux within them (Stecker and Patterson, 1996). Note that the electrode wires for both the disposable and reusable electrodes in **Fig. 20.4** have been braided together. If all of the above have been considered, and the recording still appears too noisy, the gain can be adjusted.

When the patient is properly prepped and relaxed, and all sources of biologic and electronic noise have been sufficiently reduced, data collection begins. A few tips for the novice clinician regarding data collection are summarized in **Table 20.3.** Of utmost importance is ensuring patient safety by following some simple rules with respect to electrical safety. Common sense dictates that food and drink should not be anywhere near the test equipment. Make sure that the equipment is properly grounded; most clinical systems will have their own isolation transformer. If for any reason the equipment/software malfunctions during testing, and it is necessary to reboot the system, the clinician should unplug electrodes and disconnect the patient before turning the system off and on (Netherton, Stecker, and Patterson, 2007).

Table 20.3 Consideration for Data Collection

- Except in the case of a very well-defined waveform at relatively high stimulus intensity, always replicate waveforms when performing a latency-intensity function (threshold search). For infants, it is sometimes necessary to record three waveforms to see proper repeatability.
- Develop a plan ahead of the test session to minimize down time between the end of one waveform recording and the beginning of the next.
- Mark waveform components during the test session when possible.
- During extended test sessions, periodically recheck impedances. Make adjustments and reapply electrodes if impedances spike.
- If the waveform becomes noisy because of patient movement, the recording can be paused until the patient quiets down rather than having to stop and restart again.
- Use common sense with respect to electrical safety issues.

♦ After the Test Session

Once you have obtained all the data you desire, or the patient can no longer maintain the desired state, and testing is over, the first order of business is to remove earphones and electrodes and clean off the remaining electrode paste/gel from the patient's skin. Keep in mind that the chance of skin irritation from conductive paste/gel increases with increased time the skin remains in contact with the substance. Some clinicians will use alcohol pads to remove the remaining gel/paste, although alcohol has a drying effect on the skin and may sting if there are small abrasions as a result of preparation with abrasive materials. Instead, a moistened gauze pad will often do the trick. Another handy removal agent is a premoistened cleaning cloth (e.g., baby wipes), which is far less irritating to the skin than an alcohol pad. Adult clients will probably appreciate a handheld mirror to ensure complete removal of conductive material before leaving the testing room.

The report write-up for an electrophysiologic test session is often much more complex than that of a typical hearing evaluation. The clinician should not feel obligated to have a thorough analysis of all data collected for dissemination of results on completion of the test. Because of the sensitive nature and clinical responsibility of counseling patients based on test results, you will want to have a complete analysis before providing results. This is of particular concern when a hearing loss is initially identified. It is acceptable and often preferable to inform the patient that time needs to be given to analyzing the waveforms collected and that a report will be written and sent to the referral source to explain and summarize the findings (see Chapter 21 for information regarding clinical report writing). Verify with the patient that consent has been given and information is provided in the chart for any additional individuals whom he or she would like the report sent to, including the patient. Of course, if the results are simple and unquestionably within normal limits, it is advisable to share this information with the patient and/or parents to put their minds at ease.

The last remaining task is the care and cleaning of everything that came into contact with the patient, including the chair/bed, transducers (earphones), and electrodes. If a recliner was used, depending on the upholstery material, the chair can be sprayed directly and wiped down with disinfectant after each use. If the chair/bed is upholstered such that spray cannot be used, a disposable drape over the chair back or pillowcase can be used and changed between patients. Foam inserts for insert earphones should be thrown away, and supra-aural earphones should be wiped with disinfectant cloths. Disposable electrodes can be thrown away, but care of reusable electrodes is especially important to help prolong their lifetime.

Special Consideration

When removing the foam insert ear tip, take care not to remove the plastic connector piece that connects the tip to the insert earphone tubing. Because this connector is so small and often fits snugly over the foam tip, student clinicians are especially prone to making this mistake. If the connector is inadvertently thrown away, the clinician will be unable to connect the foam tip to the tubing for the next patient.

Reusable electrodes should be cleaned as soon as possible following the test session; otherwise, electrode paste will begin to harden and adhere to the electrodes. To clean electrodes, simply use soap and water. A toothbrush is a good tool to use to scrub off any remaining paste/gel residue. If paste does harden before cleaning can occur, the toothbrush may not get paste out of the hole in the center of some disk electrodes. I have found that the blunt wooden end of cotton-tipped applicators is just the right size to pop out any hardened paste within this area. Once the electrodes are cleaned, dry them with paper toweling and hang them up somewhere safe. To disinfect electrodes between uses, soak them in a mild disinfecting liquid, but be careful not to leave electrodes soaking for prolonged periods (e.g., overnight) to maximize electrode use.

◆ Summary

This chapter contains information to aid the novice clinician in preparing for a successful electrophysiologic test session. Being prepared is half the battle; the clinician needs to account for problems that may arise during a less than optimal testing environment to have the most successful test session possible. Providing patients with information, doing an extensive chart review, preparing supplies and protocols ahead of time, and orienting patients of the procedures will do wonders to facilitate success. Having a complete understanding of what is being done, how it may affect the patient physically and emotionally, and how to best address patient concerns is important. Skills associated with electrode application and data collection procedures will come with practice and increased experience.

References

American Speech-Language-Hearing Association. (1992). *Sedation and topical anesthetics in audiology and speech-language pathology* [technical report]. Retrieved from www.asha.org/policy

American Speech-Language-Hearing Association. (2003). *Guidelines for competencies in auditory evoked potential measurement and clinical applications* [knowledge and skills]. Retrieved from www.asha.org/policy

Guillod, J. F., Hauser, C., Rufficux, P., Masouyé, I., & Harms, M. (2002). Skin injury after electroencephalography. *Archives of Dermatology, 138*(3), 405–410. PubMed

Mancuso, G., Tosti, A., Fanti, P. A., Berdondini, R. M., Mongiorgi, R., & Morandi, A. (1990). Cutaneous necrosis and calcinosis following electroencephalography. *Dermatologica, 181*(4), 324–326. PubMed

Netherton, B. L., Stecker, M. M., & Patterson, T. (2007). Mechanisms of electrode induced injury: 3. Practical concepts and avoidance. *American Journal of Electroneurodiagnostic Technology, 47*(4), 257–263. PubMed

Puig, L., Rocamora, V., Romaní, J., Saavedra, M., & Alomar, A. (1998). Calcinosis cutis following calcium chloride electrode paste application for auditory-brainstem evoked potentials recording. *Pediatric Dermatology, 15*(1), 27–30. PubMed

Schoenfeld, R. J., Grekin, J. N., & Mehregan, A. (1965). Calcium deposition in the skin: A report of four cases following electroencephalography. *Neurology, 15,* 477–480. PubMed

Stecker, M. M., & Patterson, T. (1996). Strategies for minimizing 60 Hz pickup during evoked potential recording. *Electroencephalography and Clinical Neurophysiology, 100*(4), 370–373. PubMed

Wiley, H. E., III, & Eaglstein, W. E. (1979). Calcinosis cutis in children following electroencephalography. *Journal of the American Medical Association, 242*(5), 455–456. PubMed

Zurbuchen, P., LeCoultre, C., Calza, A. M., & Halpérin, D. (1996). Cutaneous necrosis after contact with calcium chloride: a mistaken diagnosis of child abuse. *Pediatrics, 97*(2), 257–258. PubMed

Chapter 21

Clinical Report Writing

Marni Johnson Martin and Rebecca S. Atcherson

For an audiologist, effective oral and written communication skills are important factors in demonstrating one's professional competence to patients and their families, referral sources, and other professionals. Communication of test results and recommendations will occur primarily in the form of written reports; therefore, report writing should be considered a critical part of the evaluation process. This chapter provides an overview of clinical report writing as it relates to auditory electrophysiology, including the roles and responsibilities of audiologists in clinical writing, the importance of proper documentation, the purpose of clinical writing, and key aspects of the auditory electrophysiology evaluation report. In addition, sample reports are provided to assist readers in developing their own written auditory electrophysiology reports.

◆ Roles and Responsibilities of Audiologists in Clinical Writing

Like other health care providers, audiologists are required by legal and professional ethical standards to document pertinent information related to patient care. Audiology certification standards, scope of practice, and code of ethics documents address communication, documentation, and maintenance of records

(American Speech-Language-Hearing Association [ASHA], 2004, 2010; Council for Clinical Certification in Audiology and Speech-Language Pathology of the American Speech-Language-Hearing Association, 2007). In addition, the ASHA *Guidelines for Competencies in Auditory Evoked Potential (AEP) Measurement and Clinical Applications* (2003) explicitly state that audiologists performing auditory evoked potential (AEP) evaluations must be competent in data analysis, interpretation, and reporting of test results. The AEP report should include information regarding the purpose of the testing; procedural and patient influences on the testing, findings, limitations in the data collected; circumstances of the recordings; and any technical problems encountered during the testing. The guidelines also state that audiologists involved in AEP measurement should be able to organize and communicate results and identify the need for follow-up evaluations, referrals, and (re)habilitation (American Speech-Language-Hearing Association, 2003).

Special Consideration

It is extremely important that audiologists and audiology graduate students make a concerted effort in documenting their clinical encounters, test results, and recommendations and in maintaining patient records.

◆ The Importance of Proper Documentation

An individual's health care record, medical chart, or patient file chronicles his or her medical history, including procedures performed, services rendered, test and treatment outcomes, and follow-up planning. It is a permanent legal record of patient contact that serves as the primary means of communication between professionals. The health care record may be used in quality assessment reviews by accrediting bodies, including the Joint Commission on Accreditation of Healthcare Organizations (JCAHO), the Commission on Accreditation of Rehabilitation Facilities (CARF), the National Committee on Quality Assurance (NCQA), and the Council on Academic Accreditation in Audiology and Speech-Language Pathology (CAA), as well as by other local, state, and federal oversight entities (Scott, 2006). Reviewing a patient's health care record is the only reliable way to accurately recall previous procedures or services, test results, and recommendations.

It is unrealistic to think that the clinician will be able to remember every detail about every patient he or she has ever evaluated or treated over the course of his or her career; therefore, proper documentation of each patient encounter is necessary. Documentation serves as the basis for planning treatment and ensuring continuity of care, provides justification of the "medical necessity" criteria, helps protect against professional liability claims, and assists in the procurement of reimbursement from third-party payers (American Academy of Audiology, Coding, and Practice Management Committee, 2006; Scott, 2006). Therefore, it is important to remember that proper documentation of patient care is as important as the diagnosis and treatment itself; it is part of patient management. Federal changes to health care and electronic medical records, as well as computer-based files, will affect how we document patient care and clinical encounters in the future; however, one thing will not change: If it isn't documented, it didn't happen (e.g., American Academy of Audiology, Coding, and Practice Management Committee, 2006; Scott, 2006).

◆ Purpose of Clinical Writing

Writing is a skill that audiologists and audiology graduate students should not take lightly. Writing itself is a process, not a product, that develops over time; therefore, practice and experience will aid in the development of effective clinical writing skills. There is no one way to successfully convey test results and recommendations. Every patient is unique and has his or her own story to tell. As a result, templates and checklists may not be the best way to report findings. Stach (1998) said that the primary purpose of clinical report writing is to communicate results to the referral source. It is important to remember, however, that reports differ depending on the intended recipients. Patients, family members, physicians, educators, and other professionals will all be reading the report from a unique perspective with different expectations. In fact, expectations of the reader should dictate to some extent the focus, format, style, and content of the report (Gonzenbach, 2000).

Regardless of the audience, written reports need to accurately depict the patient's story. Factual information, observations, test results, and recommendations should all be presented in a clear, concise, and consistent manner (Stach, 1998). Written reports should contain only information that is relevant to the case at hand. Providing additional irrelevant information is not necessary and is often distracting to the reader. As a general rule, written reports should be patient focused and summarize evaluation outcomes and recommendations rather than emphasize details of the evaluation process or nature of the testing (i.e., test focused) (Zapala, 2008).

Methods of Documentation

In audiology, the two primary methods of documentation are SOAP note writing and report writing. SOAP note writing consists of four elements: subjective information (S), objective information (O), the assessment of the clinical encounter (A), and the treatment or management plan (P). Subjective information includes the patient's primary presenting complaints or symptoms; medical, otologic, and audiological history; and reason for the patient's visit. Relevant observations about the patient and his or her family may also be included in this section. Objective information describes the tests, procedures, or services performed together with their findings. However, conclusions drawn from outcomes of such tests, procedures, or services are not included in the objective section. The assessment portion of a SOAP note is where data obtained from the subjective and objective sections are synthesized to formulate a conclusion (e.g., diagnosis). The assessment is data driven; therefore, the same assessment should be reached by different audiologists if given the same subjective and objective information (Gonzenbach, 2000). Finally, the plan includes recommendations regarding the next steps in the management of the patient. This may include, but is not limited to, recommendation for further testing, follow-up, or referral. Zapala (2008) recommends reading the SOAP note in reverse order to check for completeness of documentation. The outcome of the clinical encounter should relate back to the plan, the plan should relate back to the assessment, and the assessment should always relate back to the subjective and objective findings. SOAP note writing may include the use of professional abbreviations and jargon as it is typically intended to be read by a colleague or other professional familiar with the terminology used. Case 1 is an example of a SOAP note for an auditory brainstem response (ABR) evaluation.

Diagnostic report writing is routinely used to describe the results of comprehensive assessments, including hearing, auditory processing disorder (APD), vestibular, and auditory electrophysiology evaluations. Diagnostic reports are frequently written in narrative form and tell the patient's story by describing relevant case history information, objective tests results, the audiologist's assessment of such findings, and resulting recommendations. The information included in the case history section of a diagnostic report is similar to the subjective portion of a SOAP note, and the information included in the results section is similar to the objective portion of the SOAP. The summary and impressions section of a written report is essentially the assessment portion of the SOAP note; however,

more detail is likely to be provided in the written report, particularly if the recipient of the report is someone unfamiliar with the tests performed and outcomes of such test measures. The recommendation section of the written report can be thought of as the plan portion of the SOAP note. It is not uncommon for diagnostic reports to be written in letter format and addressed to the intended recipient of the report, most frequently the referral source. Case 2 is an example of an ABR report written in letter format.

◆ The Auditory Electrophysiology Evaluation Report

Auditory electrophysiologic measures use complex testing equipment and require advanced skill in the administration and interpretation of such tests. As a result, audiologists and audiology graduate students have a tendency to overreport details of the evaluation process and nature of the testing (Stach, 1998). Auditory electrophysiology evaluation reports should be written in the same manner as any other audiology evaluation report, with emphasis on the outcome of the testing and recommendations made. Detailed information about the testing itself should be provided as supplemental documentation, rather than within the written report, to those who may be interested and likely to read the information. For example, copies of waveforms, test parameters, and latency values may be valuable to other audiologists or other professionals well versed in electrophysiologic testing.

Hood (1998) recommends that ABR reports be limited to a one-page summary of results. However, there is no ideal length for an auditory electrophysiology evaluation report. The length and amount of detail provided will depend on the purpose and recipient of the report. For example, someone working in a busy ear, nose, and throat (ENT) practice writing ABR reports primarily for other audiologists or ENTs will likely include technical details about test parameters and the nature of the testing, whereas someone working at a children's hospital writing reports for parents, primary care physicians, and educators will try to avoid technical, professional jargon, as it can be distracting or intimidating to the reader. From our experience, most recipients of written reports are interested in knowing what we did, what the results were, and where they go from here (i.e., what is the plan?). So above all else, know your audience and write your reports to suit their needs.

A framework for writing auditory electrophysiology evaluation reports is described in the following sections. Patient-specific reports are recommended; therefore, readers should be cautioned regarding the use of templates. It is best to create custom templates based on one's experience, employment setting, and patient population served.

Identification

A patient's personal identifying information, including his or her name, date of birth, gender, patient identifying (file) number, address, and phone number, should be included near the top of every report. Age is an extremely important variable when evaluating normative data; therefore, it is recommended that patient age in infants should be reported in weeks of conceptional age (CA), rather than gestational or chronologic age, until 60 weeks CA. Age in children should be reported in months until 36 months of age. After 36 months, age should be reported in years (American Clinical Neurophysiology Society [ACNS], 2006a,b; Newman-Ryan, 2001). As with age, gender may be an important factor in some normative studies related to auditory electrophysiology (ACNS, 2006b).

Information regarding the referral source (name and contact), evaluator (name and credentials, including degree, licensure, and certification), testing facility (name, address, and phone number), and evaluation date should always be included in the report. The test time and test or procedure numbers are not typically mentioned in hearing evaluation reports; however, this information may be useful to include on auditory electrophysiology evaluation reports (ACNS, 2006a,b; Newman-Ryan, 2001). Identifying information is typically included near the top of the report or within the letterhead (facility information).

History and Observations

This section of the written report should describe relevant background information related to the case, including a statement regarding the clinical question being investigated (ACNS, 2006b; Newman-Ryan, 2001). An overview of the patient's pertinent medical history, including current medications, is important to report, particularly if the patient is taking a sedative, hypnotic drug, or any medication that affects the nervous system. The patient's audiological history is also important to document, especially if a factor such as hearing sensitivity or middle ear status could affect the present testing. Keep in mind, however, that it is not necessary to provide a detailed explanation of the patient's medical, otologic, and audiological history if it is irrelevant to the current evaluation. Additional case history information will be located in the patient's health care record and can be accessed as needed by following the appropriate protocol (refer to your facilities' Health Insurance Portability and Accountability Act [HIPAA] guidelines).

Observations related to the clinical question being investigated are very useful to provide in the report, as they help to paint a clear picture of the overall clinical case. For example, a parent reports that his or her child exhibits no observable response to sound; however, prior to performing an ABR, you observe that the child elicits a robust startle response when you clap your hands. In this situation, your clinical observation is certainly worth noting. It is important to document the patient's behavior, particularly if it may affect the reliability of the testing (e.g., activity level or state of arousal). Body temperature should also be reported when testing sedated patients (ACNS, 2006b; Newman-Ryan, 2001).

Electrophysiology Evaluation Results

Technical data, including information related to the test conditions and environment, collection parameters, and stimulus parameters affecting test interpretation, as well as a description of the test findings, should be specified in the results section of the electrophysiology evaluation report (ACNS, 2006a,b; Ferraro, Durrant, Sininger, and Campbell,

1996; Newman-Ryan, 2001). However, more or less detail should be made available depending on the intended recipient of the report. For example, a parent will require very few if any technical details, whereas another audiologist or ENT well versed in the test measures may be interested in specifics about attainment of the test results.

Testing conditions and environment refer to how and where the testing was conducted. Was the testing performed in a quiet room, in a sound booth, at the patient's bedside while he or she rested quietly, or in the neonatal intensive care unit (NICU) with an abundance of equipment running and nursing staff or other medical personnel moving around the room? These conditions are all different from one another and may dramatically affect the testing. Collection parameters refer to the type of electrodes and electrode montage (e.g., active and reference) used in addition to the recording (filter settings, time window, and number of averages) setup. Rather than describe all of the collection parameters used in the narrative report, the option to print specific protocol information is available with most auditory electrophysiology equipment. This information can be provided as supplemental material to those interested. Stimulus parameters refer to the transducer used, type of stimuli (e.g., click or tone burst), stimulus polarity stimulus, presentation rate, stimulus intensity level, output (e.g., unilateral or bilateral), and masking, if used. Stimulus parameters should be described in narrative reports; however, they will print together with the collection parameters on most equipment. In addition to documenting the preceding test conditions and environment, collection parameters, and stimulus parameters, it is essential to report any change made in the standard test procedure or protocol, especially if it could potentially affect interpretation of the test results (ACNS, 2006b; Newman-Ryan, 2001).

Reported results should include absolute, interpeak (or interwave), and interaural latency and amplitude values. When reporting amplitude, mode of measurement (e.g., peak to following trough or preceding trough to peak, ACNS, 2006b; Newman-Ryan, 2001), waveform morphology or overall quality of the AEP, and reproducibility should be reported.

Remember the following caveat: *If you are unable to replicate, you must investigate.* Finally, it is important to note the normative data used when interpreting the results. This allows the recipient of the report to form his or her own impressions of the results obtained (ACNS, 2006b; Newman-Ryan, 2001).

Pearl

Copies of marked waveforms, latency and amplitude values, and latency-intensity functions are very useful to enclose with the written report, particularly when sending to a colleague.

Summary and Impressions

The summary and impression section of the report should include the examiner's interpretation of the evaluation. It is basically the "so what" of the testing. All too often audiology graduate students simply restate the test results. This is not the purpose of the summary and impression section, nor is it helpful to the reader. The reader should be able to obtain the examiner's professional opinion as to the normality or abnormality of the evaluation by reading this section of the report (ACNS, 2006b; Newman-Ryan, 2001). Unusual or unclear findings should always be explained. As is the case with all audiological measures, limitations of AEP testing exist and should always be reported to assist the reader in understanding the examiner's impression of the test results.

Readers are looking for an honest interpretation of the test results even if the clinical significance of such findings is unknown. It is important to keep in mind that when interpreting AEPs, sometimes a particular finding can mean different things in different clinical situations. It should be noted in the report that test results are consistent with a possible site of dysfunction; they are not diagnostic in and of themselves. Accurate interpretation requires the examiner to consider every piece of the patient's overall clinical puzzle. The patient's presenting complaints, symptoms, case history, and clinical observations need to be explained, together with the results, to fully describe the possible site of dysfunction and potential neurophysiologic cause of any presenting abnormalities (ACNS, 2006b; Newman-Ryan, 2001).

Recommendations

The summary and impressions of the report should segue into the recommendations. Upon reaching the recommendations section, the reader should have a general understanding of the overall case, as the reader has already been updated on the patient's history, test results, and interpretation of those results. At this point, the reader is interested in answering the question, Where do we go from here? The recommendations should provide the reader with the course of action or plan following the evaluation process. Recommendations should be patient specific and directly address the areas of concern. For example, recommendations may include the need for reevaluation or periodic monitoring following medical management of the disorder to confirm current findings. They may also include the need for additional electrophysiologic testing and imaging studies to further assess the brainstem and central auditory pathways. Finally, the need for otologic follow-up to examine the possibility of retrocochlear involvement may be recommended. Regardless of the recommendations made, the rationale behind each should be provided.

Sample Reports

The following sample reports illustrate the concepts discussed herein; they are not meant to be used as templates, as there really is no such thing as a "standard" patient. As previously mentioned, every patient has his or her own story to tell; therefore, the written report should reflect the specifics of the case.

Case 1 is a sample SOAP note for a neurodiagnostic ABR evaluation. Cases 2, 3, and 4 are sample pediatric ABR reports for the purpose of estimating hearing sensitivity. Cases 5 and 6 are sample adult ABR reports for the purpose of assessing neurologic integrity of the auditory system. Case 7 is a sample CAPD electrophysiology evaluation report, and Case 8 is a sample vestibular evoked myogenic potential (VEMP) report.

♦ Summary

Proper documentation of patient care is as important as the diagnosis and treatment itself. Therefore, audiologists should make considerable effort to formulate their written reports. Remember that although there is no one way to successfully convey test results and recommendations, written reports should be patient focused; presented in a clear, concise, and consistent manner; and contain only relevant information. It is more important to summarize evaluation outcomes and recommendations than to emphasize details of the evaluation process or nature of the testing itself.

> **Case 1   SOAP Note for an ABR Evaluation**
>
> **Name:** John Doe
> **DOB:** 6/25/1971
> **Date of Evaluation:** 5/1/2010
> **Patient File Number:** 11111
> **Type of Evaluation:** ABR
>
> **S:** Mr. Doe is a 38-year-old man who reported experiencing sudden hearing loss in his left ear accompanied by tinnitus and aural fullness, which began approximately 3 weeks ago. Hearing test results performed 1 week ago revealed hearing WNL (within normal limits) in the right ear with a moderate to moderately-severe SNHL (sensorineural hearing loss) in the left ear. Asymmetrical word recognition was obtained, with left ear worse than right. Significant occupational and recreational noise exposure was noted. Additional history is unremarkable at this time.
>
> **O:** ABR testing was conducted using rarefaction click stimuli presented at a rate of 11.1/s through insert earphones at 90 dB nHL (normal hearing level) in both ears. Right ear test results revealed identifiable and repeatable waves I, III, and V with absolute and interpeak latencies WNL. Waveform morphology was excellent. Left ear test results revealed the presence of wave I only. Waves III and V were not identifiable in the left ear.
>
> **A:** Normal right ear ABR; abnormal left ear ABR. Findings are suggestive of possible retrocochlear pathology in the left ear.
>
> **P:** Medical follow-up with ENT including imaging studies is recommended to rule out left retrocochlear pathology.
>
> _____
>
> Evaluator Signature and Credentials

Case 2 Pediatric Report in Letter Format: Normal ABR Consistent with Normal Hearing Sensitivity

March 1, 2010
Re: Johnny Smith
DOB: 1/1/2006
Patient #: 12345

Dear Dr. Jones,

I had the pleasure of seeing Johnny today for Auditory Brainstem Response (ABR) testing to assess his auditory system. The results suggest normal hearing sensitivity bilaterally, and I have recommended annual hearing evaluations.

Background

Johnny has Down syndrome and has been followed by our clinic in conjunction with the Ear Nose and Throat Clinic since birth. He passed his newborn hearing screening as well as several subsequent otoacoustic emission (OAE) screenings. We have seen him for several evaluations; however, he typically does not respond consistently to sound in the test booth. While this is not uncommon for children with developmental delays, at his last appointment an ABR evaluation was recommended to obtain a more complete hearing assessment. Today, Mrs. Smith reported that although she does not have concerns about Johnny's hearing, she is interested in obtaining the ABR due to the number of incomplete hearing evaluations previously attempted and the risk of hearing loss associated with Down syndrome.

Current Evaluation Results

Johnny no longer has PE (pressure equalization) tubes, and his ears were noted to be clear and healthy by Dr. Anderson in ENT Clinic today. Behavioral hearing testing was attempted. Mrs. Smith reported that Johnny responded better than during previous evaluations; however, his responses were still elevated above normal, and ear-specific information was unable to be obtained. Johnny fell asleep prior to the scheduled testing, so fortunately we were able to complete the ABR without sedation today. ABR testing was conducted using rarefaction click stimuli presented at a rate of 31.1/s through insert earphones. Repeatable responses were obtained from 70 dB nHL down to 15 dB nHL bilaterally. Absolute and interpeak latencies of waves I, III, and V were well within normal limits bilaterally, with excellent waveform morphology. Presence of the cochlear microphonic was verified using condensation polarity clicks at 70 dB nHL. These results are consistent with essentially normal transmission of auditory stimuli through the brainstem auditory pathways. In addition, ABR thresholds were measured through identification of wave V in response to 500-Hz tone bursts (low-frequency), 2000-Hz tone bursts (mid-frequency), and 4000-Hz tone bursts (high-frequency). Thresholds were at least 20 dB nHL or better for all frequencies in both ears, which is a normal result and better than Johnny's behavioral responses.

Summary and Impressions

Although an ABR is not a direct test of hearing sensitivity per se, test results are consistent with normal hearing bilaterally.

Continued

Recommendations

1. Annual hearing evaluations to monitor Johnny's hearing and middle ear status.

It is a pleasure to be included in Johnny's care. Please feel free to contact me with questions or concerns at 123–456–7890

Sincerely,
Jane Doe, Au.D.
Audiologist

Case 3 Pediatric Report: ABR Consistent with Conductive Hearing Loss

ELECTROPHYSIOLOGY EVALUATION REPORT
Name: Jack Smith
Date of Birth: 1/1/2010
Address: 225 Anywhere Drive
Anycity, Anystate 12345
Date of Evaluation: 4/1/2010
Referral Source: Dr. Olson, Pediatrician
Phone: (202) 234–1234
Patient File Number: 22225
Evaluator: Jane Doe, Au.D.

History and Observations

Jack was seen today for an auditory brainstem response (ABR) evaluation due to three failed newborn hearing screenings. Today, Mrs. Smith reported concerns about Jack's hearing, stating that he doesn't seem to respond consistently to sound. A normal pregnancy and birth were reported. Jack was slightly jaundiced at birth; however, no treatment was necessary. According to Mrs. Smith, Jack is not taking any medications at this time and is overall a healthy baby. Additional case history is unremarkable at this time.

Results

Prior to ABR testing, otoscopic examination and immittance testing were performed. Otoscopic examination revealed clear ear canals bilaterally; however, tympanic membranes and landmarks could not be fully visualized in either ear. High-frequency (1000 Hz) tympanometry revealed Jerger type B tympanograms in both ears, suggestive of possible middle ear pathology in both ears.

ABR testing was conducted using rarefaction click stimuli presented at a rate of 31.1/s through insert transducers. Jack slept quietly in his mother's arms during the testing. Wave V was identifiable bilaterally. Waveform morphology was good. Repeatable responses were obtained down to 50 dB nHL bilaterally. Additional testing was conducted using 500-Hz (low frequency) and 4000-Hz (high-frequency) tone bursts. Repeatable responses were obtained down to 65 dB nHL in both ears. Absolute latencies of waves I, III, and V were delayed in both ears; however, interpeak latencies were within normal limits based on Boys Town normative data for infants. Responses to bone-conducted click stimuli with masking presented to the nontest ear were obtained at 15 dB nHL in both ears. Copies of marked waveforms, including absolute and interpeak latencies, as well as waveform amplitudes, are enclosed.

Summary and Impressions

Although the ABR is not a direct test of hearing sensitivity, today's test results are consistent with a moderate hearing loss in both ears. Normal ABR responses to bone-conducted click stimuli together with abnormal tympanometric findings suggest that the hearing loss is conductive in nature.

Continued

Recommendations

Results from today's evaluation were discussed with Mrs. Smith, and the following recommendations were made:

1. Jack should seek medical follow-up with an ENT physician for the abnormal middle ear function and conductive hearing loss identified bilaterally.

2. Hearing reevaluation should be performed post medical management.

Please do not hesitate to contact me with any questions or concerns.

_____

Jane Doe, Au.D.
Clinical Audiologist

Case 4 Pediatric Report: ABR Consistent with Sensorineural Hearing Loss

ELECTROPHYSIOLOGY EVALUATION REPORT

Name: Jenny Jones
Date of Birth: 9/5/2009
Address: 123 Anywhere Drive
Anycity, Anystate 12345
Date of Evaluation: 10/24/2009
Referral Source: Dr. Olson, Pediatrician
Phone: (303) 321–4321
Patient File Number: 11122
Evaluator: Jane Doe, Au.D.

History and Observations

Jenny Jones was seen today for an auditory brainstem response (ABR) evaluation to confirm the bilateral hearing loss detected during her newborn hearing screening and diagnosed via ABR testing completed at Primary Children's Hospital in Anycity, AS, on 10/2/2009. ABR testing revealed a moderate to severe bilateral sensorineural hearing loss across all frequencies tested. Mrs. Jones reported a normal pregnancy and birth. There is no known family history of hearing loss. Additional history is unremarkable.

Results

Prior to ABR testing, otoscopic examination, immittance testing, and distortion product otoacoustic emissions (DPOAEs) were performed. Otoscopic examination revealed clear ear canals with normal-appearing tympanic membranes and landmarks bilaterally. High-frequency (1000-Hz) tympanometry was performed. Tracings were obtained that are consistent with normal middle ear function in both ears. However, it should be noted that normal tympanometric findings obtained in infants can sometimes be due to external auditory canal elasticity rather than to tympanic membrane compliance. Therefore, in infants, normal tympanograms do not always reflect normal middle ear function. DPOAEs were absent in both ears.

ABR testing was conducted using rarefaction click stimuli presented at a rate of 31.1/s through insert transducers. Jenny slept quietly in her mother's arms during the testing. Wave V was identifiable bilaterally. Waveform morphology was good. Repeatable responses were obtained down to 80 dB nHL in both ears, with absolute and interpeak latencies within normal limits for age. Additional testing was conducted using 500-Hz tone bursts. Repeatable responses were obtained down to 70 dB nHL in both ears. Additionally, no response was present for bone-conducted click stimuli in either ear at the limits of the equipment (50 dB). These results are consistent with a moderate to severe sensorineural hearing loss bilaterally. Copies of marked waveforms, including absolute and interpeak latencies, as well as waveform amplitudes, are enclosed.

Summary and Impressions

Although the ABR is not a direct test of hearing sensitivity, today's test results are suggestive of a moderate to severe sensorineural hearing loss bilaterally. These results are consistent with previous testing performed at Primary Children's Hospital in Anycity, AS.

Continued

Recommendations

1. Comprehensive otologic follow-up to determine the possible cause of Jenny's hearing loss.

2. Mrs. Jones expressed an interest in pursuing hearing aids for Jenny, so we will begin the hearing aid fitting process as soon as medical clearance is obtained and hearing aids, and ear molds can be ordered. Mrs. Jones reported that it is much more convenient for her to obtain hearing aids and follow-up at our clinic as Primary Children's Hospital is a 2-hour commute for her.

3. Jenny should undergo behavioral testing in 3 to 6 months to gain further information regarding her hearing sensitivity.

If further information or assistance is needed, please do not hesitate to contact me.

_____

Jane Doe, Au.D.
Clinical Audiologist

Case 5   Adult Report: ABR Consistent with High-Frequency Sensorineural Hearing Loss

ELECTROPHYSIOLOGY EVALUATION REPORT

Name: George Smith
Date of Birth: 7/15/1950
Address: 335 Anywhere Drive
Anycity, Anystate 12345
Date of Evaluation: 6/1/2010
Referral Source: Dr. Jacobs, PCP
Phone: (404) 432–4321
Patient File Number: 22222
Evaluator: Jane Doe, Au.D.

History and Observations

Mr. Smith was seen at the Speech and Hearing Center today for an auditory brainstem response (ABR) evaluation to further explore hearing test results that suggested a slight asymmetry between ears (left worse than right). Mr. Smith has normal low-frequency hearing, which gradually slopes to a moderately severe sensorineural hearing loss in the high frequencies bilaterally. Mr. Smith reported a history of noise exposure as a farmer and right-handed hunter. Mr. Smith reported experiencing tinnitus in both ears, with his left ear significantly worse than his right. He reported no problems with dizziness, ear pain, ear infections, or aural fullness. Mr. Smith's medical and audiological histories are otherwise unremarkable. Additional information regarding Mr. Smith's history may be obtained from the audiological evaluation report dated 5/14/10. Today's testing was undertaken to rule out retrocochlear pathology as a contributing factor to Mr. Smith's hearing loss.

Results

Prior to ABR testing, otoscopic examination, immittance testing, and distortion product otoacoustic emissions (DPOAEs) were performed. Otoscopic examination revealed clear ear canals with normal-appearing tympanic membranes and landmarks bilaterally. Immittance testing revealed findings consistent with normal middle ear function in both ears. Normal tympanograms were obtained, and ipsilateral and contralateral reflexes were obtained at elevated levels in the mid and high frequencies, which is consistent with a high-frequency hearing loss. Additionally, DPOAEs were absent in both ears in the mid and high frequencies, consistent with abnormal cochlear function bilaterally.

ABR testing was conducted using rarefaction click stimuli presented at a rate of 11.1/s, 31.1/s, and 61.1/s through insert earphones at an intensity level of 90 dB nHL in both ears. Testing revealed repeatable responses with good waveform morphology at 70 dB nHL and 90 dB nHL in both ears. At 70 dB nHL, waves III and V were identifiable bilaterally. At 90 dB nHL, waves I, III, and V were identifiable bilaterally. Absolute latencies of waves I, III, and V were slightly elevated bilaterally; however, interaural latencies are within normal limits. Interpeak latencies for waves I–III, III–V, and I–V were also within the normal range bilaterally. The degree of latency shift observed with rapid stimulus rate (61.1/s) was within the normal range.

Summary and Impressions

Today's findings indicate transmission of auditory stimuli through the brainstem auditory pathways that is consistent with Mr. Smith's high-frequency sensorineural (cochlear) hearing loss. ABR results do not suggest the presence of retrocochlear pathology. The slight asymmetrical hearing loss noted on the audiogram is likely due to Mr. Smith's history of noise exposure.

Continued

Recommendations

Results from today's evaluation were discussed with Mr. Smith, and the following recommendations were made:

1. Mr. Smith should see an ear, nose, and throat physician (ENT) to obtain medical clearance to further pursue amplification for his hearing loss.

2. Following medical clearance, Mr. Smith should return to the Speech and Hearing Center or to another audiologist for a hearing aid evaluation to discuss amplification options.

3. Mr. Smith should have his hearing monitored annually or earlier if a sudden change in hearing sensitivity or speech understanding is noted.

Please do not hesitate to contact me if further information or assistance is needed. Mr. Smith was a pleasure to work with today.

Jane Doe, Au.D.
Clinical Audiologist

Case 6 Adult Report: ABR Consistent with Retrocochlear Pathology

ELECTROPHYSIOLOGY EVALUATION REPORT

Name: John Jackson
Date of Birth: 6/25/1971
Address: 100 Anywhere Drive
Anycity, Anystate 12345
Date of Evaluation: 2/1/2010
Referral Source: Dr. Jacobs, PCP
Phone: (123) 456–7890
Patient File Number: 23456
Evaluator: John Doe, Au.D.

History and Observations

Mr. John Jackson returned to the Speech and Hearing Center today for auditory brainstem response (ABR) testing. ABR testing was recommended following Mr. Jackson's hearing evaluation dated 1/1/10 to further assess his auditory system, specifically neural synchrony of the brainstem auditory pathways. Test results obtained on 1/1/10 revealed an asymmetrical mild to moderate sensorineural hearing loss, with right ear worse than left. Asymmetical word recognition scores were obtained with the right ear significantly worse (35%) than the left (90%). Normal tympanograms were obtained in both ears. Acoustic reflexes (ipsilateral and contralateral) were obtained at expected levels when the stimulus was presented to the left ear but were absent when the stimulus was presented to the right ear. Distortion product otoacoustic emissions (DPOAEs) were absent in both ears, indicative of abnormal cochlear function. The combination of asymmetrical hearing sensitivity, significantly poorer word recognition abilities, and absent ipsilateral and contralateral acoustic reflexes is suggestive of possible retrocochlear pathology in the right ear. Additional information regarding Mr. Jackson's history may be obtained from the audiological evaluation report dated 1/1/10. Today's testing was undertaken to rule out retrocochlear pathology as a contributing factor to Mr. Jackson's hearing loss.

Electrophysiology Evaluation Results

Otoscopic Examination: Otoscopy revealed clear ear canals with normal-appearing tympanic membranes and landmarks visible in both ears.

Auditory Brainstem Response (ABR): ABR testing was conducted using rarefaction click stimuli presented at a rate of 11.1/s, 31.1/s, and 61.1/s through insert earphones at 90 dB nHL in both ears. Left ear test results revealed identifiable and repeatable waves I, III, and V for all test conditions with absolute and interpeak latencies within normal limits. The degree of latency shift observed with rapid stimulus rates (61.1/s) was within the normal range. Waveform morphology was good. Right ear test results revealed the presence of wave I only. Waves III and V were not identifiable in the right ear for any test condition. Copies of marked waveforms including absolute and interpeak latencies and waveform amplitudes are enclosed.

Summary and Impressions

In the left ear, test results suggest essentially normal time-based transmission of auditory stimuli through the brainstem auditory pathways. Mr. Jackson's hearing loss in the left ear appears to be cochlear in nature owing to the abnormal otoacoustic emissions findings accompanied by present left-ear (stimulus left) acoustic reflexes and good word recognition ability. In the right ear, test results are suggestive of possible retrocochlear pathology in addition to cochlear involvement. Abnormal ABR findings suggest

Continued

abnormal transmission of auditory stimuli through the brainstem auditory pathways. In addition, the asymmetrical word recognition (right ear significantly worse than left) and abnormal right-ear (stimulus right) acoustic reflex results further suggest the presence of retrocochlear pathology in the right ear.

Recommendations

1. Comprehensive otologic follow-up, preferably with a neuro-otologist, is recommended to examine the possibility of a right retrocochlear involvement. Imaging studies are recommended to further assess the brainstem.

John Doe, Au.D.
Clinical Audiologist

Case 7   APD: Electrophysiology Evaluation Report

ELECTROPHYSIOLOGY EVALUATION REPORT

Name: Jane Doe

Date of Birth: 10/15/1987

Address: 123 Anywhere Drive

Anycity, Anystate 12345

Date of Evaluation: 1/1/2010

Referral Source: Speech & Hearing Clinic

Phone: (123) 123–1234

Patient File Number: 12345

Evaluator: John Doe, Au.D.

History

Jane Doe, a 23-year-old woman, was seen at the Speech & Hearing Clinic for an auditory electrophysiology evaluation. She is currently a part-time college student and is experiencing difficulties in the classroom. Prior hearing evaluation results at this clinic revealed normal tympanometry, normal pure tone hearing sensitivity, and excellent word recognition abilities in quiet, bilaterally. Acoustic reflex testing revealed ipsilateral responses within normal limits for the left ear but an elevated response at 2000 Hz and absent response at 4000 Hz for the right ear. Contralateral acoustic reflexes, however, were absent or elevated, bilaterally. The QuickSIN test was conducted and revealed a mild signal-to-noise ratio (SNR) deficit in the right ear. The auditory processing evaluation revealed the following finding:

- Left ear weakness on Competing Words subtest of the *SCAN-3: A* (binaural integration dichotic task)

- Left ear weakness on Competing Sentences subtest of the *SCAN-3:A* (binaural separation dichotic task)

- Difficulty verbally labeling stimuli on the Pitch Pattern Perception test, but no difficulty humming stimuli (temporal ordering task)

Additional case history is significant for chronic childhood ear infections and periodic ear infections throughout her life (which her two sons are also experiencing); high-pitched tinnitus in both ears; ongoing evaluation for possible multiple sclerosis; allergies; sinusitis; migraines; and taking medications Cymbalta, Topomax, Valium, and Zanaflex.

Evaluation and Results

Auditory brainstem response (ABR): Acoustic clicks were presented at 80 dB nHL with stimulation rates of 17.7/s and 57.7/s. Electrode montage was Fz as noninverting and ipsilateral earlobe as reference. Normal waveform morphology with strong appearance of waves I, III, and V, absolute and interwave latencies within normal limits, and excellent repeatability in both ears were recorded, suggesting that auditory nerve and brainstem function appear to be intact. Increasing stimulation rate from 17.7/s to 57.7/s revealed no suggestion of abnormality for either ear. (Note: Ms. Doe reported that stimulation to the right ear was uncomfortable at the chosen intensity level but comfortable for the left ear.)

Middle latency response (MLR): 1000-Hz tone bursts were presented at 60 dB nHL with stimulation rate of 7.1/s. Electrode montage was C3 and C4 with linked earlobes as reference. Waveform morphology and peak-to-peak amplitudes for Waves Na and Pa were examined. No electrode effect

Continued

was observed for either ear of stimulation (i.e., no hemispheric differences in waveform amplitude between C3 and C4 with the same ear of stimulation). However, there was a contra-lateral ear effect in which the left hemisphere response (1.38 µV) to right ear stimulation was smaller than the right hemisphere response (0.78 µV) to left ear stimulation. The corresponding amplitude difference was 77%. An amplitude difference of 50% or more for the ear effect is considered a weak but positive finding for potential brainstem/thalamocortical abnormality.

Late latency response (LLR): 1000-Hz tone bursts were presented at 70 dB nHL with stimulation rate of 1.7/s. Electrode montage was C3 and C4 with linked earlobes as reference. Waves P1, N1, and P2 were examined. Clearly identifiable P1, N1, and P2 were within expected latencies and amplitude for both ears. There was no observable electrode or ear effect suggestive of normal cortical auditory pathway function.

It should be noted that none of these tests are "tests of hearing." Rather, they are tests of neural integrity at various points in the central auditory pathway.

Summary and Impressions

The auditory electrophysiology evaluation revealed normal ABR and LLR recordings. However, the MLR recordings point to a right ear deficit as determined by the significant ear effect when comparing hemispheric activity to contralateral stimulation. An amplitude difference between hemispheres to contralateral stimulation of 50% or more is considered a positive finding for brainstem/thalamocortical abnormality, but a weak one.

Taken together, the results of the auditory processing evaluation and the present evaluation consistently point to a right ear deficit in which the corpus callosum may be involved. This neurological deficit along with reported auditory difficulties may have a multiplicative effect, particularly in acoustically harsh environments (e.g., fast speech rate, reverberant conditions, and background noise). These findings strongly indicate that an auditory processing disorder is present.

Recommendations

As a result of the above findings, the following recommendations are being made:

1. Ms. Doe should consider formal or informal dichotic listening training.

2. Ms. Doe should consider contacting the Disability Services Office on her campus to explore services that might be available to assist her in the classroom. Services of note include preferential seating and permission to use recording devices in the classroom. Trial of an assistive listening device to enhance access to the instructor's voice may be another worthwhile accommodation.

3. Ms. Doe should begin adopting strategies to maximize communication success in her various listening environments, and to advocate for herself to ensure adequate communication access. If Ms. Doe is not currently familiar with communication strategies, clinicians at the Speech & Hearing Clinic are available to assist her.

John Doe, Au.D.
Clinical Audiologist

Case 8   VEMP Report

ELECTROPHYSIOLOGY EVALUATION REPORT
Name: Ima Dizzy
Date of Birth: 6/15/1960
Address: 545 Anywhere Drive
Anycity, Anystate 12345
Date of Evaluation: 5/1/2010
Referral Source: Dr. Jones, ENT
Phone: (987) 654–3210
Patient File Number: 34567
Evaluator: John Doe, Au.D.

History

Mrs. Dizzy was seen for vestibular evoked myogenic potentials (VEMP) testing at the request of Dr. Jones for a history of a right vestibular schwannoma and worsening balance. Additional information regarding Mrs. Dizzy's history may be obtained from previous evaluation reports.

Evaluation and Results

Vestibular evoked myogenic potentials (VEMPs) were measured initially at 95 dB nHL and decreased in 5 dB steps until a response was no longer present. The stimulus was a 500 Hz toneburst. The inverting electrode was place on the belly of the sternocleidomastoid muscle, the reference electrode was placed on the sternum, and the ground electrode was placed on the forehead. Mrs. Dizzy was instructed to lift and turn her head separately to the right and to the left while lying on an examination table.

Latencies

Right Ear:
P1 19.75 msec (2.5 SD limits = 20.53 msec)
N1 27.76 msec (2.5 SD limits = 30.30 msec)
Left Ear:
P1 17.41 msec (2.5 SD limits = 20.53 msec)
N1 28.76 msec (2.5 SD limits = 30.30 msec)

Amplitudes

Right Ear: 91.06 uV
Left Ear: 334.96 uV
Interaural amplitude difference: 57% (>47% = abnormal)

Thresholds

Right Ear: 90 dB nHL
Left Ear: 80 dB nHL
Interaural threshold difference: 10 dB nHL (>10 dB nHL = abnormal)

Continued

Summary

The results of today's VEMP measurements suggest dysfunction of the saccule and/or inferior branch of the vestibular nerve for the right ear as indicated by reduced amplitude and an elevated threshold. The VEMP for the left ear was normal.

Recommendations

1. Referral back to Dr. Jones, ENT, for medical consultation regarding today's findings.

It is a pleasure to be included in Mrs. Dizzy's care. Please feel free to contact me with questions.

———————————————————————————————

John Doe, Au.D.
Clinical Audiologist

References

American Academy of Audiology, Coding, and Practice Management Committee. (2006). *Capturing reimbursement: A guide for audiologists.* Reston, VA: Author.

American Clinical Neurophysiology Society. (2006a). *Guideline 9A: Guidelines on evoked potentials.* Retrieved from http://www.acns.org/pdfs/ACFDFD0.pdf

American Clinical Neurophysiology Society. (2006b). *Guideline 10: Guidelines for writing clinical evoked potential reports.* Retrieved from http://www.acns.org/pdfs/ACFDF29.pdf

American Speech-Language-Hearing Association. (2003). Guidelines for competencies in auditory evoked potential measurement and clinical applications. *ASHA Supplement 23,* 35–40.

American Speech-Language-Hearing Association. (2004). *Scope of practice in audiology.* Retrieved from http://www.asha.org/docs/html/sp2004-00192.html

American Speech-Language-Hearing Association. (2010). *Code of ethics.* Retrieved from http://www.asha.org/docs/html/ET2010-00309.html

Council for Clinical Certification in Audiology and Speech-Language Pathology of the American Speech-Language-Hearing Association. (2007). *2007 standards for the certificate of clinical competence in audiology, revised March 2009.* Retrieved from http://www.asha.org/certification/aud_standards_new.htm

Ferraro, J. A., Durrant, J. D., Sininger, Y. S., & Campbell, K. (1996). Recommended guidelines for reporting AEP specifications. *American Journal of Audiology, 5*(3), 35–37.

Gonzenbach, S. (2000). Preparing the clinical report. In H. Hosford-Dunn, R. J. Roeser, & M. Valente (Eds.), *Audiology: Practice management* (pp. 231–255). New York: Thieme.

Hood, L. J. (1998). *Clinical applications of the auditory brainstem response.* San Diego: Singular Publishing Group.

Newman-Ryan, J. (2001). *Auditory brain stem evoked potentials: Laboratory exercises and clinical manual.* Boston: Allyn & Bacon.</bok>

Scott, R. W. (2006). *Legal aspects of documenting patient care for rehabilitation professionals* (3rd ed.). Sudbury, MA: Jones and Bartlett.

Stach, B. A. (1998). *Clinical audiology: An introduction.* San Diego: Singular Publishing Group.

Zapala, D. A. (2008). Documentation in clinical audiology: An information management perspective. In H. Hosford-Dunn, R. J. Roeser, & M. Valente (Eds.), *Audiology: Practice management* (2nd ed., pp. 195–214). New York: Thieme.

Chapter 22

Stimulation Calibration and Generation

Samuel R. Atcherson

The purpose of this chapter is to present some basic information about how to calibrate stimuli and how to generate them, if necessary, above and beyond the capabilities of a commercial evoked potential system. Whether a person is generating and calibrating custom stimuli or simply calibrating existing stimuli, this important issue ought to be in the minds of all audiologists (and auditory researchers): We need to have a healthy skepticism about the quality of any stimulus, and we must be confident in the intensity levels we intend to use with patients. The reader should be aware that treatment of the topics in this chapter focuses largely on nonresearch evoked potential systems.

◆ Stimuli for Auditory Evoked Potentials

It is to be expected that evoked potential systems from different manufacturers will vary somewhat in terms of what stimuli are available within their recording software. Virtually all evoked potential systems generate click and tone-burst stimuli internally. However, clinicians may have the option of modifying various stimulus parameters, such as duration, rise/fall times, plateau time, and stimulus frequency, as would typically be the case for tone bursts. For evoked potential systems with auditory steady-state response (ASSR) capabilities, clinicians may have the option of modifying certain aspects of the modulated signals. Some evoked potential systems provide clinicians with access to previously generated or special stimulus files whose stimulus parameters have already been predetermined. For example, a variety of synthetic consonant–vowel (CV) speech stimuli, such as /da/, /ba/, and /ga/, may be available for cortical and cognitive potential recordings. A handful of evoked potential systems allow clinicians to generate their own custom stimuli within the software, such as click trains, two-tone complexes, and gated noise bursts, to name a few. Some manufacturers offer proprietary modules using stimulus and recording parameters that have been optimized by collaborating researchers and development teams. Finally, it is rare that relatively newer evoked potential systems do not also offer the ability to import custom stimuli so long as the imported file meets the formatting requirements of that system. Calibration is an important issue regardless of how the stimuli are generated.

◆ Calibration of Acoustic Stimuli

Ensuring that any test equipment is functioning properly should be the highest priority for audiologists to avoid test results that lead to inaccurate diagnosis, poorly generated recommendations, and unnecessary referrals. The calibration of equipment generally refers to the comprehensive evaluation in which test signals are measured against known reference values or some standard. Such calibration often takes place by a technician from a local distributor of audiology equipment, but some audiologists may feel comfortable conducting the calibration themselves, provided that they have the right equipment and resources to do so. Audiologists are quite familiar with the type of calibration when test signals generated by audiometers are checked through various transducers. Not only are test signals checked for the purity of their pure tones (e.g., little to no distortion), but they are also checked across a variety of other variables, such as linearity (levels of attenuation are checked with each dB step size) and rise/fall time of test signals, as well as through a biologic check (i.e., checking with one's own eyes and ears), for any evidence of hardware connection problems, fraying or broken cables, loose dials or buttons, and audible clicks and intermittency in test signals. Test signals used for auditory evoked potential (AEP) testing also require calibration, especially to ensure that the intensity values are meaningful, purposeful, valid, and reliable. For example, if an auditory brainstem response (ABR) wave V is recorded at a threshold of 40 dB, it is generally helpful to know that an intensity level of 40 dB on the monitor screen is 40 dB SL (sensation level) relative to the average behavioral detection threshold achieved by listeners with normal hearing for that particular stimulus. However, recall that just because the behavioral detection threshold may be at 0 dB in young, normal-hearing listeners does not necessarily mean that an evoked potential (e.g., tone burst ABR) will also be recorded at 0 dB (Sininger and Hyde, 2009) (see Chapter 14). In any case, calibration may help a pediatric audiologist in estimating thresholds on the audiogram (with correction factors) for the purpose of generating safe and audible hearing aid levels for an infant using a desired fitting prescription. In another example, calibration may help ensure that tonal or speech stimuli used for a cortical potential recording is adequately intense to achieve a large response, but at the same time does not damage the transducer and is safe for the patient.

The ANSI S3.6 Specification for Audiometers (American National Standards Institute, 2004) standard is one of the most visible standards that we have in our field for the calibration of audiometer signals. Each test tone frequency is usually presented over several seconds and has a specified reference equivalent threshold sound pressure level (RETSPL) that makes it possible to check the output levels using a sound level meter (SLM). For example, the RETSPL for a 500-Hz tone using the ER-3A insert earphone in the HA-1 2cc coupler is 6 dB SPL. When calibrating the 500-Hz tone on an audiometer, the attenuator dial is often set at a much higher level, such as 70 dB HL, to overcome ambient background noise. If the SLM reads 76 dB SPL, then the tone would not require adjustments or a correction factor, because SLM output of 76 dB minus the attenuator dial level of 70 dB equals 6 dB, which is the RETSPL. Unfortunately, ANSI S3.6 (American National Standards Institute, 2004) is insufficient for the calibration of acoustic transients such as clicks (100 µsec or 0.1 msec durations) and tone bursts (<8 msec durations).

Most SLMs usually offer one of two different time-weighting scales, fast (F) or slow (S). The fast setting will integrate a signal greater than 125 msec, whereas the slow setting will integrate a signal over 1000 msec (Yeager and Marsh, 1998). Neither of these time-weighting scales will properly integrate the SPL of an acoustic transient and will ultimately underestimate its value. There is no ANSI standard with RETSPLs for different acoustic transients. Thus, it may sometimes be difficult to make direct comparisons of data from one clinic or laboratory to another. In the absence of an ANSI standard, there are two international standards (see below) that we can use as a guide. Whether acoustic stimuli are long or short, there are several different stimulus intensity references that clinicians may encounter. **Table 22.1** shows stimulus intensity references commonly reported in AEP recordings.

Methods of Stimulus Calibration

There are two commonly used methods of stimulus calibration that a clinician can conduct with AEP stimuli. The first method is called behavioral calibration, which is often used for acoustic transients (e.g., Stapells,

Table 22.1 Commonly Seen Stimulus References Used in Auditory Evoked Potential Recordings

dB Reference	What It Stands For	What It Is and When It Is Used
dB SPL	Sound pressure level	Referenced to 20 µPa for long stimuli as measured with a sound level meter; it is based on an RMS measure over the course of the time-weighting scale
dB pSPL	Peak sound pressure level	Usually the highest measured dB SPL within a 1-s recording window; the dB pSPL for a pure tone is typically 3 dB higher than dB SPL
dB peSPL	Baseline-to-peak equivalent sound pressure level	Referencing peak-to-baseline voltage of a transient stimulus to the peak-to-base voltage of a sinusoidal reference tone using an oscilloscope through a sound level meter
dB ppeSPL	Peak-to-peak equivalent sound pressure level	Referencing peak-to-peak voltage of a transient stimulus to the peak-to-peak voltage of a sinusoidal reference tone using an oscilloscope through a sound level meter
dB HL	Hearing level	Referenced same as dB SPL for long sinusoidal stimuli; however, correction factors are applied based on behavioral RETSPL values (e.g., 0 dB HL vs 6 dB SPL for 500 Hz using ER-3A with HA-1 2 cc coupler)
dB nHL	Normal nearing level	Referenced to average normal hearing group behavioral threshold (i.e., 0 dB nHL) using desired transient stimulus presented through the evoked potential system
dB SL	Sensational level	Referenced either to 0 dB HL or 0 dB nHL, but presented at a specified suprathreshold level (e.g., 40 dB SL)

Abbreviations: RETSPL, reference equivalent threshold sound pressure level; RMS, root mean square.

Picton, and Smith, 1982). In this method, behavioral threshold is determined for each desired stimulus using the evoked potential system and relevant transducers on a group of individuals with audiometrically normal hearing. This means that the evoked potential system is used like an audiometer on as few as 5 to as many as 20 individuals. Granted, the more individuals tested, the greater the precision. Where possible, behavioral calibration should take place in an acoustically shielded sound booth. Thresholds should be obtained using a bracketing procedure. The average threshold for a particular stimulus will become the 0 dB normalized hearing level (nHL) reference irrespective of the intensity level that is on the computer screen or the intensity dial control. That is, 0 dB nHL may not always be 0 dB on the evoked potential system. Thus, if the intensity level of 10 dB on the monitor screen equals 0 dB nHL, then clinicians must subtract 10 dB at every presentation level. Alternatively,

the clinician may have the ability or option to make the correction internally within the software so that 0 dB on the evoked potential system actually equals 0 dB nHL. However, reliance only on behavioral calibration is judged to be less than ideal by many expert clinicians (e.g., Gorga and Neely, 1994; Lightfoot, Sininger, Burkard, and Lodwig, 2007).

Pearl

Clinicians should verify that 0 dB nHL on the computer screen or dial is in fact 0 dB nHL through behavioral or physical calibration, with preference for the latter.

The second method, called physical calibration, involves the use of calibration equipment to check the output levels of various stimuli presented through various transducers (e.g., Richter and Fedtke, 2005). Minimally, the equipment required includes the evoked potential system and its transducers, a signal generator (for producing reference tones), an SLM, appropriate ear couplers (2 cc for insert earphones or 6 cc for supra-aural earphones), and an oscilloscope. A calibrated audiometer could be used as the sound generator. With a high-quality sound card in a desktop or laptop computer, an oscilloscope software program may be a more cost-effective yet viable alternative to achieve comparable results as a desktop oscilloscope. For long-duration stimuli (>200 msec), a simple SPL measure will usually suffice. Burkard and McNerney (2009) indicate that if one can temporarily lengthen the tone-burst duration to several seconds, the steady-state tone should closely approximate the true SPL. Modulated stimuli for the ASSR are also long enough in duration to use the SPL reference and later convert to HL (hearing level) for direct application to audiograms. For transient stimuli (<200 msec), there are two international standards that can help guide the calibration of acoustic transients: the IEC 60645–3 (International Electrotechnical Commission, 2007) and ISO 389–6 (International Organization for Standardization, 2007); however, some find that even these standards are still lacking (Lightfoot, Sininger, Burkard, and Lodwig, 2007).

The two international standards quantify transient levels using a peak-to-peak equivalent SPL approach. That is, the peak-to-peak waveform of a transient stimulus (e.g., 100- μsec click or tone burst) through a transducer is matched to the peak-to-peak waveform of a known reference signal (e.g., 1000-Hz sine wave or matched frequency) through the same transducer. The measurement is accomplished through a calibrated SLM whose analog output is sent to an oscilloscope. Unfortunately, working with acoustic transients is a bit more complex than the international standards will account for. For example, the temporal waveform of transient stimuli from different earphones will often not be uniform about the zero baseline on an oscilloscope. Because of this, the RETSPL based on the peak-to-peak equivalent SPL approach may fall short. It is for this reason that an ANSI S.3 Bioacoustics Working Group currently led by Dr. Robert Burkard (chair) is proposing additional measures in a draft ANSI standard. In

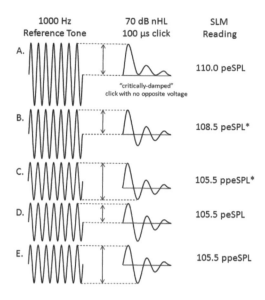

Fig. 22.1 Different waveform morphologies of a click stimulus through insert earphones and supra-aural headphones (same or different make/model). (A) Critically damped click with no voltage in the opposite polarity. (B, C) The same click with asymmetric voltages using the base-to-peak (peSPL) and peak-to-peak (ppeSPL) measurement approaches yielding different dB values and different units of measurement. (D, E) The same click with equal voltages using the base-to-peak (peSPL) and peak-to-peak (ppeSPL) measurement approaches yielding identical output but different units of measurement. The horizontal dashed lines indicate those portions of the stimulus and the reference tone that are being compared or measured. Asterisk denotes the most common voltage configuration seen with clicks. nHL, normal hearing level; SLM, sound level meter.

the ANSI standard draft, additional measures of quantifying transient levels would also include peak SPL (pSPL), baseline-to-peak peak equivalent SPL (peSPL), and peak-to-peak peak equivalent SPL (ppeSPL). The take-home message here is that depending on which approach is used, there can be a difference in level of up to 6 dB (Burkard, 1984, 2010; Burkard and Secor, 2002). **Figure 22.1** illustrates how two different measurement approaches (peSPL and ppeSPL) with various click stimulus morphologies may impact SLM readings using a 1000 Hz reference tone. The problem of relying only on the ppeSPL measurement can be seen when one compares B and C with D and E. Stimulus B and stimulus C are identical, but they do not have voltages that are symmetrical about the baseline. Stimulus D and stimulus E are identical, but unlike B and C, they do have voltages that are symmetrical about the baseline. Thus, B and C will have different peSPL and ppeSPL values, whereas D and E will not.

Another issue regarding transients has to do with the stimulation rate for earlier AEPs, such as ABR. It is generally well known that as stimulation rate increases, the transient stimulus may sound louder perceptually to one's ear as a result of temporal integration of rapidly presented stimuli. Although increasing stimulation rate (and intensity level) will improve the behavioral detection threshold for that stimulus, the ABR does not integrate this energy in the same manner. In fact, as stimulation rate increases for the ABR, the waveform morphology will begin to degrade. Thus, some guidelines for converting threshold at different stimulation rates would also be helpful in a standard. The approach that some manufacturers might take by automatically adjusting intensity level to changes in stimulation rate is strongly opposed by Lightfoot et al (2007).

The bottom line is that the inherent lack of an acceptable standard negatively impacts screening, threshold estimation, and habilitation efforts for young children. Thus, this author agrees that a standard that takes into account each of the variables described above is desperately and urgently necessary.

Pitfall

Some evoked potential systems make intensity level adjustments with increases or decreases in stimulation rate. This feature is not advisable because ABR waveform morphology generally becomes poorer with increases in stimulation rate. This in turn results in poorer, not better, thresholds.

Other Stimulus Parameters for Consideration

Today's evoked potential systems operating on digital computers offer a degree of precision that may not have been possible in an analog format. However, there can be a false sense of security in assuming that the evoked potential system and its transducers are free from calibration errors. Therefore, it is generally advisable to check not only output levels of

the stimuli, but also the quality and reliability of other stimulus parameters, such as polarity, linearity of intensity steps, rise/fall time of tone bursts, envelope functions of tone bursts, and amplitude spectra. Readers are referred to Gorga and Neely (1994) for more information on these other stimulus parameters.

Steps for Conducting Behavioral Calibration of Acoustic Transients

Use the behavioral calibration method in the event that you do not have access to the required calibration equipment discussed above. If you do have calibration equipment, it is highly recommended that you conduct the physical calibration, which is described in the next section.

1. Recruit some subjects with audiometrically normal hearing. These can be your colleagues and/or office personnel.

2. Determine the behavioral detection threshold for the click or tone burst using 20 to 30 subjects with normal hearing (as homogeneous as possible). Although Richter and Fedtke (2005) suggest using alternating stimulus polarity for the behavioral calibration, Stapells et al (1982) found no differences between rarefaction and condensation clicks using the TDH-49 transducer. Stimulation rates of 10 or 20/s are commonly used, although other rates could be used based on the clinic's protocol. Use the evoked potential system's intensity features to search for threshold using the stimulus of interest. You can use the bracketing method as if you are doing this on an audiometer. Gorga and Neely (1994) recommend that behavioral calibrations take place in an acoustically shielded sound booth.

3. For each subject, threshold will be the softest intensity level indicated by what you see on the evoked potential system's computer screen or intensity dial.

4. Calculate the average threshold across all subjects.

5. If the average threshold is at or near 0 dB on the computer screen or intensity dial, then your reference will be 0 dB nHL. If the average threshold is not at 0 dB on the

computer screen or intensity dial, then you will need to apply a correction factor (subtract or add the appropriate amount) to each presentation level you use.

Steps for Calibrating Acoustic Transients with Calibration Equipment

When calibration equipment is available, ISO 389–6(2007) is a reasonable starting point in the absence of an ANSI S3 standard for acoustic transients (Burkard, 2010; Lightfoot, Sininger, Burkard, and Lodwig, 2007). In this example, procedural steps are outlined to calibrate a click stimulus with insert earphones (see Richter and Fedtke, 2005, as a reference). The reader is directed to the ISO 389–6 (2007) standard to obtain RETSPL values for both clicks and tone bursts using a variety of different transducers (including bone oscillators and loudspeakers). There are several different suggested methods for calibrating acoustic transients; however, the one described in this example will be ppeSPL, as it works well for clicks, tone bursts, and even short-duration consonant-vowel (CV) speech stimuli. The following example is specifically for clicks to be used with **Fig. 22.2.**

1. Prepare the calibration system by first connecting a 2 cc artificial ear coupler to the SLM with the alternating current (AC) output to an oscilloscope. Next, connect the desired insert earphone into the 2 cc coupler (only one insert earphone will be tested at a time). Prepare your signal generator as well for step 3.

2. Present the click at a rate of 20/s using a single-stimulus polarity and a moderately high-intensity level (70 or 80 dB is usually sufficient). While the transient is displayed on the screen, the amplitude (usually in μV) and time settings (usually in msec) should be adjusted so that the click is clearly displayed and an approximate peak-to-peak voltage can be obtained. For example, the click might fit into a row of squares on the grid with a voltage output of 0.1 V (or 100 μV).

3. Next, present a 1000-Hz pure tone to the SLM. You may either use the evoked potential system to produce this tone (if available), or you may use any number of different signal generators. I use a calibrated audiometer and route another insert earphone directly into the 2-cc coupler. The 1000-Hz tone is then matched, in peak-to-peak voltage, as

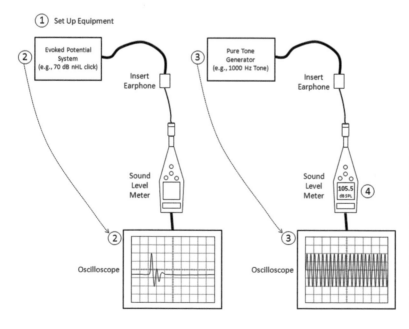

Fig. 22.2 Calibrating acoustic transients with calibration equipment. See text for descriptions of each step. All equipment is the same except when changing out the evoked potential system and its transducer with the pure-tone generator and its transducer. In step 3, the SLM should not be adjusted.

measured using the click (**Fig. 22.1**). During this time, you will momentarily ignore the SLM reading until the 1000-Hz tone has been matched to the peak-to-peak voltage of the click.

4. After the tone has been matched, the SLM reading will then be obtained. It is critical that the SLM scale not be changed during this procedure (Burkard and McNerney, 2009).

5. If the presentation level you used in step 2 was 70 dB, you will need to subtract 70 dB from the SLM reading to find out what the ppeSPL level is for behavioral threshold (or 0 dB nHL). What do you find? Richter and Fedtke (2005) reported a reference of 35.5 dB ppeSPL. Stapells et al (1982) reported a ppeSPL of 36.4 dB ppeSPL for TDH-49 headphones, which is very close to Richter and Fedtke's reference. If the values do not match the standard, you will need to apply a correction factor to all recordings or make the adjustment internally within the evoked potential system software.

> ### Pearl
>
> When performing physical calibration, be sure to use a moderately high-level stimulus and simply subtract the intensity value used from the reading on the SLM. The use of the moderately high-level stimulus ensures that ambient noise in the room will not affect the readings of the sound level meter.

◆ Generating Custom Stimuli

From a clinician's standpoint, there are a number of different ways to generate stimuli. Some commercial evoked potential systems may allow the clinician flexibility in changing various stimulus parameters such as rise/fall times, plateau time, and envelope as would be the case for creating tone bursts. Some evoked potential systems may even permit the clinician to generate click trains (a fast series of clicks), click pairs and tone burst pairs to assess auditory fusion, noise bursts with specific envelope functions, and even combine sinusoids to form two-tone complexes or beating tones. If these stimuli are generated within the software of the evoked potential system, the process of generating, saving, importing, and calibrating the stimulus for use may be a very painless process. However, there may be times when the generation of stimuli external to the evoked potential system is necessary. The remainder of this section discusses the external generation of a custom stimulus with the intent of importing into the evoked potential system.

Because today's evoked potential systems are desktop or laptop computers, the stimulus file that is generated will be in digital format, usually in the form of a "wave" (.wav) file. A .wav file is a commonly used standard audio format for different operating systems such as Windows, MacIntosh (Apple), and Linux. There are numerous other audio formats, but .wav files are commonly used in evoked potential systems. If a stimulus is recorded or generated in a different format (e.g., Audio Interchange File Format [AIFF]), it may be possible to convert that file format into a .wav files using sound-editing software or an audio file converter software that is available for download or purchase from the Internet. Audacity SourceForge. net, WavePad (NCH software Canberra, Australia), and Praat (Boersma and Weenik, 2009) are digital sound editors that can be downloaded from the Internet for free, whereas others such as MIXCRAFT Recording Studio (Oakhurst, CA), AVS Audio Tools (London, United Kingdom), and Goldwave (St. John's, NL, Canada) are also available on the internet at affordable prices. Adobe Audition (Adobe Systems Inc., San Jose, CA) is another popular sound-editing software with several useful editing and analysis features, but this software costs upwards of a few hundred dollars. If you know a speech-language pathologist or university researcher with a Computerized Speech Laboratory (CSL; e.g., KayPENTAX, Montvale, NJ) workstation, the CSL is also useful for generating custom speech stimuli given the high-quality microphone and user controls. Because most computers today have built-in sound cards, with the addition of a microphone of relatively good quality, a person could record stimuli directly into the digital audio editor software.

Regardless of the software used, the stimulus must be prepared so that it has the correct parameters necessary to be read and/or processed by the evoked potential system to which the stimulus will be imported. For example, stimuli imported to the Navigator Pro system (Natus Medical Inc., Mundelein, IL) must be digitized with a sampling rate of 48,000 Hz using a single channel (mono). The SmartEP system (Intelligent Hearing Systems Corp., Miami, FL) must be digitized with a sampling rate of 44,100 Hz also using a single channel (mono). A difference between the two systems, however, is that Navigator Pro will use .wav files, whereas SmartEP requires additional steps to convert the .wav file into their proprietary STM format. The reader is referred to the system's operation manual for determining the requirements of importing custom stimuli.

Recording and Editing a Speech Stimulus

For this example, the freely available Audacity software will be used to illustrate how to prepare a speech stimulus that might be used in a cortical potential recording. Because most computers have a sound card with microphone input, we could use a microphone of relatively good to high quality to record the word /ʃi/ ("she"). The first step in any sound-editing software is to ensure that (1) the recorded sounds can be played back through headphones or speakers; (2) the microphone levels are set so that sound can be recorded and its volume does not produce clipping; and (3) the software is set up with the correct recording parameters (e.g., sampling rate and bit rate). Again, this would be a good time to consult with the operating manual of the evoked potential system you are using. For the purposes of this example, we will assume that the sampling rate must be 44,100 Hz and that the bit rate be set to 16 bits (see Chapter 2 to review basic digital signal processing concepts). **Table 22.2** shows recommended minimal preferences in Audacity by clicking on Edit and then Preferences (or clicking Ctrl+P). After making these changes, click OK.

Now would be a good time to make sure that the speaker/headphones and the microphone are set up properly. On newer computers, the sound card input and output lines can generally be found on the back or front of the computer but sometimes can have a second set on the front of the computer. In either case, the sound output port is typically indicated by the color lime green, and the microphone input port is typically indicated by the color pink. You may find, however, that some sound cards have a single input/output port for use with a set of headphones with built-in microphone. Plugging in the speakers or headphones should be relatively straightforward, and you can adjust the volume using the standard controls on your computers or through Audacity using the Output Level Meter slider bar. Once the microphone has been properly connected and positioned (lapel microphone or standalone), a practice recording can be performed to ensure that the speaker's voice is sufficiently loud without causing clipping. A slider bar is also associated with the microphone in Audacity. If you find that nothing is being recorded while the microphone is plugged in, you may have to go into your Windows audio settings to see if your microphone has been disabled. Familiarity with the buttons and controls in Audacity and any hardware troubleshooting is beyond the scope of this chapter; therefore, external references may have to be consulted.

Table 22.2 Recommended Minimal Sound Format Preferences in Audacity

Preference Tab	Settings
Audio Input/Output (I/O)	Playback device: Microsoft Sound Mapper–Output Recording device: Microsoft Sound Mapper–Input Channels: 1 (mono)
Quality	Default sample rate: 44,100 Hz Default sample format: 16-bit
File formats	Uncompressed export format: .wav (Microsoft 16-bit PCM)

Audacity has documentation and tutorials available on their Web site (http://audacity.sourceforge.net/).

Assuming that the preceding setup, settings, and preferences have been met, we can begin recording some samples. Ensure that background noise is at a minimum by closing your door or recording at a time when there is less noise. The closer the microphone is to your mouth, the greater the chances are for better recordings with less background noise. Hit the record button and say /ʃi/ about five times in a normal but clear manner. Having multiple recordings (and possibly multiple speakers) will help ensure that a viable token can be extracted (Skoe and Kraus, 2010). After the recording is over, stop the recording and evaluate the recorded waveform. There should be no clipping as would be evidenced by maximal peaks "hitting" the top (1.0) and bottom (−1.0) of the recording window. If this is not the case, adjust the input level of the microphone and re-record your stimuli. You should also notice at this point in the far left-hand side of the recording window that your Audio Track is just as you set it up initially with the settings of Mono channel, sampling rate of 44,100 Hz, and bit rate of 16. Once you are satisfied with the recording sample, the next step is to remove any direct current (DC) offset by normalizing the entire waveform back to a baseline of zero. DC correction helps to balance the amplitude on both sides of the zero baseline. DC offsets can be caused by hardware problems and/or software A/D conversion problems. In any case, DC offsets are generally not a big problem, but severe DC offsets can produce unwanted audible clicks and pops. To correct for any DC offset, Audacity has a normalize function. Following DC correction, it may be necessary to remove existing ambient noise within the recording. There are generally two approaches if noise removal is warranted: (1) simply reducing the overall amplitude can reduce or eliminate the ambient noise without noticeably altering the desired stimulus; or (2) Audacity has a noise removal function that is a useful three-step process. First, select one or two seconds of ambient noise, which can be found in the areas between the words you recorded. Next, go to the noise removal function under the Effect menu and click on "Get Noise Profile." Finally, select the entire recording

(Ctrl+A) and go back to the noise removal function and click on "Remove Noise." In your recording, you may immediately be able to see that most of the ambient noise is removed and replaced by a flat line around the zero baseline. Undo the noise removal, and redo it using the Preview function and slider bar to determine whether more or less noise removal is needed. After noise removal, the next step is to play back your five recorded stimuli and judge which one sounds best. You may wish to call on colleagues to obtain their judgment as well. After selecting the best stimulus, you will need to trim away the remaining recorded stimuli leaving only the stimulus you've chosen. In Audacity, there are several different ways to trim unwanted parts of the waveform. You will need to experiment with different techniques using the different buttons or functions from the Edit menu. To improve your trimming precision, you may need to use the zoom buttons. After trimming, you may want to amplify or attenuate the overall level a few decibels by clicking on the Effect menu and selecting "Amplify." Finally, you will want to save your stimulus file. See **Fig. 22.3** for an example of the final /ʃi/ stimulus token. In Audacity, all recordings are saved initially as projects. To create a .wav file using the project, you will need to click on the File menu and select "Export as WAV... ." Assuming you made the changes shown in **Table 22.2**, your stimulus should be ready to import into your evoked potential system. If you have discovered after the fact that you require a different sampling rate, open your stimulus file in Audacity and then go to the bottom left-hand corner of the Audacity window to change the project rate (e.g., 22,050, 10,000, or 48,000 Hz). When you save or export your stimulus by changing the project rate, the temporal information of your stimulus will be preserved. In other words, the stimulus will have been resampled to the new project rate. If, however, you do not change the project rate, and simply change the rate, the temporal information of your stimulus will be altered.

When the stimulus is imported to the evoked potential system, it will most likely be by default that the stimulus trigger coincides with the onset of the stimulus. As with any stimulus, calibration is necessary to ensure that the stimulus is audible, at a desired intensity level, and

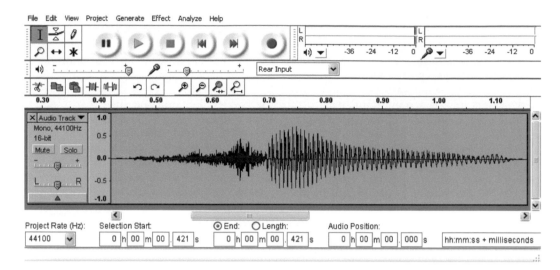

Fig. 22.3 Example stimulus recorded and edited using Audacity. (See text for detailed description.)

is safe for the patient. Because the duration of this stimulus is 421 msec, the intensity in dB SPL can be evaluated with an SLM using the fast (125-msec) time-weighting scale.

◆ Summary

This chapter focuses on some basic principles of stimulus calibration and stimulus generation. As discussed, acoustic transients are somewhat troublesome because SLMs have time weightings that often exceed the duration of a brief stimulus such as a click or tone burst. Thus, the SLM will underestimate the intensity of acoustic transients. Both behavioral and physical calibration methods can be used, but physical calibration is preferable. The physical calibration of acoustic trends usually will be measured as peSPL or ppeSPL and should be related meaningfully back to the intensity level on the computer screen or intensity dial of the evoked potential system. It should never be assumed that 0 dB nHL or 0 dB HL is actually behavioral threshold unless it is calibrated either behaviorally or physically. Acoustic stimuli that have long durations, whether sinusoidal or complex, may simply be measured in dB SPL. If the long-duration stimulus is a sinusoid or has a narrowband of spectral energy, it may easily be converted to dB HL with the appropriate transducer RETSPL value. When generating custom stimuli, clinicians will need to produce reasonably clean stimuli that meet the requirements of their evoked potential system. After importing custom stimuli, clinicians should calibrate in the manner expected for all other stimuli available. Taking the time to check one's evoked potential equipment will go a long way in obtaining reliable and valid clinical data.

References

American National Standards Institute. (2004). *Specifications for audiometers*. ANSI S3.6–2004. New York: Author.

Boersma, P. & Weenink, D. (2009). Praat: doing phonetics by computer (Version 5.1.05) [Computer program].

Retrieved January 19, 2012, from http://www.praat.org/

Burkard, R. (1984, Jan). Sound pressure level measurement and spectral analysis of brief acoustic transients. *Elec-*

troencephalography and Clinical Neurophysiology, 57(1), 83–91. PubMed

Burkard, R. (2010). Update on a standard for the calibration of acoustic transients. ASHA Audiology Connections, 15. Retrieved from: http://www.asha.org/uploadedFiles/10AudConn.pdf

Burkard, R., & Secor, C. (2002). Overview of auditory evoked potentials. In J. Katz (Ed.), Handbook of clinical audiology (5th ed, pp. 233–248). Baltimore: Lippincott Williams & Wilkins.

Burkard, R., & McNerney, K. (2009). Introduction to auditory evoked potentials. In J. Katz, L. Medwetsky, R. Burkard, & L. Hood, (Eds.), Handbook of clinical audiology (6th ed). (pp. 222–241). Philadelphia: Lippincott Williams & Wilkins.

Gorga, M. P., & Neely, S. T. (1994). Stimulus calibration in auditory evoked potential measurements. In J. T. Jacobson (Ed.), Principles and applications in auditory evoked potentials (pp. 85–97). Boston: Allyn & Bacon.

International Electrotechnical Commission. (2007). Electroacoustics—Audiometric Equipment—Part 3: Test signals of short duration (IEC 60645-3). Geneva: Author.

International Organization for Standardization. (2007). Acoustics—reference zero for the calibration of audiometric equipment—Part 6: Reference threshold of hearing for test signals of short duration (ISO 389-6). Geneva: Author.

Lightfoot, G., Sininger, Y., Burkard, R., & Lodwig, A. (2007). Stimulus repetition rate and the reference levels for clicks and short tone bursts: A warning to audiologists, researchers, calibration laboratories, and equipment manufacturers. American Journal of Audiology, 16(2), 94–95. PubMed

Richter, U., & Fedtke, T. (2005). Reference zero for the calibration of audiometric equipment using "clicks" as test signals. International Journal of Audiology, 44(8), 478–487. PubMed

Sininger, Y. S., & Hyde, M. L. (2009). Auditory brainstem response in audiometric prediction. In J. Katz, L. Medwetsky, R. Burkard, & L. Hood, (Eds.), Handbook of clinical audiology (6th ed., pp. 222–241). Philadelphia: Lippincott Williams & Wilkins.

Skoe, E., & Kraus, N. (2010). Auditory brain stem response to complex sounds: A tutorial. Ear and Hearing, 31(3), 302–324. PubMed

Stapells, D. R., Picton, T. W., & Smith, A. D. (1982). Normal hearing thresholds for clicks. Journal of the Acoustical Society of America, 72(1), 74–79. PubMed

Yeager, D. M., & Marsh, A. H. (1998). Sound levels and their measurement. In C. M. Harris (Ed.), Handbook of acoustical measurements and noise control. Melville, NY: McGraw-Hill.

Chapter 23

Evidence-Based Practice in Auditory Evoked Potentials

Radhika Aravamudhan, Yell Inverso, and Tina M. Stoody

The incorporation of evidence-based practice (EBP), also commonly referred to as evidence-based medicine (EBM), has become the focus of clinicians, hospitals, and university instruction for several years now. Although this is not a new concept, it has only been recently that EBP has become the cornerstone to how we as clinicians approach our work. Whether or not clinicians are actively engaged in research activities, it has become increasingly important for them to be avid consumers of research so that they can integrate the available knowledge base with their clinical expertise to make informed decisions regarding treatment plans. EBP in its simplest form is the use of quality evidence to shape clinical decision making. We must ask ourselves, How do we as responsible health care providers determine the most effective and efficient testing protocols, methods, and treatment plans for our patients? EBP demands that practitioners abstain from relying solely on expert opinions and anecdotal clinical experience when addressing individual patients and patient populations, and instead rely on the highest available level of evidence in the clinical decision-making process. We make the distinction, though, that EBP does not replace the role of clinical judgment; if anything, it enhances it. Even though EBP is the recommended approach to all clinical care, the process of finding and interpreting all available evidence is not always straightforward.

This chapter is designed to provide a brief, practical overview of the EBP process and how best to obtain and evaluate the available evidence. Let us begin by defining "best available evidence." When there is a lot of basic science and translational research that is conducted in any area, you need to find and evaluate the evidence that is directly applicable for your patient. The result of sorting through research and finding the evidence that is best applicable to the patient is what we mean by "best available evidence." After locating the most applicable evidence, you will want to assess the accuracy and precision of the various research methods used. Furthermore, the process requires the ability to extrapolate the results from the research study and apply the findings to your patient. Although this sounds like a daunting task, Sackett et al (1996), explain that EBP is not an unattainably high standard that cannot be practiced in everyday clinical situations. Even though EBP is not always the easiest or most convenient way to determine the course of care for your patients, its use in the health sciences, audiology included, should be the standard to determine best practices.

◆ Steps in Evidence-Based Practice

One of the approaches used to obtain the best available evidence is a "bottom-up" approach. According to Sackett et al (1996), "Evidence based medicine is not restricted to randomized trials and meta-analyses. It involves tracking down the best external evidence with which to answer our clinical questions" (p. 72). The bottom-up approach begins with formulating a question that you are interested in understanding.

Formulating a Well-Defined Clinical Question

The first step in EBP is to formulate a well-defined clinical question. Such clinically driven questions are often referred to as PICO, based on the four key components of the question: (P) the patient (or population) of concern; (I), intervention, prognostic factors, or exposure; (C), comparison treatment or diagnosis; and (O), outcome or desired outcome. For example, if you would like to know whether there is evidence supporting the use of a bone-anchored hearing aid (Baha) over conventional amplification to improve speech recognition in an adult patient with a history of recurrent middle ear pathology and a mixed hearing loss, the four components of the question would be:

P: Adult patients with mixed hearing loss and recurrent middle ear pathology

I: Use of Baha

C: Use of conventional hearing aids

O: Better speech perception scores in quiet

Once the clinical question is formed, you can use the same terms from the PICO components to search for relevant literature.

Searching for Relevant Literature

The first important aspect in searching for literature is to find one or more appropriate search engines and databases. Literature searches can be performed using various databases, such as MEDLINE, PsychInfo, and EBSCO. Although there are countless databases, some require a subscription for use. Therefore, PubMed will be used throughout this chapter as it is a public database accessible to anyone with an Internet connection and Web browser by going to the following Web address: http://www.ncbi.nlm.nih.gov/pubmed. The terms used to search are usually a combination of terms from the clinical question formulated using the PICO format. There is no paucity of literature to help in answering clinical questions; on the contrary, it is perhaps the abundance of information readily available that can lead to confusion and ultimately irresponsible decision making. As an example, put yourself in the shoes of a patient seeking your care. Based on the full and thorough clinical protocol that you or your employer has established, you are prepared to make a recommendation for an intervention. When discussing appropriate technology (for this example, bilateral digital behind-the-ear [BTE] hearing aids), your patient unfolds the pieces of paper he had been concealing in his pocket. He informs you that he has been "thoroughly" researching hearing loss and technology options online prior to this appointment. This is a proactive and responsible action on the part of the patient, right? A patient or family member taking the time to research hearing and technology (for this example) can be a useful indicator of a patient or family's motivation and seriousness about their hearing. However, when given the chance to look at the "evidence" your patient has brought, you see that the patient's information was printed off Web sites in the public domain, such as http://www.Wikipedia.com. Because there is no peer-review process, similar Web sites that allow nonexperts to post site content, as well as discussion boards, are among the lowest levels of evidence. The goal of this chapter is not to warn consumers to avoid the Internet. On the contrary, the Internet has increased the individual practitioner's access to evidence exponentially. However, it is to provide the reader with information as to how to make the best use of the peer-reviewed evidence available to make well-informed clinical decisions.

Evaluating the Evidence: Source and Levels of Evidence

An understanding of the level, quality, and applicability of the evidence you use to make clinical decisions is of the utmost importance. It is your responsibility as a practitioner not only to keep up to date with the emerging literature in your scope of practice, but also to evaluate systematically the strength of the evidence you are reviewing. The publication of a study in a peer-reviewed scientific journal is not reason enough to incorporate its findings into your daily practice. Individual studies are generally assessed along two dimensions: level of evidence and study quality.

Level of evidence refers to a hierarchy of study designs or types of evidence. The stronger the design of a particular study, the higher the level of evidence. There are many published hierarchies, and although no one is used universally, the concepts are similar. **Table 23.1** presents one example of a hierarchy of levels of evidence. In general, a meta-analysis, or systematic review, of any topic is considered the highest level of evidence. The next acceptable category of evidence comes from randomized, controlled trials (RCTs), followed by cohort studies and case–control studies. The lowest level of evidence comes from case series/case reports. When searching for research to answer a clinical question, it is important to evaluate and focus on those studies with the highest levels of evidence. One thing to keep in mind

Table 23.1 Levels of Evidence

Level of Evidence	Type of Study
1a	Systematic reviews of randomized control trials/meta-analyses
1b	Individual randomized control studies
2a	Control study without randomization
2b	Quasi-experimental research
3	Correlational research or case studies
4	Expert opinion based on clinical experience

Note: The lower the number assigned, the stronger the level of evidence (e.g., level 1a is the highest and level 4, the lowest).

is that audiology is a still a relatively new field; therefore, there are fewer systematic reviews or meta-analyses published within the field in general. At the time this chapter was written, a PubMed search using the terms *meta-analysis* AND *auditory evoked potential* found only 18 results. Combining *meta-analysis* AND *auditory evoked potential* AND *auditory brainstem response*, the results shrank to five. As our information base grows, the amount of research with higher levels of evidence is certain to increase.

> **Pitfall**
>
> Not all search engines include all journals. For example, PubMed and MEDLINE do not currently index articles for the *Journal of Speech-Language Pathology and Audiology.* Based on the previously described PubMed search with the terms *meta-analysis* AND *auditory evoked potential* AND *auditory brainstem response*, an important literature meta-analysis on auditory brainstem response threshold estimation using tone bursts by Stapells (2000) would have been missed. The Stapells meta-analysis was found in an ordinary Internet search engine (e.g., Google) with the search terms *auditory brainstem response meta-analysis*.

Once the relevant literature is found and deemed to be appropriate based on the level of evidence produced by the study's design, the next step is to critically appraise the merits of your findings.

Critical Appraisal of Articles

Critical appraisal of research is the process of systematically examining the relevance of the study, validity of the methodology, and reliability of the results and ultimately the clinical applicability of the results as it pertains to your day-to-day practice. This appraisal is imperative in making informed decisions for your patient. The process of critical appraisal may seem tedious and time consuming; however, it helps to close the gap between research and practice. Often an article can appear to have a great deal of clinical applicability based on its title, or even the topics covered in its introduction section. However, it is important to examine the validity, both internal and external, of any research study before applying its findings to your patients. *Internal validity* refers to the confidence that the reader can place in the causal relationship between variables in a study. More specifically, it is the extent to which the independent variable being investigated produced the observed effect. Internal validity is achieved if the effect on the dependent variable is due only to variation of the independent variable(s). Take a simple study of the progress that patients show after 6 months of hearing aid use. The reader would need to evaluate closely whether the study was designed in a way that hearing aid use was the only variable that had an effect on a user's progress. If, however, some of the study participants happen to be enrolled in aural rehabilitation classes, and this is not a controlled part of the study, the internal validity of the study has been compromised. This is because the reader cannot surmise if the progress that the study reported was really based on the use of amplification, and not due to the therapy services that some of the participants received.

External validity is also a very important concept in determining whether a study applies to your patient population and whether it should be considered for use in your clinical decision-making process. External validity relates to the generalizability of a study's findings. Can you, generalize the findings of a particular study or group of studies beyond the sample investigated (e.g. to patients in your own audiology practice)? One of the broadest examples of population external validity relates to pediatrics versus geriatrics. If a study is completed investigating the treatment of a disorder, and the study population is older adults, attention must be paid before considering the same treatment for a pediatric patient in your facility.

Evaluation of external validity requires one to pay close attention to certain methodological items, including sample size, effect size of the results, and possibility of any conflicts of interest (Ioannidis, 2005). Small sample size can be a limitation or weakness in many studies. Unfortunately, small sample size plagues a large body of research in the area of audiology and auditory evoked potentials because we are often working with clinical populations, with limited accessibility to patients who exhibit a specific clinical manifestation (i.e., there are not many individuals who possess a given disorder/trait available to the researcher(s) to include in the study). Also, although it is always best to have larger samples, sample size is not always a weakness. A sample of 20 individuals may be more than enough, depending on the type of analysis being done. However, studies with smaller sample sizes are said to lack power. What this translates to is that it is often difficult to obtain statistical significance in a study without an appropriately large sample size. Effect size is an important tool in interpretation of relationships found in a given study, but it may or may not be reported within the research. If the effect size is available, it helps to provide information about the strength of a relationship between two variables in addition to any statistical significance found. Finally, conflicts of interest are related to certain author affiliations. Is the author in any way benefiting from the research outcomes? An example of a potential conflict of interest is a hearing aid company employee publishing a study showing the benefits of new technology for that company. In addition to the aforementioned items, there are a few other questions that a good consumer of research will ask when critically appraising a particular study or body of evidence. These questions are summarized in **Table 23.2.**

The benefit of EBP is highly dependent on how we use it in everyday clinical practice. We can examine how to adopt the use of EBP clinical electrophysiologic testing and interpretation with a few case examples.

Special Consideration

The EBP process gives the impression that published case studies have no place in clinical practice. Group studies that reflect "averages" may have little value to the individual patient. Case studies involving repeated measurements can be quite valuable in the clinical decision-making process (Barlow and Hersen, 1984).

Table 23.2 Questions to Ask When Critically Appraising Research Design

Question	Why This Information Is Important
Was the assignment of patients to treatment and control groups randomized?	A randomized study is one that randomly places participants into different treatment/control groups. This reduces bias by providing an equal chance for each individual to be in each group. Sometimes random assignment is not possible if the goal of the study is to compare certain disordered populations.
Were all patients who enter the trial properly accounted for at the end of the study?	All subjects need to be accounted for. If there was subject attrition (not all subjects completed the study), then the authors need to account for those individuals.
Was there any blinding in the study (single- or double-blinded study)?	Blinding helps avoid bias to some extent by the various investigators in the study. If the individual analyzing the data has a given expectation about the results, it could bias his or her interpretation of the results. If the participants are aware of the treatment, it may also bias their responses. Blinding can help reduce these biases.
Aside from the experimental intervention, were all groups of patients treated equally?	All the conditions need to be the same except for the one under investigation. Along with this, baseline similarities are very important to consider effect size and the truth in the results (e.g., were all possible confounding variables controlled for?).
Was there a control group?	Do not confuse this with controlling for confounding variables within the subject population. If a researcher wants to look at the effectiveness of different treatments, a control group would be one that receives no treatment.

Case 1: Diagnostic Testing for Auditory Neuropathy Spectrum Disorder

Patient History

A 3-year-old female patient had a significant language delay, difficulty following verbal instructions, and very concerned and frustrated parents. Her parents reported that the child passed her newborn hearing screening (NHS) and responds, usually with tears, to loud sounds; however, they feel very strongly that she does not hear sometimes. The test used for hearing screening at the birthing hospital was otoacoustic emission (OAE) testing. The parents had an appointment with an otolaryngologist, who felt that the child's NHS results and clear response to loud sounds indicated normal hearing. The parents were still concerned and therefore brought the child for a full audiological evaluation.

Audiologic Test Battery

Otoscopy revealed bilateral ear canals free of cerumen and debris and tympanic membranes which appeared translucent and unremarkable. Tympanometry results were within normal limits, indicating appropriate compliance bilaterally. Acoustic reflex testing could not be completed because of the child's inability to tolerate the stimuli or remain quiet for the procedure. Speech audiometry using supra-aural headphones was attempted employing conditioned play audiometry without success. Using a visual reinforcement audiometry procedure, responses to speech stimuli were obtained in each ear at 25 dB HL with moderate reliability. Because of the child's inability to respond consistently to pure-tone stimuli using conditioned play audiometry, visual reinforcement audiometry (a two-tester paradigm) was used to obtain a pure-tone audiogram. Minimum response levels of 35 and 30 dB HL were obtained for 2000 Hz in the right and left ears respectively, and responses were recorded for 500-Hz stimuli at 35 dB bilaterally. The responses were slightly higher than ideal with respect to the speech thresholds that were previously obtained, and the reliability of the test results was overall deemed questionable. The child was able to sit still and remained quiet on her parent's lap, watching a silent cartoon on a computer. This "quiet" time allowed the audiologist to complete two runs, per ear, of distortion-product otoacoustic emission (DPOAE) testing. The DPOAE were present in both ears at two test frequencies, although the responses were not robust. The results of the diagnostic DPOAE were suggestive of abnormal outer hair cell (OHC) function, which contrasted with the results of the child's NHS and the behavioral results. Because of the incomplete and somewhat confusing information, the patient's inability to respond consistently, and the discrepancies between test results and the parent's reports of the child's listening abilities, the audiologist considered recommending a sedated auditory brainstem response (ABR) evaluation. The goals of the ABR are to learn more about the integrity of the child's auditory pathway through the brainstem and to further rule out the audiologist's anecdotal suspicion of auditory neuropathy spectrum disorder (ANSD).

Evidence-Based Approach

Clinical Question

The clinician question is as follows: (*P*) In children who have inconsistent audiometric test findings, difficulty acquiring spoken language, a history of both present and absent OAE results, and reports of parental concern (*I*), will a sedated ABR (*C*) add diagnostic information to rule out a diagnosis of ANSD and further clarify the type and severity of this child's hearing loss (*O*) and result in a diagnosis, and ultimately a treatment plan, that will enable this child to acquire speech and language?

Continued

Literature Search

A review of the available literature provides a wealth of information regarding diagnosis of ANSD. The use of behavioral pure-tone testing and speech perception testing in quiet is believed to be the least effective method of evaluating a child who may have ANSD (Davis and Hirsh, 1979; Hood, Berlin, Morlet, Brashears, Rose, and Tedesco, 2002; Kraus, Ozdamar, Stein, and Reed, 1984; Starr, Picton, Sininger, Hood, and Berlin, 1996). Hood et al (2002) found that ANSD is characterized by normal or once-normal OHC function and dyssynchronous neural responses. Traditionally, ANSD is diagnosed by an absent or abnormal ABR to a high-intensity click stimulus in the presence of normal OHC function, typically determined by present, robust, and repeatable OAEs. It is further recommended that the clinician complete middle ear muscle reflex (MEMR) testing (Berlin, Morlet, and Hood, 2003; Hood et al, 2002), as MEMRs would be expected to be absent both ipsilaterally and contralaterally in both ears for patients with bilateral ANSD. There are several complicating factors in the diagnosis of ANSD that are not often discussed anecdotally or in many textbooks. A thorough review of the literature reveals particular ABR protocol requirements for the definitive diagnosis of this disorder, specifically, the stimulus polarity used for recording the ABR. The use of alternating polarity is recommended at times to obtain cleaner waveforms or to minimize the possibility of a frequency-following response (FFR). This recommendation can be found in commonly referenced textbooks (Hall, 2004, 2007). However, in the most recent literature, which is of a higher level of evidence, it is shown that if you use only alternating polarity, meaning you do not do at least one run of the ABR with condensation (positive) and one run with rarefaction (negative) polarity, you are in danger of misreading the cochlear microphonic (CM). The CM follows the characteristics of the external stimulus. There will be a reversal of the direction of the CM with changes in polarity of the stimulus. Therefore, a comparison of responses obtained with condensation and rarefaction polarity stimuli will show an inversion of the peaks of the CM waveform (Berlin et al, 1998; Hood, 1998; Hood et al, 2002). The peaks of the ABR should not reverse, so if all of the peaks in the waveform reverse, then only a CM is being seen, and the ABR is in fact absent, allowing the clinician to distinguish between cochlear and neural components.

Additionally, stimulus intensity and its effect on response latency can aid in differentiating between cochlear and neural responses. The waves of the ABR increase in latency and decrease in amplitude when stimulus intensity decreases (Hall, 2007). However, the latency of the CM does not increase in latency as the stimulus intensity decreases (Hood, 1998); therefore, a comparison of response latency at decreasing intensities can be used to distinguish cochlear from neural responses.

Further information presented by Berlin et al (1998) and Hood et al (2002) suggests a third way to differentiate between cochlear and neural responses to aid in the diagnosis of ANSD. The latency of the CM does not shift in response to masking presented to the same ear, while the compound action potential (CAP), which is wave I of the ABR, shows a decrease in amplitude and an increase in latency during simultaneous masking to the same ear (Dallos, 1973). For an in-depth discussion of this topic and examples of responses showing these characteristics, the reader is referred to Berlin et al (1998) and Kumar and Jayaram (2006).

At the time of writing this chapter, a search on PubMed using the search terms *auditory neuropathy spectrum disorder* AND *auditory brainstem response* yielded just five results. Each of the results is relatively recent (publication dates of 2007–2011). The first article (James, 2011) involves neonates, which is not the target population for this PICO question. The third result (Meyer et al, 2010) focuses on genetic mutations, which are not directly related to our question. The fifth result (Beutner, Foerst, Lang-Roth, von Wedel, and Walger, 2007) focused more on risk factors for ANSD rather than diagnosis methods. This search leaves us with two references: "Audiological results in a group of children with auditory neuropathy spectrum disorder" by Mo et al (2010) and "Multi-site diagnosis and management of 260 patients with auditory neuropathy/dyssynchrony (auditory neuropathy spectrum disorder)" by Berlin et al (2010). Mo and colleagues (2010) analyzed ABR, OAE, and behavioral audiometric data for 48 infants and young children, concluding that absent or severely abnormal ABR with present

Continued

OAEs are the most reliable test measures to detect ANSD during early childhood. Berlin et al (2010) summarized test results for more than 200 individuals diagnosed with ANSD; 85% of these individuals were 12 years of age or younger. Pure-tone behavioral thresholds ranged from within normal limits to profound hearing loss, and all of the participants showed absent or abnormal ABR with present OAEs.

Conclusion/Recommendation

By consulting the evidence, we learned that the use of behavioral testing alone in the diagnosis of ANSD is inappropriate. Many of the behaviorally obtained audiometric patterns can manifest as a variety of configurations and often as an auditory processing disorder (APD, see Case 2). Also, the common electrodiagnostic description of ANSD as the presence of OAEs and the absence of an ABR is not sufficient, depending on the child's documented history and the ABR protocol. In this case study, the child once had present OAEs; however, at the time of testing, the OAEs were suggestive of abnormal OHC function. The use of CM testing ultimately revealed that the cochlea was receiving sound and processing it with some regularity but that the ABR was absent. The ABR waveforms, if evaluated only with alternating polarity, may have been incorrectly evaluated as present. The literature suggests, however, that you must record at least two runs of the ABR using one positive and one negative polarity to determine whether the CM reverses and whether the ABR waves stay appropriately upright. ANSD is not a subjective diagnosis; it is rooted in electrophysiology. When the clinician keeps a close eye on the literature and is willing to adjust his or her day-to-day protocols to obtain the most reliable results, the patients and their family will benefit greatly.

Case 2: Electrophysiologic Tests for Auditory Processing Diagnosis

Patient History

A 10-year-old boy presented with academic difficulties, particularly related to understanding directions and materials covered in the classroom. The school nurse made a referral for a hearing evaluation, and the child's parents made an appointment with an audiologist.

Audiological Test Battery

Pure-tone and speech audiometric procedures revealed thresholds and word recognition scores consistent with normal hearing abilities. Following this, the audiologist suspected a possible APD. Results from a behavioral test battery were marginal for APD. The audiologist wanted to see whether adding electrophysiologic testing to the diagnostic battery would be beneficial.

Evidence-Based Approach

Clinical Question

The clinical question is as follows: (P) In children with normal hearing and marginal behavioral test results suggesting APD (I), will electrophysiologic testing (C) add diagnostic value in to behavioral test results (O) in diagnosing CAPD?

Literature Search

When looking for information online, it takes some practice and a little time to figure out the best terms to use to narrow down a literature search. A literature search on PubMed using the terms *evoked potentials and auditory processing disorders* yielded 768 results, which is far too many to sort through. Adding *and ABR* to the search cut the results down to 54. Because the use of speech-evoked ABR has been a more recently discussed method to measure an individual's ability to process more complex stimuli (e.g., speech signals), the search term was changed from *and ABR* to *and speech-evoked ABR*. A search using the terms *evoked potentials* AND *auditory processing disorders* AND *speech-evoked ABR* yielded 23 results. Playing with the search terms enabled us to narrow down our field of research from 768 to 23 results, a much more manageable number.

Another way to narrow down your findings is to set limits within your search. By clicking on the "limits" function at the top of the PubMed search page, the search was confined by language (English only), subjects (humans only; no animals), publication date (within the last 5 years), and availability of links to full text. One can even limit searches to reveal only articles with links to free full text, but we advise against this, as it will very likely eliminate an excellent body of evidence. Using the limits of English language, human participants, research published within the last 5 years (January 2006 to January 2011), and full-text available, the results are narrowed down to five studies.

Some of the research was not specifically evaluated because the focus was not specifically APD (e.g., specific language impairment, Friedreich's ataxia, autism spectrum disorder, and acquired immunodeficiency syndrome). The focus of one of the remaining studies is the use of the ABR and middle latency response (MLR) to investigate binaural hearing effects in normal listeners (Weihing and Musiek, 2008). The relationship to auditory processing is the common complaint that individuals with APD often have difficulty understanding speech in compromised listening environments (i.e., hearing in noise). However, because these researchers used normal listeners and did not directly relate their assessments to diagnosis of APD, their findings are not able to help us answer our question. The last remaining study, written by Banai, Abrams, and Kraus (2007), provided information about the speech-evoked ABR as a diagnostic tool for evaluating abnormal auditory processing at the level of the cortex.

Continued

To investigate speech-evoked ABR further, a new search was performed using the terms *click and speech-evoked ABR* with no limits imposed. The new search yielded 46 results. By limiting the search to publications within the last 5 years and those published in English, the results were reduced to just 10. Again, some of the research was not directly related to our question, so we needed to read through the abstracts before deciding on delving further into each study. When a given study proves to be valuable, a few things can be done to find similar research. In PubMed, when you click on a result to expand it in a new window, there are "related citations" listed in the right-hand column of the page. Another option is to search for other articles authored by the same individuals. We found that Karen Banai had authored several papers on the speech-evoked ABR. Banai and colleagues (2005, 2007, 2009) have shown that ABR responses using clicks are usually normal in individuals with learning, reading, and/or auditory processing deficits.

Although the research showed that there is a difference in encoding of speech signals when the patient has an auditory processing problem, critical evaluation of these articles found that the effect sizes were small as were the sample sizes. However, the results were consistent among the studies that used speech ABR and its correlation to the presence of a speech-encoding/auditory processing problem. Considering the consistency of these findings, it is reasonable to include the use of speech ABR in the diagnostic protocol if resources permit. But inclusion of this test cannot replace any of the behavioral tests that are a part of the original test battery.

Conclusion/Recommendation

Even though sensitivity and specificity measures are not available yet for speech ABR as a diagnostic tool for APD, there is preliminary evidence to include this in the diagnostic battery. Electrophysiologic tests are able to distinguish between children and adults with normal auditory processing abilities and the individuals with auditory processing deficit (either in isolation or along with other learning disabilities). Especially when individuals are suspected of having neurologic involvement, electrophysiologic tests can be very helpful. Even though electrophysiologic tests cannot be used as diagnostic tests in isolation, it has become increasingly important to include these tests in the test battery, along with behavioral APD testing.

♦ Summary

It is the educated practitioner's responsibility to include evidence-based practice it in the care of patients. When making clinical decisions, the practitioner acts using his or her experiences, previous education, and intuition. The evidence-based practitioner utilizes these tools, but also remembers that clinical decisions, big and small, should be based on the four key components of PICO: (*P*) the patient (or population) in concern; (*I*) intervention, prognostic factors, or exposure; (*C*) comparison treatment or diagnosis; and (*O*) outcome or desired outcome. To answer PICO questions, it is imperative to critically appraise the wealth of literature in the field. You must evaluate the quality and applicability of evidence by determining the level of the evidence you seek and read. Additionally, it is important to systematically critique evidence, evaluating its internal and external validity.

References

Banai, K., Abrams, D., & Kraus, N. (2007). Sensory-based learning disability: Insights from brainstem processing of speech sounds. *International Journal of Audiology, 46*(9), 524–532. PubMed

Banai, K., Nicol, T., Zecker, S. G., & Kraus, N. (2005). Brainstem timing: implications for cortical processing and literacy. *Journal of Neuroscience, 25*(43), 9850–9857. PubMed

Banai, K., Hornickel, J., Skoe, E., Nicol, T., Zecker, S., & Kraus, N. (2009). Reading and subcortical auditory function. *Cerebral Cortex, 19*(11), 2699–2707. PubMed

Barlow, D. H., & Hersen, M. (1984). *Single case experimental designs: strategies for studying behavioral change.* New York: Pergamon Press.

Berlin, C. I., Bordelon, J., St John, P., Wilensky, D., Hurley, A., Kluka, E., et al. (1998). Reversing click polarity may uncover auditory neuropathy in infants. *Ear and Hearing, 19*(1), 37–47. PubMed

Berlin, C. I., Hood, L. J., Morlet, T., Wilensky, D., Li, L., Mattingly, K. R., et al. (2010). Multi-site diagnosis and management of 260 patients with auditory neuropathy/dys-synchrony (auditory neuropathy spectrum disorder). *International Journal of Audiology, 49*(1), 30–43. PubMed

Berlin, C. I., Morlet, T., & Hood, L. J. (2003). Auditory neuropathy/dyssynchrony: its diagnosis and management. *Pediatric Clinics of North America, 50*(2), 331–340, vii–viii. PubMed

Beutner, D., Foerst, A., Lang-Roth, R., von Wedel, H., & Walger, M. (2007). Risk factors for auditory neuropathy/auditory synaptopathy. *Journal for Oto-Rhino-Laryngology, Head & Neck Surgery, 69*(4), 239–244.

Dallos, P. (1973). *The auditory periphery.* New York: Academic Press.

Davis, H., & Hirsh, S. K. (1979). A slow brain stem response for low-frequency audiometry. *Audiology, 18*(6), 445–461. PubMed

Hall, J. (2004). ABRs or ASSRs? The application of tone-burst ABRs in the era of ASSRs. *Hearing Review, 11*(9), 22–30, 60.

Hall, J. (2007) *New handbook for auditory evoked potentials.* Boston: Allyn & Bacon.

Hood, L. (1998). Auditory neuropathy: What is it and what can we do about it. *Hearing Journal, 51*(8),10–18.

Hood, L. J., Berlin, C., Morlet, T., Brashears, S., Rose, K., & Tedesco, S. (2002). Considerations in the clinical evaluation of auditory neuropathy/auditory dys-synchrony. *Seminars in Hearing, 23*(3), 201–208.

Ioannidis, J. P. A. (2005). Why most published research findings are false. *PLoS Medicine, 2*(8), e124. PubMed

James, A. L. (2011). The assessment of olivocochlear function in neonates with real-time distortion product otoacoustic emissions. *Laryngoscope, 121*(1), 202–213. PubMed

Kraus, N., Ozdamar, O., Stein, L., & Reed, N. (1984). Absent auditory brain stem response: Peripheral hearing loss or brain stem dysfunction? *Laryngoscope, 94*(3), 400–406. PubMed

Kumar, U. A., & Jayaram, M. M. (2006). Prevalence and audiological characteristics in individuals with auditory neuropathy/auditory dys-synchrony. *International Journal of Audiology, 45*(6), 360–366. PubMed

Meyer, E., Michaelides, M., Tee, L. J., Robson, A. G., Rahman, F., Pasha, S., et al. (2010). Nonsense mutation in TMEM126A causing autosomal recessive optic atrophy and auditory neuropathy. *Molecular Vision, 16, 650–664.* PubMed

Mo, L., Yan, F., Liu, H., Han, D., & Zhang, L. (2010). Audiological results in a group of children with auditory neuropathy spectrum disorder. *Journal for Oto-Rhino-Laryngology, Head and Neck Surgery, 72*(2), 75–79.

Sackett, D. L., Rosenberg, W. M., Gray, J. A., Haynes, R. B., & Richardson, W. S. (1996). Evidence based medicine: What it is and what it isn't. *British Medical Journal, 312*(7023), 71–72. PubMed

Stapells, D. R. (2000). Threshold estimation by the tone-evoked auditory brainstem response: A literature meta-analysis. *Journal of Speech-Language Pathology and Audiology, 24*(2), 74–83.

Starr, A., Picton, T. W., Sininger, Y. S., Hood, L. J., & Berlin, C. I. (1996, June). Auditory neuropathy. *Brain, 119*(Pt 3), 741–753. PubMed

Weihing, J., & Musiek, F. E. (2008). An electrophysiological measure of binaural hearing in noise. *Journal of the American Academy of Audiology, 19*(6), 481–495. PubMed

Index

Distortion-product otoacoustic emissions
(DPOAEs), 94, 96, 192
Documentation
evaluation results in, 322–323
history in, 322
identification in, 322
importance of, 320
impressions in, 323–324
intraoperative monitoring and, 283, 284f, 285f
methods of, 320–321
observations in, 322
overview of, 321–322
purpose of, 320–321
recommendations in, 324
roles and responsibilities in, 319
samples, 325–339
summary in, 323–324
DSP. *See* Digital signal processing (DSP)

E

Early Hearing Detection and Intervention (EHDI),
189, 189t. *See also* Newborn hearing
screening (NHS)
EBP. *See* Evidence-based practice (EBP)
EEG. *See* Electroencephalogram (EEG)
Efficiency, test, 191, 191t
Electrical outlets, 3
Electrically evoked middle latency response
(EMLR), 126–128
Electrocochleogram (ECochG), 3, 4t
action potential in, 59, 183
amplitude utility, 30t
analysis technique for, 29t
as auditory evoked potential, 57–58
as transient, 28
clinical applications, 63–65
cochlear microphonic in, 58–59
component labeling, 183–184
components of, 58–59
electrode montage for, 60–61, 61t, 179–180,
179f, 180t
electrode types and, 175–177, 177f
extratympanic, 59–60
for auditory brainstem response wave I
enhancement, 184
for auditory neuropathy spectrum disorder, 63,
186
for Meniere disease, 64
in history of auditory evoked potentials, 5
in intraoperative monitoring, 184–186
interpretation, 182–184
latency utility, 30t
preparation for, 177–181
recording, 59–62, 178–179
recording parameters, 61
stimulus parameters, 61–62
subject effects in, 62–63

summating potential in, 59, 183
synchrony in, 47
transtympanic, 59–60
troubleshooting, 184, 185t
tympanic membrane electrodes in, 176–177,
177f, 180–181, 181f
Electrode(s), 18–21
application, 310–314
array, 21–22
dermatologic reactions to, 313–314
impedance, 18
in auditory brainstem response, 74–75,
211–212, 211f, 241–242
in auditory steady-state response, 113
in electrocochleogram, 60–61, 175–177, 177f,
179–180, 179f, 180t
in frequency-following response, 92
in late auditory evoked potential, 141t
in vestibular evoked myogenic potentials,
166–167, 290–291
number of, *vs.* number of channels, 19–21
placement, 18–19, 20f, 20t
sites, 12–13, 13t, 14f, 18–19, 20f, 20t
supplies, 312t
switching, 223–224
tympanic membrane, 176–177, 177f
types, 18, 19f
Electroencephalogram (EEG)
alertness on, 2, 9
auditory evoked potentials and, 2
auditory evoked potentials *vs.*, 2
epochs, 16
evoked potentials *vs.*, 9–10
signal, 9
Electromyogram (EMG), in vestibular evoked
myogenic potentials, 168
EMG. *See* Electromyogram (EMG)
EMLR. *See* Electrically evoked middle latency
response (EMLR)
Endogenous potentials, 3, 4t, 52
Endolymphatic hydrops, vestibular evoked
myogenic potentials in, 293–294
Enlarged vestibular aqueduct, 294
EP. *See* Evoked potentials (EP)
Evidence
evaluating, 355
levels of, 355, 355t
source of, 355
Evidence-based practice (EBP)
article appraisal in, 355–356
case studies, 358–362
evaluating evidence in, 355
literature search in, 354–355
overview of, 353–354
question formulation, 354
steps in, 354–356
Evoked potentials (EP), 9–10, 43, 44. *See also*
Auditory evoked potentials (AEPs)

Index